WHAT TO DO WHEN
YOUR BABY
IS PREMATURE

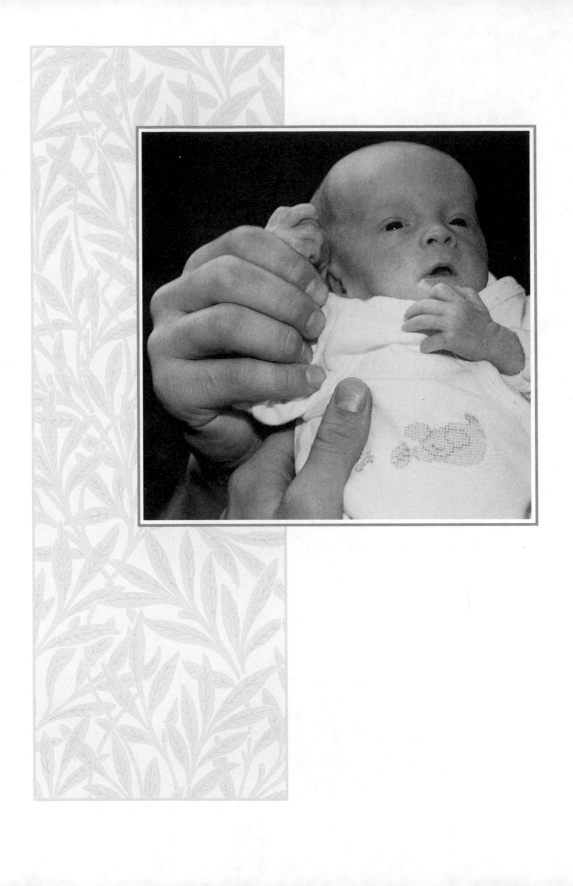

WHAT TO DO WHEN YOUR BABY IS PREMATURE

A Parent's Handbook for Coping with High-Risk Pregnancy and Caring for the Preterm Infant

Joseph A. Garcia-Prats, M.D., and
Sharon Simmons Hornfischer, R.N., B.S.N.

THREE RIVERS PRESS • NEW YORK

Published by Three Rivers Press, New York, New York.
Member of the Crown Publishing Group.

Random House, Inc., New York, Toronto, London, Sydney, Auckland
www.randomhouse.com

THREE RIVERS PRESS is a registered trademark and the Three Rivers Press colophon is a trademark of Random House, Inc.

Printed in the United States of America

Design by Helene Wald Berinsky

Library of Congress Cataloging-in-Publication Data
Garcia-Prats, Joseph A.
What to do when your baby is premature : a parent's handbook for coping with high-risk pregnancy and caring for the preterm infant / Joseph A. Garcia-Prats and Sharon Simmons Hornfischer.—1st ed.
p. cm.
Includes bibliographical references and index.
1. Infants (Premature)—Care. 2. Pregnancy—Complications. 3. Infants (Premature)—Growth.
I. Hornfischer, Sharon Simmons. II. Title.
RJ250.G37 2000
618.92'011—dc21
99-086497

ISBN 0-8129-3109-2

10 9 8 7 6 5 4 3 2 1

First Edition

This book is dedicated to the many parents who responsibly deal with so many difficult and happy situations involving their premature infant/s. Likewise it is dedicated to the obstetric and neonatal physicians and nurses, respiratory therapists, and social workers who strive so hard to bring ethical and happy endings to these many prematurely born patients.

—Joseph A. Garcia-Prats, M.D.

To my son, David James, who came into this world ahead of schedule, on a wing and a prayer, and made us the family that we have always dreamed about.

To my husband, Jim, whose belief in and support of this project helped catapult it into reality. We couldn't ask for a better husband or father.

To Grace Ann, my daughter, who was born at full term within days of this manuscript's due date. Thanks for your exquisite timing—and for sleeping through the night at six weeks.

To our youngest, Henry Hutchins, who arrived just in time to get his name in print. Hutch, you complete our family

To my wonderful mother, Mavis Lee Simmons, who taught me everything I know about motherhood. And in memory of my father, Robert Wyatt Simmons, for his ready smile and love of family.

—Sharon Simmons Hornfischer

When I first saw you, kid, you were tiny and thin
And slimy and red and your head was mushed in.
I said to your mother, "He looks kind of sloppy,
And two pound four ounces ain't big for a crappie."

But something about you, the look in your eyes,
Said you fully intended to grow to full size.
They slapped your backside and you let out a cry,
And I said, "We will keep him, at least we shall try."

Some babies are born in nine months, by the clock.
Some babies are born, and they sit up and talk.
Some babies are born, and no doctor is there.
But some babies come in on a wing and a prayer.

Poor little fetus as big as your hand.
Poor little fish thrown up on dry land.
Who came in late April though he had till July,
Too small to live and too precious to die.

They shipped you downstairs to the big Neonatal
Intensive Care Unit's computerized cradle
And attached you to wires and stuck you with tubes
Monitored closely by digital cubes.

And thanks to the latest neonatal therapeusis
And regular basting with greases from gooses
And hot chicken soup intravenously fed
You did not fade away, you grew up instead.

We'll always remember the months that you spent
With tubes in your head in the oxygen tent
And the mask on your face, the wires attached,
Sweet little baby who was only half hatched.

I'm sure you'll grow up and mature and extend
To six feet six inches and become a tight end.
But I'll always remember each doctor and nurse in
The NICU who helped make you a person,
The kid who crash landed, who was carried away,
Who survived it, this bundle we bring home today.

—GARRISON KEILLOR

Acknowledgments

I would like to thank my obstetric and neonatal colleagues for their advice regarding the many topics covered in this book. I would like to particularly thank Carol Turnage-Carrier, M.S.N., R.N., for her advice and input in our chapter dealing with developmental care.

—JOSEPH A. GARCIA-PRATS, M.D.

This book started off innocently enough. My husband and I were enjoying the excitement of our first pregnancy, anticipating parenthood. One minute, we were picking out nursery wallpaper, then, all of a sudden, *bam*—I'd been told I was having a high-risk pregnancy. The next thing I knew, I was being whisked to the hospital for an emergency delivery at thirty-two weeks. Thrown into the surreal world of the neonatal intensive care unit, I found that my medical background was little help to me. I was an experienced registered nurse, and I was still thrown for a loop. We felt pretty helpless. What were our son's chances? What should we expect? How should we care for him? If someone with my background was struggling with these questions, I thought to myself, how must non-medically trained parents feel?

The idea for the book came about as a result of our discovery that none of the books on the market integrated a complete discussion of high-risk pregnancy with a full treatment of the experience of premature delivery. My husband, a published author himself with years of experience in the book business, and Joe Garcia-Prats, a family friend, the father of ten boys, and a respected veteran neonatologist, decided that we could all team up and fill this void, write a book for parents and families caught up in the experience of high-risk pregnancy and premature birth. So this is exactly what we did. We found a need and filled it.

This has been an exciting project to be involved with. I was able to combine my educational and professional background and my first-hand experience, collaborate with an experienced and compassionate neonatologist and an equally compassionate and publishing-savvy husband, and bring a project to completion that I hope will help many, many people for years to come.

Of course, a project of this magnitude does not happen without the guidance and support of many. First, I would like to thank my literary agent, Jim Hornfischer, who also happens to be my husband. His dedication and passion were things that only the father of a preemie could have. I would like to thank my editor, Betsy Rapoport at the Crown Publishing Group, for her support of the project from day one. Her strong vision for this project was inspiring, and her editorial genius shows throughout the book. Betsy, you have been a joy for a first-time author to work with. Thanks also to editorial assistant Stephanie Higgs for her valuable help.

I would like to thank my coauthor, Joe Garcia-Prats, M.D., not only for his contribution to this project, but also for his years of service in neonatology—past, present, and future. Joe, you have made a difference in the lives of so many.

I would like to thank neonatologist George Sharp, M.D., for his valuable comments on the manuscript. Your input and support were greatly appreciated. Thank you for your many and continued contributions to the field of neonatology.

I also wish to thank neonatologist Dr. Donald Kelley for his skill and compassion during the delivery and six-week NICU admission of my son. Additionally, to the whole NICU medical and nursing staff at Seton Medical Center in Austin, Texas: you are quite a team. What you do for children and their families on a daily basis is truly awe-inspiring.

A very special thanks to obstetrician Dr. Chris Seeker and his wonderful staff for their guidance, care, and compassion. You will always hold a special place with our family.

I cannot thank enough the dozens of women and couples who shared their stories in the following pages. Their generosity will make this journey easier for others who may happen to travel down this road. Thanks to each and every one of you.

Thanks also to Dr. Julian De Lia, Mary Slaman-Forsythe, Mara Stein, Ph.D., Deborah L. Davis, Ph.D., Susan Davenport, R.N., Candace Hurley, Sara McKinney, and Annie Douglas for their generous contributions to this project.

Finally, and most important, I would like to thank our wonderful family for their support during my stint on bed rest and during those long days and weeks in the NICU. Jim and I will always remember the love that you showed by the phone calls, flowers, packages, meals, visits, and prayers. We count our blessings daily, knowing how lucky we are to have each and everyone of you on our team.

—SHARON SIMMONS HORNFISCHER

Contents

Introduction

The park is alive with children. A sunny, breezy Saturday afternoon finds a green field buzzing with their playtime activities. At the face-painting table, young cheeks are round canvases for bright roses, yellow balloons, and green dinosaurs. The small petting zoo set up in the shade of a large live oak is a hotbed of activity as parents watch their little ones interact, with growing confidence, with a tolerant Shetland pony and her sidekick, a black pygmy goat. An inflatable moonwalk playhouse is a-jiggle with the energies of half a dozen kids bouncing the day away. And a swing set stands in full motion with small legs propelling themselves in playful arcs.

It could be any playground in the country, really, except that on this Saturday the park is the site of a special sort of reunion—Seton Medical Center's Annual Neonatal Reunion Party. The children participating in the reunion share the unique bond of having been born prematurely. Some are hardy veterans of this annual occasion in Austin, Texas—seven-, eight-, and nine-year-olds who have been returning year after year to frolic with friends who were once their incubator neighbors in the neonatal intensive care unit (NICU). Others are babies approaching their first birthdays who are only now beginning to catch up with their full-term sisters, brothers, and cousins, only beginning to appreciate the fun of the festivities taking place around them.

These children were born as much as four months early. Some once weighed scarcely more than a pound. For the first weeks and months of their lives, their "home" was a neonatal special care unit full of beeping, microcircuit-driven, high-tech equipment, tended to by a topflight medical staff keeping tabs on it all. During their time here, their parents were little more than visitors—frequent visitors, to be sure, but visitors nonetheless. When the lights went out, mom and dad went home to bed. More often than not it was a member of the neonatal nursing staff who fed them in the predawn hours. These babies were so busy saving their energy to grow that they took little interest in their surroundings. Most of their energy was concentrated on staying warm and growing, gaining weight, and drawing breath well enough and often enough so that they could eventually go home.

On this day in the park, their days in the NICU seem a lifetime away. These preemies have grown into bright-eyed little children. There is little Carly, full of curiosity and spirit. From the smile on her parents' face, you wouldn't know that once upon a time she had been among the neonatal ward's smallest inhabitants at 2 pounds 1 ounce.

"We saw so many healthy babies and children," her mother, Gini, said. "Sure, there were some children there who had lasting problems. But the most important thing was, they were there. It was really healthy for my husband and me to see."

Ty, Elliot, and Jason are lined up like a baby bobsledding crew in their triple stroller. When the triplets were born six and a half weeks premature, their father might have had trouble imagining that just two years later they would form their own three-man soccer team.

Diane, almost ten years old now, stands by and tolerates her father boasting, once again, that when she was in the NICU she held the unit's record for the highest ventilator pressure ever given to a newborn. Those days are a distant memory as she looks away in decidedly preteen embarrassment. "Whatever, Dad."

The reunion has gathered together hundreds of happy endings. "This is a celebration," organizer Lynda Shanblum said. As well it should be. Though they are not in all cases perfect endings (a certain small percentage of children born prematurely will have difficulties ranging from learning disabilities to cerebral palsy to physical or mental disabilities even more severe), in just about every instance the children overcame obstacles and confronted difficulties that most infants (and even many adults) are never called upon to face. The children living with disabilities are all the more worth celebrating because of the great odds that

they have overcome just to be here. These children celebrate every day with their dedicated, loving, and nurturing parents and families who understand better than anyone the full extent of their children's triumph.

For the more than four hundred thousand premature babies born every year—a little more than 11 percent of all births in the United States—the good news today is that advances in technology and medical know-how over the past thirty years are allowing the majority of premature babies to go on to lead normal, healthy lives. All of them don't, to be sure. Disability of one form or another continues to be a reality for a minority of premature infants, most of whom are among the very smallest preemies born at birth weights of less than 1,500 grams (3 pounds 5 ounces) and at less than twenty-eight weeks' gestation. Some never survive their severe immaturity. For most, however, high technology, when applied by compassionate, skilled neonatal medical professionals, offers a reprieve that children only a few decades ago had no chance to receive.

In 1969 only 50 percent of babies with birth weights between 1,000 and 1,500 grams (between 2 pounds 3 ounces and 3 pounds 5 ounces) survived their first year. By 1985 our rapidly progressing understanding of prematurity, its causes, and its remedies boosted that survival rate to 85 percent. Today it stands at over 90 percent. Among the very smallest preemies, those weighing less than 750 grams (1 pound 10 ounces) at birth, the improvement has been even more dramatic. In 1969 less than 4 percent of these babies survived. By 1985—before the 1969 survivors were even out of high school—the survival rate had spiked nearly sevenfold to 25 percent. Today the survival rate for very premature infants (twenty-four weeks' gestation) is climbing toward 50 percent.

In the sixties it was thought that the best care a preemie could receive was to be left in isolation. "You were to feed them and put them in an incubator to keep them warm, but beyond that it was hands off while the heavens considered their fate," wrote Jeff Lyon in his excellent book *Playing God in the Nursery*. "It was so crude it was almost biblical," Lyon quoted Dr. L. Joseph Butterfield of Children's Hospital in Denver as saying.

Today, leaving preemies alone has its place, but as a general rule preemies are actively managed with a variety of techniques developed and first applied just in the past few decades. A condition known as *hyaline membrane disease* (HMD), also known as *respiratory distress syndrome* (RDS), baffled doctors until the late 1950s. The advent of techniques for maintaining air pressure in the infant's airways and air sacs within the lungs has led to startling reversals in the mortality rate from RDS. In 1969 doctors at the University of California at San Francisco began implementing a technique called *continuous positive airway pressure* (CPAP), which was designed to keep the tiny air sacs in the infant's lungs from collapsing in on themselves. The survival rate there for preemies with birth weights below 1,500 grams shot up almost overnight from 11 percent to 83 percent. Other innovations made by doctors in the United States, Europe, and Australia improved preemies' prospects still further. Sophisticated medical ventilators that adjust their pressure to the continuously changing needs of the baby, artificial surfactant to help the lungs, phototherapy to treat neonatal jaundice, maternal steroid injections to promote fetal lung maturity, new methods for intravenous feeding—all have forever strengthened the survival prospects for premature and low-birth-weight infants. These improvements in the care of preemies have cut the overall infant mortality rate dramatically in this country. Although approximately 11 percent of all infants are born prematurely, 75 percent of all infant deaths are the direct or indirect result of prematurity. Thus even a small change in the rate of prematurity can have a large effect on overall mortality.

There is still a long way to go. According to the National Center for Health Statistics, in 1996 prematurity/low birth weight was the second leading cause of infant mortality (occurring at a rate of 100.3 for every 100,000 live births), ahead of sudden infant death syndrome (78.4) and behind birth defects (164). Nonetheless, the improvements medicine has made in the care of premature infants over the past three decades are far-reaching. Thirty years ago all you might have been able to hear at that park in Austin was the wind in the trees. But several decades' worth of advancement in the medical arts have allowed that park to hum with the energies of hundreds of healthy young children who began life prematurely. It is often said that premature infants enter the world early to get started on some as yet unknown ambition. Whatever their goals, every year finds them coming back to the reunion. Another year, another celebration of life.

≫

We have written this book for parents of babies born earlier than thirty-seven weeks' gestation, for mothers who are at high risk of premature labor or delivery for whatever the cause, for parents whose full-term infants have had neonatal complications, and for any parent concerned with the later-life implications of these complications. In the pages that follow we strive to recognize the emotional as well as the clinical side of premature labor and premature birth. Though we draw upon a wealth of recently published statistics on premature and low-birth-weight babies that have been assembled by nationally and internationally recognized researchers, we color the statistical picture with the testimony of couples who collectively have experienced virtually every aspect of premature delivery.

We recognize that the term *premature* encompasses a wide range of possible scenarios, from high-risk infants born at twenty-four weeks weighing slightly over a pound to babies born just a few weeks early at thirty-six weeks. We intend this book to be a resource useful to parents regardless of the circumstance they or their child(ren) find themselves in. At the same time, we have structured the book to provide information targeted to preemies in specific age brackets. The needs of the twenty-four-weeker are very different from those of the thirty-six-weeker. Even so, parents of both babies will experience similar emotions, fears, and anxieties. They will go through the same process, from visiting their babies in the NICU to dealing with the emotional and logistical challenges that go with bringing a child into the world ahead of his time. While recognizing the special needs of babies of different gestational ages, we also acknowledge the common experience parents of preemies have, from the initial feelings of shock, denial, and concern to the joy of bringing a flourishing, healthy infant back to the hospital for her one-year reunion with her former NICU-mates.

For parents who are confronting the possibility of a very premature delivery, coupled with a higher than average likelihood that their child will have some form of developmental problem, we intend this book to be a resource and also a source of comfort. The comfort may come from the knowledge that you are not alone in your anxiety and fear. It may also come from the knowledge of the progress neonatal medicine has made in the last few decades, of the great strides it continues to make, and of what that progress means for babies with developmental difficulties in terms of an improved likelihood of living a healthy, fulfilling life, their disabilities notwithstanding.

Please allow us to introduce ourselves. As deputy medical director of nursery services at Houston's Ben Taub General Hospital, Joseph A. Garcia-Prats, M.D., has cared for preemies for more than twenty years. Along the way he has witnessed most of the changes that have revolutionized the field of neonatology over the past several decades. In addition to this clinical experience, he is also an associate professor of the section of neonatology, Department of Pediatrics, and the Center for Ethics, Medicine and Public Issues at Baylor College of Medicine.

Being the father of ten sons has deepened Joe's understanding of the parent/child bond (an understanding that is articulated in his previous book, *Good Families Don't Just Happen,* coauthored with his wife, Catherine Musco-Garcia-Prats, and Claire Cassidy).

Sharon Simmons Hornfischer is a registered nurse with experience in pediatrics and hospital emergency nursing and has also worked as a health educator for parents and other health professionals. She is the mother of a boy born eight weeks prematurely in 1997, who took his first steps as the manuscript of this book was nearing completion, and of a daughter born full-term just two days after the publisher's original deadline for the manuscript of this book. Sharon's own time in the hospital before and after an emergency cesarean section has given her a patient's-eye view of the preemie experience:

"When I was admitted," Sharon said, "the nurses and doctors knew that I was an RN. Figuring that I therefore understood everything that was going on, they would often gloss over important explanations of procedures and protocols designed to help a cesarean patient in post-op, not to mention a new mother of a preemie. But I was so ill from my preeclampsia that my medical background might as well not have existed. There were days when I didn't even feel competent to take an aspirin by myself. I think that this combination of clinical and personal experience gives me a helpful perspective on the concerns and fears of parents of premature infants."

We hope that this book will be helpful to you in providing both sound medical advice and the compassion that comes from having lived the experience ourselves in several different capacities. We have both come to appreciate and even marvel at the resilience of newborn infants and their dignity as patients and humans. We have seen enough to know that the outcomes are not always as we would wish them to be. But we have also seen the inner personal and spiritual strength that comes to the surface in the face of adversity— strength that will serve you well regardless of the particular outcome of your experience with prematurity. The relative scarcity of general information on prematurity has motivated us to write this book. We hope our effort will help you and your family better understand the experience of prematurity and cope with the inevitable fears and concerns that arise when the unexpected occurs.

WHAT TO DO WHEN
YOUR BABY
IS PREMATURE

1

"WHAT'S HAPPENING TO ME?"
The Causes of High-Risk Pregnancy

WHAT YOU WILL FIND IN THIS CHAPTER

- Confronting and coping with the shock of a high-risk pregnancy

Causes of high-risk pregnancy—an overview

- Preexisting (chronic) conditions that can lead to high-risk pregnancy or premature delivery
- Other conditions that can cause prematurity
- Pregnancy-induced conditions that can lead to high-risk pregnancy or premature delivery
- Other causes of high-risk pregnancy

Confronting and Coping with the Shock of a High-Risk Pregnancy

Your first inkling that something was wrong may have come when you saw your doctor midway into your pregnancy and his or her normally reassuring attitude was suddenly tinged with barely perceptible concern. A routine medical checkup may have revealed that your blood pressure was up, or that you were gaining weight too fast, or that your blood sugar was too high. You might have discovered that you were the mother of multiples. Any of these may have come as a total shock to you. Or perhaps you knew from the day you learned you were pregnant that premature delivery was a possibility. The situation unfolds a little bit differently for everyone.

When Gini discovered she was headed for a premature delivery, she was only beginning to get started working on her new daughter's nursery.

"I was lying in my doctor's office examination room, and I heard my husband talking to a nurse out in the hall. The nurse was explaining to him that I needed to be transferred to the hospital right away. It's ten weeks from when the baby's coming. That can't be right, I thought. I had no idea that I wouldn't carry Carly to term. The nursery wasn't set up. I was on spring break from teaching, and that was the week I was going to start working on it. We were not at all prepared. Of course, since it took two months for our daughter to come home from the hospital, we later had plenty of time to get prepared."

Daryl, a thirty-year-old attorney who had an incompetent cervix, remembered her sudden acquaintance with the complete disruption that a high-risk pregnancy can cause in a busy life. "At twenty-five weeks, I was visiting family in New York for a week, and I was having this feeling as though my belly were too low. I felt as if I had to hold it up. I had a slight watery discharge, but nothing that caused me any concern. When I saw my doctor, he found that I was 3 centimeters dilated. After doing the sonogram, he said to me, 'Your life is about to change dramatically. Oh, and by the way, it's a boy.'

"I didn't realize how serious it was at first. In hindsight, I'm glad the doctor didn't tell me. He told me that my amniotic sac was bulging into my cervix—a dangerous situation because it could burst at any time, leading to a premature delivery. He admitted me to the hospital and said, 'Hopefully you'll be there fourteen weeks.'

"*Hopefully?* I thought. He didn't explain to me what any of this meant. We didn't discuss prematurity. But all kinds of things were flashing through my head. I had just gotten back from vacation, and I had a great deal of work to catch up on. All of a sudden my next six weeks of plans needed to be canceled."

No matter what your circumstances were when you discovered that your pregnancy had somehow run off the rails, your reaction may very well have been, "What's happening to me?" After the initial surprise passed and the possible ramifications of a premature delivery began to take shape in your mind, you may have progressed from questions to declarations: "This *can't* be happening to me!"

Liz, from Maryland, is an avid competitive swimmer who experienced a partially abrupted placenta at fifteen weeks. "I was so healthy, I never expected this to happen to me. I planned to swim till the day I delivered. I never dreamed I would have a complicated pregnancy. There was no indication of it in my medical history. The whole bottom just fell out of my world."

The surprise is entirely understandable. From the time the obstetrician first calculates your baby's expected due date, it's only natural to dream of a full-term pregnancy, a short, on-time labor with no unpleasant surprises, and a smooth, happy transition to life with a new baby. You might already have been planning the phone calls you'll make, picturing balloons and cigars being delivered, and envisioning a new life with a healthy, full-term baby as the center of your new family. Unless you had a known health condition that put you at high risk for prematurity, you probably have not spent a great deal of time worrying about the problems that can bring about a preterm delivery. So when the unexpected occurs, it is only normal to wonder, What's wrong with me?

You're likely reading this book for one of a small number of reasons. You may have been told that your pregnancy is not progressing as planned and that your baby may be born prematurely. Or you may have been admitted to the hospital and are reading this book while on bed rest. Perhaps you are suddenly experienc-

"I was feeling awful but didn't know why"

SHARON HORNFISCHER: "I'll never forget it. At the end of my second trimester, I was seeing my OB/GYN for a routine prenatal checkup. Frankly, I was feeling awful but didn't know why. I was tired. Even minor exertions were making me short of breath. My ankles were starting to swell. And I was generally feeling overwhelmed by life. I thought to myself: This is all just par for the course for a normal pregnancy. Having heard my sisters and friends discuss their pregnancies in the past, I thought this was just part of the 'wonder of pregnancy.' I sure didn't want to look like a wimp by complaining.

"But at this routine appointment, while I was having my blood pressure checked, the nurse suddenly got this concerned look on her face. She asked another nurse to recheck my blood pressure. When the reading was confirmed, they told me that my reading was 150 over 96. They called in my obstetrician, who reassessed me. He soberly informed me that I was beginning to develop pregnancy-induced hypertension. He said that while my baby and I were doing fine for now, I was facing a potentially serious medical problem that could, in time, pose risks not only to me, but to my baby as well.

"I couldn't believe what I was hearing. This can't be happening to me, I thought. My husband is six feet six. I'm five nine. We're strong, healthy people. We always pictured ourselves having a child in the 10-pound-plus range. We often said that if a cesarean were needed, it would only be because our baby was too big.

"I couldn't believe my own body could be letting me down like this."

ing premature contractions and are all at once facing fears that you never knew existed. You may have already given birth to a premature infant and are wondering what your chances are of having it happen again. You may be concerned about the chances for your premature baby to develop normally. Or it may be that your full-term infant is having neonatal complications that will require him or her to stay in the special care nursery or neonatal intensive care unit for a period of time.

We intend this book to be a useful resource for readers in any of these categories. Recognizing that every pregnancy—whether it results in premature delivery or not—is a unique experience for every mother, we nonetheless hope to answer as many questions as possible. Premature delivery encompasses a wide range of potential medical issues—many of which medicine does not yet fully understand. Yet the emotional repercussions that mothers experience have a certain uniformity, fear and guilt foremost among them. We hope that by explaining what medicine knows about prematurity, and by detailing the possible outcomes of prematurity and how they can best be managed, we will assuage the fear and guilt that parents naturally experience.

PREGNANCY RISK FACTORS AND COMPLICATIONS IN THE UNITED STATES, 1997		
Medical Risk Factor/ Complication	Number of Mothers Affected (All Ages and Races)	Rate per 1,000 Births
Anemia	77,334	20.2
Diabetes	101,176	26.4
Genital herpes	31,550	9.0
Hydramnios/ oligohydramnios	50,025	13.0
Hypertension, chronic	26,378	6.9
Hypertension, pregnancy associated	141,235	36.8
Eclampsia	12,782	3.3
Incompetent cervix	10,208	2.7
Previous preterm or small-for-gestational-age infant	46,152	12.0
Renal disease	10,886	2.9
Uterine bleeding	24,463	7.0
Premature rupture of membranes	108,831	28.3
Dysfunctional labor	106,157	27.6

Source: Centers for Disease Control and Prevention, National Vital Statistics Report, vol. 47, no. 18, April 29, 1999, pp. 53–54.

Gini hadn't spent much time worrying about prematurity when she stepped into the shower prior to leaving for a routine doctor's appointment one day. When she stepped out of the shower ten minutes later, her pregnancy had taken on an entirely new dimension.

"By the time I got out," she said, "I couldn't see."

Earlier that day, when she was working on the computer, she had started seeing little fuzzy spots. Thinking that it was because of the long hours she was putting in looking at the computer screen, she "blew it off." But soon enough her symptoms were becoming so severe that she had to take notice.

"It was weird. I saw some flashing lights, then everything just kind of gradually darkened. I put my glasses on, got dressed, and walked out into the living room, where my husband, Scott, was having a business meeting. I couldn't see their faces. I couldn't tell who was who, although I recognized the shirt Scott had on. It was a sign of high blood pressure, and I didn't even realize it at the time. All the way to the doctor's office, I kept my eyes closed. I didn't even want to know if it was really true that I couldn't see."

Blurred or lost vision is one of the signs of *pregnancy-induced hypertension* (PIH). Also known as *preeclampsia* or *toxemia of pregnancy*—discussed in greater detail later in this chapter—it is a potentially serious complication of pregnancy that often leads to preterm delivery. The onset of such unusual symptoms can be gradual. Or it can be sudden and frightening. Preterm labor is especially notorious for arriving without warning and turning a normal pregnancy, overnight, into a struggle to adjust to dashed hopes and expectations. "Everything was fine until I went into labor," said Melissa, the twenty-seven-year-old mother of Emma (full-term) and Erin, a twenty-six-week preemie born at 2 pounds 1 ounce in 1996. "I had considered every other possibility except that she would be born early." Prematurity is certainly not the first thing on the minds of most expectant mothers as they make their way through pregnancy. It's a natural by-product of optimism to believe that such things happen only to those proverbial "other people."

Today many women have learned perhaps too well "what to expect when they're expecting." Innumerable books and magazines describe the latest step-by-step program for having the idyllic full-term pregnancy and are full of photos of cherub-faced, full-term infants. In a world of sophisticated, high-tech therapies, it's easy to think that pregnancy and childbirth are processes that can be measured, controlled, and brought into line with our orderly twenty-first-century lives. It's easy to have the illusion that pregnancy's mysteries are solvable at last. Since you're reading this book, you may already know that's not always the case.

Pregnancy is a delicately choreographed biological and genetic minuet that we are only beginning to comprehend. While we have become quite skilled at measuring and managing many of its steps, there remain mysteries that may never be solved.

- "Why did my blood pressure suddenly increase?"
- "Why am I having contractions now?"
- "Why did my placenta implant too low?"

Questions like these don't always have the definitive answers we have learned to expect from modern medicine. Even the most skilled obstetrician sometimes has to throw up his or her hands and cite the mysteries of creation and the limits of scientific inquiry. But while it is frustrating not to be in control, not to know the cause of, consequences of, and cure for every possible symptom or circumstance under the sun, there is ultimately something healthy about recognizing the limits of our knowledge and control. Sometimes things just happen, things that could not possibly have

been foreseen or prevented. Science may have all of the questions. But answers take time to discover.

We will nonetheless try to offer you as many of the answers as modern medicine has to the perplexing questions that arise in the course of a high-risk pregnancy. Before we get to those answers, however, we have to confront the first question that comes to mind when you have been told that your pregnancy may end in a premature delivery.

"What did I do wrong?"

When you're faced with premature delivery, it's only natural to feel the sense of guilt that compels such a question. "Among high-risk mothers, there's this unconscious belief that they're faulty," said Dr. Mara Tesler Stein, a Chicago-based clinical psychologist who works with mothers with high-risk pregnancies. "Some parents are relieved that their child is in NICU, because the 'good people' can take care of him. Even at discharge, they're thinking, My baby survived fifteen weeks in NICU, now I'm going to take him home and do him in."

For ninety-nine out of one hundred parents, the answer is, you have done nothing wrong. While it is natural to wonder what has gone awry with your body, unless the threat of prematurity arises from drug or alcohol abuse or some other explicit lifestyle choice, there are no grounds to blame yourself and in most cases no reliable way of predicting when, where, or why a high-risk pregnancy will develop.

What has gone wrong with your body? If you knew the cause, you reason, you might be able to do something about it. Or at least, knowing the cause, you might feel less guilty

Choosing Your Caregiver

If you are in premature labor but had no advance warning that you were at risk, you may need to make some changes in the kind of doctor you're seeing. What kind of physician would best serve your needs from this point on? If you have already been seeing an obstetrician (or midwife) for your until now normal pregnancy, that person should be your first phone call. Discuss with her whether she should be your primary physician for your now high-risk pregnancy. But if you have not yet seen a physician for your pregnancy and you suspect you're in premature labor, then an emergency room is the best place to go to get immediate care. Ask the emergency room physician to summon an obstetrician to consult with you as soon as possible. After the emergency situation has passed, you can make arrangements for your longer-term care.

Since you are about to undergo numerous medical evaluations that may require complex treatment decisions to be made, you need to have the benefit of the best-informed medical mind available. Some would argue that if you're in preterm labor—especially when your baby's gestational age is less than thirty-two weeks—you may want to discuss with your OB/GYN the need to consult a perinatologist, who is an obstetrician specializing in high-risk pregnancies. A possibly better alternative would be to have your obstetrician consult a perinatologist. This arrangement would allow you to maintain your relationship with the obstetrician you've been seeing up until now, if you have one, and still have the special expertise of a perinatologist at your disposal. If the complexity of your problem demands more intensive attention, your obstetrician may decide to turn over all aspects of your care to the perinatologist.

If you think something may be wrong with your pregnancy, talk to your doctor about it. Don't be worried about feeling stupid or coming across as panicky. If your obstetrician subtly or overtly makes you feel silly or irrational for voicing your concerns, you might want to find another one.

Liz, from Maryland, shared with us her views on selecting an OB: "Choosing an obstetrician is one of the most important decisions a woman makes. She and her husband should find a physician who includes them in decisions about her care. A woman should feel as though her obstetrician knows her and all aspects of her pregnancy and always acts in her and the baby's best interests. She should know what is in her medical file and have anything she doesn't understand explained to her."

You can help your obstetrician by being a good "historian" of your pregnancy. Accurately and promptly report any concerns or signs and symptoms, and make sure your reports are detailed enough to be useful to your doctor.

about your perceived responsibility for your condition. We have yet to meet parents who didn't experience a sense of guilt that they somehow "caused" their child's prematurity. "If only I ate better." "If only I exercised more [or less]." "If only we hadn't had sex in my second trimester." "If only I hadn't pushed myself so hard at work." Any number of things can be blamed for the unexpected occurrence of prematurity by parents eager to latch on to cause and effect in the face of great uncertainty. Christine, a thirty-three-year-old Denver mother who had six high-risk pregnancies, including two miscarriages, said: "You have these thoughts in the back of your head: I shouldn't have picked up that 5-pound bag of sugar . . . I shouldn't have taken my kids to see that movie . . . I shouldn't have run around for six hours straight cleaning the house late at night." Although these thoughts are natural, it may surprise you—and, we hope, comfort you—to know that physicians simply don't yet understand all of the causes of premature delivery. For instance, the chemical trigger of preterm labor remains undiscovered. The factors that cause pregnancy-induced hypertension remain shrouded in mystery as well.

In the absence of a solid explanation, it's understandable if speculation becomes the order of the day. That long, stressful weekend at the office may appear to you to be the straw that broke the camel's back. Or maybe that weekend in the city, when you walked twenty blocks on a nice sunny day, seems like a possible suspect. Realize, however, that this is just guilt talking. Guilt can take on many shapes and forms, often irrational ones. So don't jump to conclusions and beat yourself up.

"People have to be willing to admit that [prematurity] is a possibility," said Leslie, a mother from Queens, New York, who delivered a 2-pound-2-ounce boy via cesarean at twenty-eight weeks owing to a placental abruption. "We have to educate women about their bodies. I have this great doctor, but she never said to me, 'Oh, you have to watch out for these things—lower back pain, rhythmic contractions . . .' If women could just become educated as to what's going on with their high-risk pregnancies, it would cut down preterm labor drastically. I don't think I was properly educated."

A close, trusting relationship with your obstetrician can go a long way toward dispelling these unjustified feelings of guilt. If you have a good relationship with your OB, confide your fears and concerns. Listen to the answers—and know that you are doing the best thing possible for yourself and your child by following your doctor's advice. The good, empathetic counsel of a medical professional can be the best remedy for irrational fear and guilt.

Gain as much information as you can from your physician. Consider also talking to a friend or family member who is medically savvy or, better yet, has been through a difficult pregnancy herself. When all else fails, educate yourself. Knowledge is power, and there are few better ways to dispel fear of the unknown than to inform yourself about as many aspects of prematurity as you can.

- Go the library and consult books on high-risk pregnancy. They can range from the very technical to the very basic. Choose the one that suits you best.

- Log on to the Internet and find a medical Web site from a well-established, reputable health organization (see Appendix C). Even if you're on bed rest, you may be able to use a laptop computer (check with your doctor first). Caveat emptor: We've seen a lot of suspect health information on the Web. Chat rooms where parents with high-risk pregnancies share their experiences can offer you some insights.

- Talk to a friend, relative, or acquaintance who's been there before. It's amazing how fast you will bond with someone else who has experienced prematurity. An organization called Sidelines is a free national support network for women with high-risk pregnancy. You can find them on the Internet at www.sidelines.org.

- At all times remember that you are the best advocate for yourself and your baby. Trust your instincts. Take action. And avoid keeping your fears to yourself.

While a little knowledge can indeed be a dangerous thing (if it is incomplete, inaccurate, or taken out of context—see "Separating Fact from Fiction about High-Risk Pregnancy," following)—our view is that parents should learn as much as possible about their babies' conditions. There is so much good information available today that it will make your preemie experience only go more smoothly if you understand something about the obstacle course in front of you.

Causes of High-Risk Pregnancy—An Overview

While they are not always easy to pinpoint, isolate, or control, a variety of conditions can lead to preterm delivery. Through proper medical management (gone into in more detail in chapter 2) you can maximize your chance for a good outcome. Still, about the best you can hope for, once you have been diagnosed with a high-risk pregnancy likely to result in premature delivery, is to forestall delivery for as long as possible to ensure the health of your newborn. If you have a "find it, fix it" attitude about medicine, you will have to adjust to the frustrating uncertainty of a high-risk pregnancy. Statistics show that your child can benefit significantly from the addition of even a few days to his or her time in the womb.

The remainder of this chapter outlines the most common causes of a high-risk pregnancy, in order to give you a better understanding of what's happening to you.

Preexisting (Chronic) Conditions That Can Lead to High-Risk Pregnancy or Premature Delivery

CHRONIC HYPERTENSION (HIGH BLOOD PRESSURE)

More and more women today are starting their families in their thirties and forties, a time when

Separating Fact from Fiction about High-Risk Pregnancy

There is always going to be a well-intentioned friend or relative eager to share with you her "expertise" on what may have caused your prematurity. Trying to be helpful, she may repeat any number of myths she's heard through the pregnancy rumor mill. For example, she may tell you that you shouldn't have

- had sex in the third trimester.
- eaten that plate of seafood—didn't you know that seafood is bad for a pregnancy?
- slept on a hard mattress.
- flown in an airplane during your second trimester.

Kerrin encountered some frustration in dealing with family members who had certain ideas about how her pregnancy should go. "My family is full of opinionated women," she said. "All of them had full-term pregnancies. I had to tell them, 'You had full-term pregnancies, but this is different.' There were times when I had to bite my tongue and do my own thing. And there were times when they had to do that, too."

The bottom line is that friends and family members offering advice to you, no matter how well-intentioned they are, will probably just increase your anxiety level by being too helpful by half. Their good wishes and desire to help will often be subverted by their lack of information about high-risk pregnancy. It is best to take any questions or concerns you have to your physician. Train yourself to give wives' tales and myths the old grain of salt. If it doesn't come from your doctor or another authoritative source, tune it out.

chronic health conditions are more prevalent than they were in earlier life. *Hypertension,* or *high blood pressure,* is prominent among them. People who suffer from chronic hypertension have elevated blood pressure levels all the time. The normal adult blood pressure range is between 110 and 150 for the "upper," or systolic, number and between 60 and 80 for the "lower," or diastolic, number. When your diastolic number is consistently above 90, you are considered to have hypertension. Chronic hypertension is present all of the time, as opposed to pregnancy-induced hypertension (PIH), a condition that is brought on by pregnancy itself and usually goes away after the pregnancy has ended. (We go into more detail about pregnancy-induced hypertension [PIH] later in this chapter.)

The risk that hypertension poses to your baby arises from its principal effect during pregnancy: to constrict the bloods vessels that nourish your baby in the womb. Hypertension can affect the placenta by constricting the blood vessels within it, thus reducing the supply of oxygen and nutrients to the infant. This may increase the possibility that your baby will have *intrauterine growth retardation* (IUGR). Babies with IUGR may be born small for their gestational age and may have a wasted appearance in relation to that of other preemies born at the same gestational age. Additionally, these babies when born early may be at risk for other conditions of prematurity, depending on their gestational age at birth. (See chapter 7, "Special Concerns in the NICU.")

High blood pressure can harm the mother, too, leading to kidney and liver failure and possibly, in extreme cases, seizures (eclampsia). (For further information on high blood pressure in pregnancy, see the section on pregnancy-induced hypertension/preeclampsia, page 23.)

TREATMENT. Chronic hypertension is usually treated with a combination of close monitoring by a physician, rest, exercise (if medically appropriate), diet, and medication. It usually can be managed quite effectively with compliance and close medical attention. However, if a woman with chronic hypertension is thinking of becoming pregnant, the treatment picture changes. First, she will be automatically considered a high-risk pregnancy, whether her baby is delivered at term or prematurely. She will follow more rigorous precautions throughout her pregnancy, and every symptom will be reviewed thoroughly. The "condition" of pregnancy will possibly exacerbate her condition. And pregnancy-induced hypertension will most likely develop over time, compounding the effects of chronic hypertension, making a serious condition progressively more serious. A full-term delivery may not be possible. This is not to say that a successful pregnancy is not possible; with very close medical attention and

strict compliance, it often is. But make no mistake: This is a high-risk situation for both mother and baby, and thus it needs to be taken very seriously. If you have chronic high blood pressure, you will need close medical attention from your obstetrician and possibly even a perinatologist.

What to Do If You Have Chronic High Blood Pressure and Are Thinking of Having a Baby

Consult your high blood pressure specialist as soon as possible. This could be a cardiologist, an internist, or an endocrinologist. The earlier you do this, the more time you will have before conceiving to get your mind and body in optimal health for the strenuous road ahead. You may want to use an obstetrician who has considerable high-risk pregnancy experience, or a perinatologist. Pregnancy will place additional strain on a body that is already functioning in a state of stress. You need to recognize this and find a physician you are comfortable seeing frequently. He or she will be able to discuss your individual health concerns as well as their potential consequences on your baby. You will be monitored much more closely and more frequently than a woman who is not in a high-risk situation. It is important that you do what you can to make sure that ongoing communication is taking place between your obstetrician and your blood pressure specialist. When you begin seeing the second specialist, make sure he or she understands the need to coordinate your care with another doctor. Expressly confirm the specialist's willingness to stay in regular touch with your other doctor, for the sake of your health and your baby's.

Gini, a mother of a thirty-one-week preemie

living in Austin, said, "After having a bout with PIH in my first pregnancy, I developed chronic hypertension. My husband and I, in consultation with my doctor, decided that we would nevertheless try to have another baby, even though we knew that our chances of having a second child born prematurely was high. We decided to take an informed risk. My doctor managed me very closely throughout my pregnancy. In the end we were rewarded with a baby girl born at thirty-one weeks' gestation, 2 pounds 10 ounces. We were just thrilled."

Your hypertension will pose a number of risks to you as well as your infant. Because of the potential seriousness of the consequences, your blood pressure will need to be monitored carefully by your obstetrician throughout your pregnancy. Your physician will probably decide upon a "safe" range for your blood pressure readings based on factors such as your overall state of health and your prepregnancy "baseline" pressure reading. Your physician will request blood and/or urine tests in order to monitor your kidney and liver function. Elevated blood pressure levels can damage the small capillaries in these organs, reducing their effectiveness as filters of your blood. This can lead to buildups of proteins that are usually filtered through healthy kidneys and livers. These proteins in large amounts can act like toxins to the body (thereby accounting for the name that PIH previously went by, *toxemia*). Protein tests—which you may be able to perform yourself with a home urine test—can help your physician assess the extent to which your elevated blood pressure is damaging these vital organs.

You will also be assessed for headaches or blurred vision. These are additional signs and symptoms of vascular damage caused by the el-evated pressure. In its most severe cases, hypertension can lead to stroke, loss of vision, seizures, and even death. This is not to scare you away from building the family you long for if you are a chronic hypertensive. Rather, we wish to emphasize the risks associated with chronic hypertension primarily to underline the importance of high-quality medical care and thoughtful planning when you have any chronic condition. At your physician's direction, you will want to get your body in optimal condition for the additional demands of pregnancy.

✒ Tips for Managing High Blood Pressure during Pregnancy

The following treatments for hypertension, along with your physician's individually tailored medical plan, can increase your chances of a successful pregnancy.

MEDICATION. If you were on medication to control your hypertension before you became pregnant, your physician may change your medication to one that is proven safe for your developing fetus. Aldomet is currently the antihypertensive medication of choice for pregnant women. There are other drugs. Just be sure to check with your physician before taking medication of any kind while pregnant.

Note: If you plan to breast-feed, you will also need to consult your physician to be sure your medications don't "cross over" to the baby through your breast milk.

REST AND RELAXATION. Get plenty of it. Your body is under a lot of stress during pregnancy, and this is especially true during a high-risk pregnancy. Take frequent breaks during the day. Take a load off. Put your feet up. This can also reduce the *edema,* or swelling, often associated with pregnancy in general and hypertensive pregnancy in particular. Try to filter out of your life anything that causes you stress. Even if your job doesn't include heavy lifting, the psychological strain of working under stress can exacerbate your hypertension. Though your physician may not put you on bed rest (thereby forcing the issue for you), you should consider ways to minimize your exposure to these "stressors."

DIET. A good diet is critical to a healthy pregnancy. Pregnancy requires you to take in an additional three hundred calories per day and increases your need for protein by 30 percent. If you have hypertension, your appetite will be as strong as the next pregnant woman's. However, it is important that you resist the urge to eat everything in sight. Since sodium has been found to increase blood pressure and increase fluid retention, which can cause swelling of the extremities, you should be cautious about consuming unnecessary quantities of salt. Your physician may well place you on a low-sodium diet if you have hypertension. You will want to maintain or increase your fluid intake, as this aids in flushing your system of extra fluid as well as toxins. Other than that, your diet should include plenty of calcium, fruits, and vegetables—especially the green leafy ones that are high in iron—and lots of protein, vitamins, and minerals.

EXERCISE. Though exercise is important during a normal pregnancy—mild to moderate exercise, directed by your physician, can re-

duce blood pressure, and good overall physical fitness can help you through the rigors of labor—it may be harmful if you have chronic hypertension. With a high-risk pregnancy, it is not always advisable to subject your body to the additional strain a workout imposes. Engage in it only as prescribed by your physician.

Debra, who was twenty-nine when she had her first pregnancy, worked as an accountant for a large manufacturing company. Her doctor put her on modified bed rest at twenty weeks—which allowed her to be on her feet up to six hours a day, "as long as I didn't do anything stupid." Whenever possible, however, she would avoid exercise. "I wasn't taking the stairs at work, and I was getting picked on by people who thought I was hurting my baby. 'You're supposed to be exercising. It's good for the baby,' they would say. They thought I was setting up my child for a sedentary life. I would really get upset. I'm feeling guilty because you read about how beneficial exercise is, and these people are making me feel more guilty. But being mad at them wasn't good for me or the baby."

BED REST. If your doctor prescribes bed rest, take it seriously. Going on bed rest and taking good care not to overexert yourself is one of the precious few ways you can personally and directly influence your odds of having a successful pregnancy outcome. If your doctor deems it to be medically appropriate, you may be allowed to remain at home while you are on bed rest. A more serious condition can warrant admitting you to the hospital, where more sophisticated technical monitoring of you and your baby can be done.

Daryl, who spent five weeks on bed rest for

incompetent cervix, recalls the peculiar difficulty of being required to do nothing for an extended period of time. "My doctor knew me for five years. He knew I would have a hard time with this. What I wanted to know was, 'What can I do?' His answer was, 'Nothing. You can do nothing. You just have to lie there and do nothing.' I felt that shouldn't be too hard. If someone told me all I would have to do to have a healthy baby was lie there and do nothing, I would have thought, That's easy. But it was really hard."

Your physician will decide what level of bed rest is appropriate for you based on your individual circumstances: your overall health, your blood pressure level, your ability to handle stress, your responsibilities at home (for example, if you have other children), your proximity to the hospital, and your ability to be monitored from home.

See chapter 2 for a more extensive discussion of bed rest.

HOME MONITORING. With the increasing availability of computers and modems today, many women are able to use technology to remain home on bed rest. A relatively simple computerized console can be placed next to your bedside and send test results to your physician via a fax modem. Usually your physician will arrange this with a third-party firm that performs home monitoring with its own specially trained nursing staff. A company representative, usually a registered nurse, will schedule a time that is convenient and come out to your home and set up the equipment. At the same time she will instruct you, and any family members who might be assisting you, on its use.

> ### "I felt like an overinflated tire"
>
> SHARON HORNFISCHER: "You may develop a feeling for when your blood pressure is up. When I was on home bed rest due to pregnancy-induced hypertension, I got to where I could sense when my pressure was elevated. I could feel the pressure building within me, the way an overinflated tire must feel. Also, my emotions would become very volatile. I would have ups and downs for no apparent reason. I would laugh at something absolutely ordinary. Then I would cry an hour later because of the same ordinary event. Although some of this sort of thing can go along with hormonal changes that are routine during any pregnancy, this was different. I would check my pressure, and sure enough it would be up. From the intensity of it all, I got to the point I could tell that these emotions were related to my high blood pressure. This is not to say that you shouldn't continue to check your pressure. It's simply to say, try to tune in to what your body is trying to tell you."

CLOSE MEDICAL ATTENTION. Stay in close medical contact with your doctor's office. Keep all appointments. Monitor your blood pressure as directed. Report any unusual signs or symptoms.

LISTEN TO YOUR BODY. This is one of the most important things that you can do. Remember: You know your body better than anyone else, even your physician. You understand when it is trying to tell you something. Listen to it and heed its advice, even if your symptoms seem like small changes that just feel a little out of the ordinary.

DIABETES

It wasn't all that long ago that diabetic women who became pregnant had a very risky road to travel, not only for themselves, but also for their unborn children. But today, with careful monitoring and strict medical compliance, more and more women are enjoying successful pregnancies and healthy babies. Thanks to the great progress in home monitoring of glucose blood levels and the strides in patient education made in the past few years, as well as the development of better hypoglycemic agents and more effective ways to administer them (such as the portable insulin pump), diabetes is not the threat it once was. However, if left unmanaged, diabetes can still lead to significant problems for the mother as well as the baby. These can include such conditions as intrauterine growth retardation (IUGR), congenital disorders of the nervous system, heart, or skeletal systems, or an abnormally high birth weight or even stillbirth. Diabetes can also increase the risk of PIH, increase vulnerability to infection, and lead to increased fetal size, which can complicate a vaginal delivery.

Like hypertension, diabetes takes both chronic and pregnancy-induced (or gestational) forms. The general idea governing the treatment and monitoring of the two different types of diabetes is substantially the same. However, we will discuss them separately; gestational diabetes is treated later in this chapter, under pregnancy-induced conditions that can lead to prematurity. Common signs and symptoms of hypoglycemia and hyperglycemia are also listed in this section.

If you have chronic diabetes, be it type I (juvenile diabetes) or type II (adult-onset diabetes), it is imperative that you consult your doctor about your plans to start a family well before you get pregnant. Close medical attention and following through on medical recommendations will increase your chances for a successful pregnancy. For some women with a history of diabetes, pregnancy may still not be the wisest option. Others may find that their physician gives them the green light to start a family. In either case, once you are armed with sound medical advice, you will better be able to make the right choices for yourself.

TREATMENT. If you are a diabetic, chances are you have been closely medically managed throughout your lifetime. You may have previously discussed with your physician the risks associated with pregnancy. If so, you may already have made plans for diabetic care during pregnancy. The goal in managing diabetes is always to stabilize the blood sugar to a normal level. A normal blood glucose is usually 80 to 120 mg/dl.

The main difference during pregnancy will be an even stricter regime of monitoring and controlling your blood sugar. Today there is a wide variety of home blood sugar monitors on the market. Check with your physician or your hospital's diabetes educator to see if this is recommended for you and if any particular monitor is recommended over another. If the physician recommends home monitoring, his or her office will assist you in getting the needed education on monitoring as well as on overall diabetes management. These monitors need to be recalibrated routinely. You can be taught to do this, but if you're unsure about the technique, have this maintenance performed to ensure accurate readings. Some diabetics are able to control their sugar levels with diet and exercise alone. Others may need medication to assist in controlling their blood sugars during pregnancy.

If you require insulin or oral hypoglycemic agents for blood sugar control, your physician may need to adjust your insulin dose throughout your pregnancy. If you are on an oral hypoglycemic agent and you're not pregnant, you will need to change to insulin during the pregnancy, because oral hypoglycemic agents aren't safe for the baby. Additionally, you will have more frequent doctor visits during the pregnancy. At these appointments you will have additional bloodwork as well as frequent urinalysis testing to detect for excess sugar that could be spilling over into your urine. (See "Signs and Symptoms of Diabetes," page 28.)

Given the increased risk to fetal development that diabetes imposes, additional ultrasound monitoring of your baby's growth and development may be indicated during your pregnancy. If your diabetes proves to be difficult to control, you might be admitted to the hospital for the final weeks of your pregnancy. This way your baby's condition can be watched and early induction of labor or a cesarean delivery can be performed if necessary. Often babies of diabetic mothers who are not under close glucose control are large for their gestational age, and often a bigger baby will require a cesarean delivery.

Whatever the situation, it is very important that you along with your physician monitor your overall health as well as your blood sugar levels very closely during pregnancy and take appropriate action to adjust diet, exercise, and medication as necessary.

KIDNEY DISEASE

Proper functioning of the kidneys is crucial to the health of a mother and her fetus. Kidneys damaged by kidney disease can bring on elevated blood pressure, leading to a number of problems that can cause preterm labor and delivery. Most women with mild to moderate renal disease tolerate pregnancy well and have a successful obstetric outcome, without adverse side effects on the underlying kidney problem. The good news is that attentive care can minimize the risks to mother and baby.

TREATMENT. Mothers with a history of kidney disease should inform their obstetrician so that their kidneys can be monitored throughout the pregnancy. There are several ways to do this. The most common is the urine test that is performed at most of your doctor's visits. Blood tests that assess kidney function (BUN, creatinine) can also be followed.

HEART DISEASE

Just as with the other chronic conditions we mentioned, if you have a heart condition, you should be followed very closely by a medical specialist, usually a cardiologist. You should discuss with her your thoughts on becoming pregnant and discuss whether she, along with your obstetrician, feels that this is a safe course of action. Today, with close medical supervision, many women who were once unable to get pregnant because of the risk of cardiac failure are able to safely bear children. Because there are so many different cardiac conditions, we won't attempt to discuss each one. But we will give you the good advice to discuss your condition and plans to start a family with both your obstetrician and cardiologist.

TIPS ON MANAGING
CARDIAC CONDITIONS IN PREGNANCY

- Follow doctor's orders
- Take medication as prescribed
- Follow a heart-healthy diet (low sodium, low fat, low cholesterol)
- Exercise per medical orders
- Rest
- Avoid alcohol and smoking

SIGNS AND SYMPTOMS
TO REPORT TO YOUR PHYSICIAN
IMMEDIATELY

- Cough
- Dyspnea, shortness of breath
- Edema
- Heart palpitations
- Excessive fatigue

Other Conditions That Can Cause Prematurity

Although this list is by no means comprehensive, here are some other, less common conditions that can lead to premature delivery. If you have any of them, be sure to inform your obstetrician. This way you can discuss and follow any special medical advice.

AUTOIMMUNE DISORDERS

Your body's immune system is extraordinarily effective at fighting off infection, kicking in and generating disease-killing antibodies whenever you have a cold, flu, or other unwanted alien presence in your body. But sometimes the autoimmune system gets carried away with its power and takes action when you don't want it to. When an *autoimmune disease* (also called *connective tissue disease*) is present, the body doesn't recognize certain normal tissue, muscle, or cellular growth patterns as normal. Considering them foreign, the autoimmune system fights against them. In other words, the body fights itself.

Autoimmune disorders are fairly rare, and until the last ten to twenty years little has been known about them. We mention them here briefly because they typically occur in women more commonly than in men, and when they occur in women of childbearing age, they may increase the chance of high-risk pregnancy, premature delivery, and in some cases even fetal death.

In this section we discuss several of the most common disorders and how they can affect pregnancy. If you have been diagnosed with an autoimmune disease or just want more information, consult your physician.

✖ Antiphospholipid Syndrome

Sometimes referred to as "lupuslike syndrome," antiphospholipid syndrome is a potentially serious condition that causes women who have it to experience frequent pregnancy loss. If you have this condition, you are at an increased risk for developing preeclampsia and blood clots

Autoimmune Diseases That Can Affect Pregnancy

- Antiphospholipid syndrome
- Hashimoto's disease
- Graves' disease
- Idiopathic thrombocytopenic purpura (ITP)
- Myasthenia gravis
- Rheumatoid arthritis (RA)
- Systemic lupus erythematosus (SLE)

known as *deep vein thrombosis (DVT)*. Additionally, the placenta is at risk for developing blood clots, which could prove fatal to the fetus if left untreated. Though its cause is unknown, it is signaled by the presence in the blood of lupus anticoagulants and anticardiolipin antibodies. If you have a history of recurrent pregnancy loss, your chances of having antiphospholipid syndrome is around 5 to 10 percent. The risk increases to 30 to 40 percent if you have lupus.

TREATMENT. Prenatal visits are very important, especially for women with autoimmune disease, and as with most high-risk pregnancies, they will be more frequent. You may be seen once every week or two once you reach your second trimester. To assist your physician in closely monitoring your infant, you may also receive monthly ultrasounds. At the same time your ultrasound is performed, your physician may also do a Doppler study, which gives her a picture of the blood flow between the placenta and fetus. If the placental blood flow has been compromised, your physician may recommend

Finally, an Answer

LeeAnn had two miscarriages, a full-term pregnancy, and four more miscarriages before she finally discovered the cause of her problems. Late one night while driving in her car, she heard a radio commercial that grabbed her attention. *"Have you had miscarriages with no explanation . . . ?"* After all she had been through, having seen doctor after doctor who after endless tests told her, "Nothing is wrong—you are perfectly normal," LeeAnn decided to follow up with this radio voice and get tested for autoimmune disease.

Soon thereafter she was diagnosed with antiphospholipid syndrome. She was relieved to discover the cause of her string of miscarriages, even though dealing with it meant additional burdens for her when she became pregnant for the eighth time. Because of other complications (she was put on full bed rest right at the beginning), her doctor had already prescribed terbutaline, which she received in a continuous dosage, via a pump. The heparin she required to manage her autoimmune disorder was delivered via pump as well. "Having the two pumps made life really interesting," she said. "One would beep when it was out of meds, and since they were both the same type of pump and made the same sound, I could never tell which one was beeping. It's like when you have a pager go off and you can't find it. This was all during my bed rest, and I was just going crazy. Now that I look back on it, it was pretty funny."

When LeeAnn made it to thirty-seven weeks, her doctor concluded that the baby was safe. "I disconnected my meds, took my daughter to gymnastics, and within an hour I was feeling contraction after contraction. I woke up at seven A.M. because I felt as though a horse had kicked me in the stomach. By the time I got to hospital, I was 8 centimeters dilated. I don't know how I slept through all that, but I did.

"We named our daughter Victoria, because she was our victory."

that you increase your fluid intake, which increases your blood volume for your baby's benefit. She may also put you on bed rest, because the less blood and oxygen you consume, the more reach your baby via the placenta.

It is still critically important to follow your physician's directions very closely. Problems with the placenta cannot be cured or stopped until delivery. And only through close medical management will your physician know when delivery is imminent.

🌿 Thyroid Disease

The thyroid, a gland located in the throat below the larynx (voice box), secretes hormones that are vital to metabolism and growth. Thyroid hormones regulate oxygen consumption by cells, and thus the metabolic rate of tissues, and they are necessary for the normal growth and development of children. Two types of thyroid disorders are autoimmune in origin: Hashimoto's disease (hypothyroidism) and Graves' disease (hyperthyroidism). Although we discuss these under autoimmune disorders, there are many other types of thyroid disorders caused by such things as infection. If you have concerns regarding other types of thyroid disorders, consult your physician.

Hashimoto's disease (hypothyroidism) is caused by underactivity of the thyroid gland. Hypothyroidism, or low thyroid hormone levels, can cause any of the following symptoms: excessive dry skin, extreme fatigue, constipation, weight gain, and hair loss. If you have or are concerned about any of these conditions, consult your physician.

Graves' disease (hyperthyroidism) is caused by overactivity of the thyroid gland. Hyperthyroidism, or an overactive thyroid gland, can cause you to experience any of the following symptoms: weight loss even in the presence of a healthy appetite and diet, diarrhea, nervousness, tremors, and in some cases *exophthalmos,* or the appearance of bulging eyes.

TREATMENT. The treatment for thyroid disorders will depend on whether you have hyper- or hypothyroidism. With hypothyroidism women often have trouble conceiving or complications with the pregnancy, though once this is diagnosed and managed, the chances of successful pregnancy are increased. Synthroid is the medication most commonly used to treat hypothyroidism in pregnancy. Hyperthyroidism, on the other hand, does not generally affect a woman's ability to get pregnant, though in severe or uncontrolled cases it may lead to preterm births. There are several medications for the treatment of Graves' disease, and they may not all be safe for use during pregnancy. If you have a thyroid disorder and are on medica-

tion for it, be sure to consult your physician if you are pregnant or are thinking about becoming pregnant.

With either of the above-mentioned thyroid conditions, proper medical management should enable you to have a successful pregnancy.

Idiopathic Thrombocytopenic Purpura (ITP)

Idiopathic thrombocytopenic purpura (ITP) is an autoimmune disorder of unknown origin that causes your body to treat your blood platelets (cells that assist in the forming of clots) as foreign objects that need to be destroyed. Since platelets are essential for blood clotting, this condition will leave you with low platelets and thus at risk of developing a blood-clotting disorder and bleeding. Because the antibodies involved in ITP can cross the placenta, your baby is also at risk for developing bleeding. However, there is little danger to your baby while she is in utero. The protective confines of the uterus and amniotic fluid make it unlikely that any trauma would occur that would cause your baby to bleed.

MANAGEMENT DURING PREGNANCY. Your platelet level will be monitored very closely in the presence of this condition. Fortunately, since your body needs very few platelets to clot effectively, a slightly low platelet count often does not cause serious problems. Excessive bruising can occur, however. If your platelets drop to a dangerously low level, your care provider may administer platelets intravenously or may place you on medications such as steroids, immunoglobulin, or other immuno-suppressive medications to help slow the destruction of platelets.

Your baby's platelet count at birth and method of delivery are important factors to consider when ITP is present, since low platelet count interferes with blood clotting, which can lead to excessive bleeding during the trauma and stress of delivery. Your doctor will want to minimize the risk of injury to the baby during delivery. If a cesarean is necessary, great care will be taken to control bleeding and minimize tissue damage. After delivery your baby's platelets will be monitored closely. If necessary, immunosuppressant medications may be given to bring the platelet count back up to where it should be.

🌿 Myasthenia Gravis

Myasthenia gravis is an autoimmune disorder that affects the muscles and skeletal system. With myasthenia the risk of preterm delivery may be increased, though the reason is unknown. Muscle weakness and extreme lethargy are classic symptoms of this disorder. Other symptoms may include drooping eyelids, double vision, and difficulty speaking, swallowing, and clearing the mouth and lungs of secretions. Pregnancy does not appear to affect the long-term prognosis of this condition. During pregnancy the condition may remain the same, become worse, or appear to be in a remission of sorts. There is really no way of determining which women with myasthenia gravis will be adversely affected by pregnancy.

MANAGEMENT DURING PREGNANCY. Your physician should stay in close contact with your neurologist to coordinate the management of your myasthenia. You will need to be closely managed medically throughout your pregnancy to coordinate and adjust any medication you might be taking. Successful treatment is usually achieved with medications such as physostigmine. Sometimes, as the condition worsens, a treatment called *plasmapheresis,* which washes the antibodies from the blood, facilitates recovery from acute attacks.

Although myasthenia gravis cannot usually be cured, treatment can minimize the symptoms of the disease so that you can lead a more normal life. But remember the importance of assisting your OB/GYN and your neurologist in the coordination of your care.

🌿 Rheumatoid Arthritis (RA)

Rheumatoid arthritis is a chronic, and sometimes deforming, autoimmune disorder. It manifests itself through inflammation of synovial joints. The exact cause is unknown, but for some reason the immune system begins to form antibodies that create a chronic inflammation of the joints. Pregnancy does not appear to contribute to the progression of the disease.

MANAGEMENT DURING PREGNANCY. The majority of women with RA experience normal pregnancies. The major concern is assuring that any medications you routinely take for RA are safe to take while pregnant. These and other concerns should be addressed to your physicians, both OB/GYN and rheumatologist.

🌿 Systemic Lupus Erythematosus (SLE)

Often referred to simply as *lupus, systemic lupus erythematosus (SLE)* is a multisystem inflammatory disorder characterized by autoimmune antibody production. This results in inflammation of connective tissue in various organs of the body. The signs and symptoms of the disease will depend on which organs or systems are affected, but the most common symptoms are fever, malaise, weight loss, skin rashes, and joint pain. The exact cause of SLE is unknown, but there are indications that it may be related to a variety of factors that are immunologic, environmental, hormonal, and genetic in nature.

The ability to become pregnant with lupus is not the potential problem. Staying pregnant is. As with other autoimmune disorders, as the body produces antibodies, it fights against itself and potentially the fetus, so the risk of miscarriage or pregnancy complications is increased. Additionally, premature delivery is a possibility due to lupus-related complications such as poor placental function, increased risk for preeclampsia, and compromised maternal health. If you have lupus, your pregnancy will automatically be considered high-risk. The actual risk for miscarriage has been found to be between 15 and 40 percent.

MANAGEMENT DURING PREGNANCY. If you have lupus and are planning to become pregnant, it is highly recommended that you discuss your condition extensively with your physician prior to conception. Proper medical management can increase your chances for a successful pregnancy. You may have frequent prenatal visits, frequent ultrasounds, and frequent laboratory studies and may need to have your medications adjusted often throughout the pregnancy. Additionally, it is thought that if you are able to become pregnant during a prolonged period of remission, you will have better chances for a successful pregnancy.

Pregnancy-Induced Conditions

Whereas chronic conditions are the known risks that a mother brings with her into pregnancy, other conditions don't become apparent until pregnancy is well under way. Pregnancy places your body under strain in a way that it has never before experienced. It is thus impossible to predict with any degree of confidence how you will respond to it.

The following complications of pregnancy account for a large percent of all premature births. But in many cases of premature delivery, there is still no reasonable explanation whatsoever. Medicine has invented the label *idiopathic causes* to describe unknown factors that result in prematurity. This is a fancy way of saying that medical professionals have no idea why they happen. But we feel it is important both to relate what medicine knows and to understand cause and effect wherever possible. The disciplines of neonatal and perinatal medicine are still in their infancy, and our understanding of these causes is improving every year. Until we arrive at a place where we have answers for almost all of the incidents of preterm delivery, women who have no history of pregnancy-threatening health problems and no high-risk lifestyle will continue asking the question we began this chapter with: "What's happening to me?"

PREGNANCY-INDUCED HYPERTENSION (PIH)

Unlike chronic hypertension, *pregnancy-induced hypertension (PIH)* is a condition where a woman develops hypertension (generally defined by the lower, "diastolic," blood pressure reading being consistently above 90) as a result of her pregnancy. Usually occurring around the twenty-sixth to thirty-second week, PIH will often be noticed by the physician at a routine prenatal visit during an otherwise uneventful, healthy pregnancy. Though the cause of pregnancy-induced hypertension remains largely a mystery, statistics indicate an increased incidence of PIH in women under the age of eighteen and over thirty-five. It is more common in women who are pregnant for the first time.

Though the term *preeclampsia* is commonly used interchangeably with pregnancy-induced hypertension, preeclampsia is more accurately understood to be an extreme case of PIH. Since the term *eclampsia* means seizures brought on by high blood pressure levels, preeclampsia is a case of PIH that is nearing the seizure threshold, typically involving diastolic blood pressure readings well over 100.

Preeclampsia is thought to be associated with the following factors:

- Mother's age is under twenty or over thirty
- Preexisting diabetes mellitus, heart disease, kidney disease, or autoimmune disorders
- History of poor nutrition
- Multiple pregnancy
- First pregnancy
- Sixth or greater pregnancy

Also known as *toxemia,* PIH is a relatively common disorder of pregnancy. It affects some 6 to 7 percent of all pregnancies, manifesting itself through high blood pressure, headaches, and a buildup of excess levels of protein in the body. Other symptoms may include rapid weight gain coupled with swelling of the ankles, hands, or feet (known as *edema*), blurry or darkened vision coupled with flashing lights before your eyes, dizziness, and even right upper abdominal pain. Most commonly found in first pregnancies and after the twentieth week of gestation, PIH is a serious complication that has the potential, if untreated, to develop into full-blown eclampsia, whose symptoms include seizure, brain hemorrhage, and coma.

Though PIH is usually a complication of first pregnancies, it is possible to have some degree of elevated blood pressure in future pregnancies. If you had PIH in an earlier pregnancy, your physician will monitor your blood pressure especially closely to check for its recurrence. If it does recur, it will probably recur later in your pregnancy and be less severe. Of course, it is still very important to monitor and properly manage any incidence of PIH.

While pregnancy-induced hypertension poses a serious threat to the health of the mother, it also endangers the baby. PIH is associated with constriction of blood vessels in the placenta and uterus. Because the constricted vessels do not carry as much blood and nutrients to the fetus through the placenta, the fetus of a mother with PIH tends to grow more slowly than normal. An infant's birth weight can be 10 percent or more below what the growth chart predicts for gestational age, a condition known as *intrauterine growth retardation (IUGR)*. Babies affected by IUGR may very well go on to develop normally, and in that sense the name sounds worse than it is. An important yardstick for measurement of IUGR's severity is the growth and development of your baby's head. The placenta applies its nutrients first toward the growth of the head. The most fortunate infants who have IUGR have heads that have continued to grow as predicted by their gestational age, despite the slower rate of growth of the rest of their body. In cases like this, the IUGR is "asymmetric"—the head is large in proportion to the rest of the body.

In cases where the growth disturbance has been long-standing, the IUGR may be symmetric—that is, the head has been affected by the IUGR along with the rest of the body. This more serious condition is often due to an illness in the fetus that may be the result of genetic abnormalities, infection, or toxin.

Other possible results of preeclampsia include the onset of premature labor, stillbirth, low blood platelet counts, or placental abruption.

The onset of preeclampsia can be sudden, typically occurring after the twentieth week of pregnancy. A consistent blood pressure reading above 140/90 generally indicates preeclampsia. Preeclampsia is also suspected if your systolic blood pressure reading (the upper number) rises twenty points or more above your prepregnancy baseline blood pressure level, or if the diastolic reading (the lower number) climbs fifteen points or more above that baseline. Preeclampsia can manifest with just a few of the symptoms we have mentioned or all of them. Thus it is important to watch out for any indications of preeclampsia as just described.

CAUSE. The cause of PIH remains a mystery to science. Its cure is simple (if not particularly helpful to a woman who wants to get rid of her PIH right away): birth of the baby. In almost all cases, delivery of the infant ends the symptoms of preeclampsia. In some cases, elevated blood pressure levels can last for as long several months after birth. In still other instances, PIH may mark the onset of chronic hypertension.

Statistically, PIH has a higher incidence in mothers who are teenagers or over the age of thirty-five; have a history of hypertension, kidney disease, or diabetes; or have a family history of preeclampsia.

PIH can vary in severity from woman to woman. Some get it as early as their twenty-fifth week and are able to continue their preg-

SHARON HORNFISCHER: "Owing to a severe case of PIH, I delivered my son at thirty-two weeks' gestation. After the delivery, while I was resting in the labor and delivery ward, the medical staff kept telling me that my pressure would be going down within days. I would be feeling much better soon, they said. But I didn't. In fact, I felt much worse. My vision became blurry, and I started seeing amber-colored spots. My blood pressure stayed elevated and at times was even higher than it was before my son was born. I was in the hospital for ten days. After about three weeks I got my full vision back, and after about eight months—by which time my doctor and I were starting to think that I was turning into a chronic hypertensive—my pressure went back to normal and I was able to get off my medicine."

nancy close to term. Others may suddenly encounter difficulties late in their last trimester and develop an explosive condition that can result in an emergency situation. PIH in this context can be either slow or fast progressing, with varying degrees of risk for maternal and fetal complications.

TREATMENT. If tests reveal you have PIH, your condition will usually be managed with a combination of bed rest, diet, and medication.

Home monitoring can be a very practical way for your doctor to keep a close watch over your vital signs while allowing you to remain in the comfort of your own home. If your blood pressure or urine protein levels reach high

enough levels, you will be hospitalized. (See chapter 2 for more details on bed rest, diet, and blood pressure medications.)

Medications will typically include blood pressure medications such as Aldomet. If your PIH is severe and your doctor expects delivery imminently, you may be given steroid medications to assist your baby's lung maturation. See chapter 2 for further details.

Close monitoring of urine protein levels is essential to tracking the progress of the condition, so you'll need to collect your urine for analysis. In addition to quick urinalysis checks for protein, your physician may order a twenty-four-hour collection of urine for testing. This twenty-four-hour assessment is a much more accurate reading of your condition, and you will probably need to collect several twenty-four-hour specimens as your condition progresses. Your physician is attempting to hold off delivery as long as possible and maintain maternal and fetal health, but when the parameters for delivery are reached, your physician will proceed with delivery. The type of delivery will depend on several factors:

- Emergency nature of delivery
- Fetal or maternal distress
- Cervical dilation, if any
- Mother and baby's ability to withstand the additional stress of labor

If maternal or fetal distress is occurring, a cesarean delivery may be your only option. Alternatively, delivery may be induced by your obstetrician if time and your overall health allows. Since eclamptic seizures can take place after delivery, you'll be monitored closely for up to seventy-two hours after birth.

HELLP Syndrome

Severe cases of preeclampsia can combine with other conditions to bring on *HELLP syndrome*. The name of this potentially very serious condition derives from its diagnostic elements: **he**molyic anemia (characterized by breakdown of red blood cells), **e**levated **l**iver transminases (liver compromise or failure), and **low p**latelet count (inability of the blood to clot). Most often occurring in the third trimester and most often in first pregnancies, HELLP develops in about 15 percent of women who have preeclampsia. However, it may begin as early as twenty weeks and recur in subsequent pregnancies. The cause of HELLP, as with preeclampsia, is not known. HELLP syndrome is diagnosed by blood tests for clotting factors and liver function. In its most mild form, HELLP requires observation and rest. In other situations—fewer than one in twenty-five cases—it can be life-threatening to mother and baby.

The most serious symptoms of HELLP—high blood pressure, protein in the urine, and swelling—are similar. However, HELLP may first reveal itself through symptoms that are more closely akin to gallbladder disease, gastritis, acute hepatitis, or other conditions. These include headache, nausea and vomiting, epigastric tenderness, and right upper quadrant pain (the result of liver distension). The most common cause of maternal death from HELLP syndrome is liver failure. However, this can be prevented if the symptoms are caught in time.

TREATMENT. As with preeclampsia, the only known treatment for HELLP syndrome is delivery of the baby, regardless of the infant's gestational age at birth.

HELLP Syndrome: *"My wedding ring became a distant memory"*

A thirty-seven-year-old consultant for a Big Six consulting firm, Marie was hospitalized at thirty-four weeks with HELLP syndrome. Just shy of thirty weeks into her pregnancy, she had started noticing edema (swelling) in her feet and hands. By 33½ weeks the swelling and water retention had made her wedding ring "a distant memory." Her newfound sources of amusement included watching her swollen, water-filled feet jiggle when she walked. ("Hey, you gotta have something to laugh about!" she said.) But this well-informed mom had few illusions. Her condition was growing dangerous. She noticed that her blood pressure was rising, and four days after her doctor first noticed the swelling, Marie was given medical instructions to leave work and go on full bed rest.

Marie had cable TV installed in her bedroom to help deal with "the stir-crazies." She found comfort in researching her condition. "The on-line support I found was literally a lifesaver," she said. "Through the Internet I learned enough about what could happen with HELLP that I knew not to argue with my doctor whenever she would tell me something needed to be done." E-mailing her friends helped her leaven her difficult situation with humor. "Hi, I've been exploring preeclampsia as an alternative to a healthy pregnancy," she wrote to one friend. But enduring the maddening uncertainty that comes from a constantly changing medical picture that HELLP syndrome presents was no laughing matter.

GESTATIONAL DIABETES

Like PIH, *gestational diabetes* develops during pregnancy and is normally "cured" by delivery. While a mother with gestational diabetes may not develop a severe form of diabetes, diagnosis and management of the condition is nonetheless important. Even a mild form of diabetes can pose a risk to the baby if it is not properly monitored and controlled. If your sugar level is too high, your baby is also receiving excess levels of sugar. This can cause problems for the baby, especially after delivery: at that time his or her blood sugar level will still be high, and the baby's pancreas (which produces insulin) may be "fooled" by this high level and produce too much insulin. Therefore any baby of a mom with gestational diabetes or any baby with irregular sugars at birth will be monitored very closely. (See chapter 7, "Special Concerns in the NICU.")

Further discussion of diabetes can be found on page 16.

"How will I know if I have diabetes?"

Around the time of your fifth-month checkup, your physician will perform a *glucose tolerance test (GTT)*. This test determines whether you are able to metabolize sugar effectively in pregnancy. Before your GTT appointment, your physician will recommend that you fast for eight to twelve hours. At the doctor's office you will be asked to drink a glucose solution, then after an hour's wait your blood glucose level will be drawn. Your physician will determine either that you passed the test or that further testing is necessary to determine whether a diagnosis of gestational diabetes is appropriate.

For Kelly, a thirty-year-old former emergency room nurse and the proud mother of two boys, pregnancy was completely normal for five months. "It was great up until that point," she said, "but in the sixth month I started to swell a little bit. My glucose tolerance test came back high, and I was diagnosed with gestational diabetes at twenty-eight weeks. The swelling was really bad; my hands and feet looked like little balls."

When another glucose tolerance test confirmed her condition, Kelly was placed on insulin and began seeing her doctor on a weekly rather than monthly basis. "I had no family history of diabetes whatsoever. It was really strange," she said.

Signs and Symptoms of Diabetes

FREQUENT URINATION (POLYURIA). Because of the excess glucose in the body, sugar is not properly metabolized. As the infant's kidneys struggle to reabsorb the sugar, excessive water is removed from the body as urine.

EXCESSIVE THIRST (POLYDYPSIA). The frequent urination that diabetes often causes can also lead to dehydration and thirst.

HUNGER PANGS (POLYPHAGIA). This is caused by tissue loss and a state of starvation that arises from the inability of your body's cells to properly utilize the blood glucose.

WEIGHT LOSS. Since the body is unable to properly utilize blood glucose and instead burns fat and muscle tissue in order to generate energy, weight loss occurs in most women who have diabetes.

TREATMENT. Diet modification may be all that's needed to manage your diabetes, or you may need to be placed on medication to control your diabetes. Insulin is the only safe medication to lower blood sugar during pregnancy. The oral hypoglycemic agents that are safe when not pregnant are not considered safe for the baby. If it's needed, your physician will send you to a diabetic educator for consultation, education, and possibly even instruction in insulin administration.

TWINS, TRIPLETS, AND OTHER MULTIPLE PREGNANCIES

If you have been blessed with a multiple pregnancy, you may well be stunned by your good fortune. At the same time, you may feel somewhat overwhelmed as you contemplate not only the slightly more complicated road to delivery

---

It's very important for the diabetic and her family to be familiar with the signs and symptoms of both *hypoglycemia* and *hyperglycemia*. Sometimes when a diabetic attack strikes, the diabetic is not in a position to recognize the symptoms or take action for their treatment. Thus it is a good idea to post the signs and symptoms in a place where your family can see them and become well informed about what to look for.

Hypoglycemia (Low Blood Sugar)	Hyperglycemia (High Blood Sugar)
• Nervousness	• Thirst
• Shakiness	• Excessive urination
• Weakness	• Dry mouth
• Hunger	• Increased appetite
• Sweating	• Exhaustion
• Cool, clammy, or pale skin	• Nausea
• Blurred or double vision	• Hot, flushed skin
• Headache or disorientation	• Abdominal cramps
• Shallow respiration	• Rapid, deep breathing
• Irritability	• Headache
• Coma	• Drowsiness
• Seizures	

At the first noticeable sign of any of these symptoms, contact your physician immediately. If you do have gestational diabetes, blood tests will become a regular part of your prenatal checkup. Your blood sugar will need to be monitored carefully up until the moment you deliver.

ahead of you, but the parental responsibilities that will grow steadily from day one. From the moment they're conceived, twins and other multiple fetuses are at relatively higher risk for premature delivery. Their shorter average gestation period is largely a function of the tight quarters the little ones occupy in the womb, which like any finite space has a certain limit to what it can hold. As a result, the average birth weight of multiples is less than that of singletons, although in most multiple deliveries the combined weight of the babies exceeds the weight of the largest single delivery. Even in the absence of additional medical complications, twins on average are delivered approximately between thirty-five and thirty-seven weeks; triplets at thirty-three and thirty-five weeks; and quadruplets at approximately twenty-nine weeks.

Your uterus is designed naturally to expand as your pregnancy progresses. However, as a result of a multiple pregnancy, pressure on the uterine walls can rise well above the normal capacity of the uterus, sometimes leading to prematurity.

Mothers of multiple fetuses often have greater odds of developing complications of pregnancy such as PIH and premature rupture of membranes (PROM), as well as an increased chance of developing premature labor. There are other conditions that are less common in multi-

Jody and Trevor's Fourfold Blessing

"We're going to be a major caravan everywhere we go," said Jody, thirty-one, from a town outside Houston. She and her husband, Trevor, are the proud parents of quadruplets. Along the way, they experienced the full range of emotions, from seeing an infertility specialist, to the shock of discovering Jody was pregnant with multiples, to the challenge of adjusting to a home that became, overnight, three times as populous as it was the day before. "It's been a major blessing," she said. "I can't imagine not having four at this point."

Because the lining of her uterus wasn't thick enough, Jody needed three cycles of Clomid before an egg would implant. Jody got pregnant on their first try after the last round of treatment, at the end of June. When Jody went in for an ultrasound at six weeks, her doctor could easily make out the forms of three tiny fetuses. "But he said, 'You know, they look a little crowded.' And sure enough, he looked a little closer and there was a fourth one.

"We knew we could handle three. But after he found the fourth, we went out to eat at IHOP, and I don't think we said a word to each other. We just looked at each other, speechless. We didn't know what to say. It sort of takes your breath away. What's going to happen to my body? What's going to happen to our lives? I thought, I'm responsible for bringing home four babies safely. I wondered if I could really do it.

"My perinatologist was great. She was so matter-of-fact. She said, 'If you do what I tell you to do, this is going to work.' At this planning session she told me about the risk of hypertension, gestational diabetes, intrauterine growth retardation, and premature labor. She said, 'Be prepared: you will be on bed rest at some point in your pregnancy.' "

Because an ultrasound at twenty weeks showed that one of the babies' heads was pushing directly on her cervix, the doctor decided to make good on that promise. "It wasn't that much of a change. I already wasn't doing chores. Trevor was doing most of the heavy stuff. The doctor said I could do things around the house, but that she didn't want me running around the mall. Trevor and I still took walks. I did a lot of sitting and drinking. I spent a lot of time in the recliner, napping. I drank gallons of water every day. Other than that, I really didn't do a lot the whole time."

At twenty-two weeks she went on a stool softener for constipation. "Having four babies sitting on your body parts was making things a little hard for me," she said. As time went by, the babies started getting bigger, but her appetite decreased. "The doctor wanted me to eat as much as I could. But it was getting hard. I wasn't really that hungry. They were taking up so much room in my stomach."

On Christmas Eve 1998, just before midnight, the home monitoring service that had been enlisted to keep track of Jody's contractions counted eight contractions in an hour. Since Jody had quadruplets and was only at twenty-eight weeks, they were cautious and had her hospitalized. She was given two shots of Brethine to stop her contractions, which elevated her heart rate to 130—"I felt like I was going to jump out of my skin"—and was monitored for nine hours. In the meantime, urine tests revealed the presence of a bladder infection, and it was found that she was dehydrated, all of her water drinking notwithstanding. "With the babies growing so fast it didn't matter how much I drank—the babies took it." Jody was given antibiotics for the infection and sent home on Christmas morning. "After three days of taking Brethine pills every four to six hours, my body got used to it. But it was still hard for me to keep my hands steady writing thank-you notes," Jody said. "The original goal my doctor set was for me to reach thirty-two weeks, and I was determined to do that no matter what."

On January 5, well into her twenty-ninth week, "things were starting to get uncomfortable" for Jody. "I was borderline hypertensive, and my contractions were hitting the limit." She was admitted to a level III facility (a hospital with an NICU) and began receiving weekly steroid injections (for five weeks) to speed her infants' lung maturation. "In some ways this was comforting because the nurses were so wonderful. On the other hand, I was thinking, There's no going back. It's going to happen now."

Jody was surprised, however, when her doctor told her, "I really think you can go longer than thirty-two weeks. It would be really good for the babies if you could go two more weeks." Jody recalled, "At first that was a major blow. Two more weeks seemed like an eternity. We did an ultrasound, which showed that all the babies were close to 3 pounds. I thought, If that's what it takes to get them over 3 pounds, that's what I'll do. I told my doctor, 'Okay, I'm in this for the duration.' "

At thirty-four weeks they had a date set for the cesarean. "My doctor said to me, 'You're on the verge of major hypertension and kidney shutdown. You're not sick yet, but you could be at any moment. We could try to make it to thirty-five weeks, but it would be day-to-day.' " Jody felt she had pushed herself hard enough. "I said I couldn't go any longer."

Jody delivered her four children—15 pounds 8 ounces of baby—via cesarean section without complication. Each child had a neonatal team consisting of a neonatologist and a respiratory therapist awaiting him or her on delivery.

Jared, 3 pounds 3 ounces: "A scrapper," in the words of his mother, he was the first to come home after two and a half weeks in the NICU. As of his first birthday, Jared was at 21 pounds, the largest of the four.

Brian, 4 pounds 15 ounces: Brian had premature lung disease, fluid in his lungs, and he needed oxygen. "Let me tell you, I felt it when she pulled him out," Jody said. "He was pushing on my windpipe, then all of a sudden I felt, Oh my, I can breathe. Ironically enough, Brian was born with breathing trouble." Brian came home after eighty-six days in the NICU. Now, Jody said, "You'd never know he was ever sick. At 17 pounds, though, the largest at birth is now the smallest of the four.

Holly, 3 pounds 9 ounces: She needed tube feedings for a while, and a few days under bililights (lights to help bring down bilirubin; see page 136), but she came home after three weeks in the NICU. "She's our little show-off," said Jody. "She's the shortest of the bunch, but at 19 pounds she's holding her own just fine."

Jenna, 3 pounds 13 ounces: She took longer to learn how to suck and came home from the NICU in less than three weeks on a heart monitor because of her apnea. Now her mother calls her one-year-old "the leader of the pack. She was the first to roll over and crawl—she's always trying something new."

ple pregnancies, such as twin-to-twin transfusion syndrome (TTTS) and failure to thrive of one or more of the fetuses. These conditions and other complications of carrying multiples should be discussed with your physician. For these reasons, if you're expecting multiples, you will most likely be followed more closely and have more frequent prenatal visits than your friends or coworkers who are having singleton births.

TREATMENT. While multiple pregnancy is not itself a malady or condition that requires "treatment," mothers of multiples will have to be very closely monitored by their prenatal care provider given the potential higher risks involved. As Jody and Trevor's story illustrates (see pp. 32–32), the presence of multiple fetuses can be detected by ultrasound around the sixth to eighth week of pregnancy. Your physician may also be able to determine if you are carrying multiples earlier in your pregnancy if he or she detects a higher than average level of *human chorionic gonadotropin (HCG)*. This level is obtained through a routine blood test performed when first testing you for pregnancy. A combination of bed rest and modified (reduced) physical activity may be necessary at some point during pregnancy to relieve the extra stress and weight placed on the body of a woman carrying multiples.

Jody successfully carried her quads until her thirty-fourth week of gestation. Back in her twenty-eighth week her physician placed her in the hospital for bed rest and close observation. "I know that this made the difference," she said. Six precious weeks, four healthy kids.

Twin-to-Twin Transfusion Syndrome (TTTS)

Twin-to-twin transfusion syndrome is one of the most dangerous and least understood complications affecting multiple pregnancies. A disorder of the placenta that affects the blood flow to the infants, TTTS occurs in roughly 10 percent of identical twin pregnancies (or about 15 percent of the 66 to 75 percent who are monochorionic). It is thought to affect some three thousand pregnancies each year, or roughly six thousand babies annually. Of these six thousand "TTTS babies," about four thousand may die unless treated. Many who survive suffer from neurological damage, including cerebral palsy. If TTTS is treated, however, survival chances for these babies can improve significantly.

TTTS occurs when blood passes disproportionately from one baby to the other through connecting blood vessels within their shared (monochorionic) placenta. The twin receiving too much blood, the "recipient," is thus at risk of heart failure due to her overworked cardiovascular system. The twin receiving too little blood, the "donor," shares her blood flow with the recipient twin but does not receive an equivalent return blood flow, causing her to be small and at risk for possibly fatal conditions associated with low blood volume, such as kidney failure.

In its most extreme form, diagnosed in midpregnancy and untreated, TTTS has an 80 to 100 percent mortality rate.

MANAGEMENT OF TTTS

Today there are several interventions/treatments that may be available. How TTTS will be managed in a particular case will depend on several factors, including the severity of the disorder, the gestational age at diagnosis, the presence of hydrops, or developmental defects in the twins. TTTS can occur at any time during a monochorionic twin pregnancy. Usually the earlier it is developed, the more severe it is. In its mild form there may be no need for treatment, and the condition may not even be diagnosed until after birth. In more severe cases, however, a procedure called *serial therapeutic amniocentesis* or a special type of *intrauterine feto-*

scopic laser surgery designed to stop the shared blood flow between the imperiled twins may be required in order to have a chance of saving the pregnancy.

Laser surgery is still considered experimental. It should be noted that while these interventions offer hope in many cases of TTTS, they are not without their risks. For more information about TTTS, contact the Twin-to-Twin Transfusion Syndrome Foundation (see Appendix C). This organization can give you the most current information about the condition and the latest therapies.

Serial Therapeutic Amniocentesis

The excess blood flow to the recipient twin causes him or her to have excess amniotic fluid (*polyhydramnios*) and suffer the effects of an overloaded cardiovascular system. If this excess fluid is not "siphoned off," the extra weight and pressure placed on the uterus places the mother at risk of premature labor and delivery.

Serial therapeutic amniocentesis resembles the more common diagnostic amniocentesis during a non-high-risk pregnancy. However, instead of withdrawing a small amount of fluid for karyotype testing, the physician removes all of the excess fluid (usually 500 to 2,000 cc, or ½ to 2 liters). Removal of fluid through amnio reduction can prolong the pregnancy until the babies are mature enough for delivery or other treatment options can be explored.

Intrauterine Fetoscopic Laser Treatment

Intrauterine laser surgery deals directly with the cause of TTTS by blocking the flow of blood through the shared vessels in the placenta. The twins undergoing this procedure have a handicap rate of 5 percent, versus 10 to 20 percent for TTTS twins who receive serial amniocentesis alone.

The following story about TTTS is not intended to gloss over the often grim truth about this syndrome and its high mortality rate, but simply to let you know there may very well be hope if you are diagnosed with TTTS.

❧

LAURA'S STORY

Laura was twenty-five during her second pregnancy. Everything was going along as usual until her eighteenth week, when a routine ultrasound diagnosed twins.

"The ultrasound took over an hour, and this seemed like a long time, but I just figured it was because there were two babies. I remember I kept asking the technician about the ultrasound, and she wouldn't say anything. At the end of the hour the doctor came in. 'Oh, this is a really bad day. Your twins have this condition. It's not good, and it is almost always fatal.' He told me I could terminate the pregnancy or wait for the babies to be delivered. But most likely if they did survive, they would be handicapped. The doctor mentioned that 'there is a doctor out west doing this procedure,' but he said that my placenta was in the wrong place."

A neonatologist whom Laura's mother worked for suggested they get a second opinion. The second doctor was more familiar with TTTS. "Though he was not optimistic, he knew the statistics and knew we were in a bad situation, but he was also familiar with the new intrauterine fetoscopic laser surgery for TTTS, so he made the referral to the TTTS Foundation (see Appendix C).

"When I first contacted the TTTS Foundation, I was so distraught about the diagnosis that I spent an hour crying to the employee who happened to answer the phone. It was so wonderful to have someone to talk with. Unfortunately, at the time I called, the doctor was out of the country. So it was my job to stay pregnant until he could get back. To keep me pregnant in the meantime, my doctor performed two amnio reductions. He withdrew 500 cc of fluid the first time and a week later took an additional 700 cc. The pressure from the excess fluid was placing me at an increased risk of going into preterm labor."

The amniocenteses were successful, and Laura was able to hold off labor and keep the twins safe. Then, two weeks after the initial diagnosis, she became the fifty-second patient to undergo fetoscopic laser surgery. It was a success. The doctor found fifteen to twenty vessels connecting the twins. "After approximately a week convalescing in the hospital, I flew back home and remained on modified bed rest for the duration of my pregnancy (with the exception of biweekly trips to my local perinatologist for fetal monitoring and ultrasound). I also received two steroid shots a week from week twenty-eight to thirty-two, to aid in fetal lung maturation. I was lucky because I was healthy myself. I didn't have any trouble with bed rest.

"The girls were born at thirty-six weeks, following sixteen weeks of bed rest. Leah, my donor twin, was 4 pounds at birth and was mildly anemic. Julianne, my recipient twin, was 5 pounds 3 ounces at birth and was very red in color relating to the extra red blood cells. Today they are perfectly fine. At a recent three-year checkup they were even noted to be advanced as far as their learning abilities. Quite wonderful news to parents who were once told that if they survived, they would be handicapped.

"We got lucky, and we know it.

"What causes twin-to-twin transfusion syndrome?"

We do not know why TTTS happens because we do not know why an embryo splits to make identical twins in the first place.

What we do know is that if the embryo splits after four days from fertilization, the twins will share a common placenta. The TTTS complications occur as a result of the connected blood vessels in the common placenta. These complications are unpredictable and completely out of anyone's control. Prevention before actual diagnosis is not possible.

Early signs of TTTS can include the following:

- Unusually large uterus (for dates)
- Sudden rapid weight gain
- Ultrasound findings that show
  single placenta with a thin membrane between the twins
  same-sex babies
  polyhydramnios (too much fluid) in one baby's sac
  oligohydramnios (too little fluid) in the other baby's sac
  difference in growth between the babies (growth discordance)
  evidence of heart failure (hydrops)

Normally the *cervix* (the neck of the uterus) stays tightly shut, sealed with a mucous plug, keeping the fetus snugly held in the uterus until the start of labor. If your cervix is "incompetent," however, it may begin to open prior to the actual onset of labor. This most often occurs at the end of the first trimester or at the beginning of the second. An opening may form that allows the amniotic sac containing the fetus to sag or bulge into the vagina. This exposure of the amniotic sac increases the likelihood of rupture, which early in pregnancy can induce miscarriage as a result of the loss of amniotic fluid or the onset of an ascending bacterial infection. When this happens prior to the thirty-seventh week of pregnancy, premature delivery is a significant risk.

If you are one of the estimated 1 to 2 percent of pregnant women who are diagnosed annually with incompetent cervix, you probably discovered this condition only *after* you experienced an unsuccessful pregnancy. By the time it is first detected, it is often too late to do anything about it. Though a high-risk pregnancy is very difficult to endure, anyone diagnosed with cervical incompetence today is fortunate that there are medical procedures that can dramatically increase the chances for a successful pregnancy.

CAUSE. The causes of a weakened or "incompetent" cervix range from your genetic makeup to your own prenatal exposure to DES (diethylstilbestrol—see box on page 37). Other known causes include stretching from previous vaginal deliveries, abortions, prior cervical

Are You a DES Daughter?

In the 1950s and 1960s, a synthetic estrogen hormone known as *diethylstilbestrol* (DES) was widely prescribed to prevent miscarriage. It is now well-known that daughters of women who took DES have a significantly higher incidence of anatomical irregularities of the uterus, cervix, and vagina and are thus at greater risk of premature delivery. DES has been the subject of extensive litigation since its unfortunate side effects became known.

Kerrin, a thirty-three-year-old mother from Massachusetts, had to do some digging before finally discovering that her own problems with conception and miscarriage probably stemmed from the fact that she was a "DES daughter."

In April 1993 she had an ectopic pregnancy that required not only removal of one fallopian tube, but twenty-four hours of chemotherapy because the tube removal did not entirely remove the fetal tissue. Four months later she became pregnant with twins after a cycle of in vitro fertilization (IVF). However, her doctor soon discovered to his shock that she had nothing left of her cervix. "As soon as I became pregnant, it shortened right up, flush with the bottom of the uterus," Kerrin said. Before he could even give her a cerclage, he would have to "build" a cervix to stitch. He performed the delicate operation successfully. Though she was on the verge of losing her pregnancy at any moment, the stitch held. But at twenty weeks one of the twins was straddling the stitch. "They were afraid I would bleed to death," she said. "I don't remember really well what happened next. I remember them saying there was a lot of bleeding. They cut the stitch and dilated me and pulled them out. They didn't survive."

Because of the persistence of Kerrin's difficulties, her obstetrician now suspected DES as the cause. Desperate to find out the cause of her difficulties, Kerrin asked her mother about the circumstances of her own pregnancy and birth. Her mother said that three months into her pregnancy with Kerrin, when her mother was just nineteen, she was told her baby felt small. Her doctor said he was going to give her a special vitamin to help her grow. Kerrin got access to her medical records and verified that her mother had received DES. "When I told my mother about it, she said, 'No, they just gave me vitamins.' She felt really horrible. She had a lot of guilt. But I don't blame her for a moment. It was like what I did. I did IVF for my daughter because I wanted to have a baby. If something happens down the line that affects my daughter, I will know that I was only trying to have a child."

After yet another pregnancy gone wrong—in April 1994 she lost a third pregnancy at seven weeks owing to a blighted ovum ("It's one of those things that happens," she said)—Kerrin took the summer off and in November once again succeeded in becoming pregnant through IVF. Three days after the pregnancy test showed positive, knowing now that Kerrin had been exposed to DES, her doctor put her on full bed rest.

"I was living in my bedroom with a dormitory refrigerator," she said. "I was on bed rest all throughout the Oklahoma City bombing and the O.J. trial," she said. "Talk about a captive audience. It was tough. You can't escape the TV. You can only read so many books and learn so many hobbies."

At thirteen weeks she underwent an unusual type of procedure called an *abdominal cerclage*, in which her uterus was surgically lifted out and tied shut above the cervix. "I was the first person in Boston to have this done," she said. Remarkably, with Kerrin's history of complications, no difficulties were associated with her innovative procedure. She did, however, have other scares. At nine weeks she was hospitalized overnight with food poisoning. At twenty-four weeks kidney stones caused her so much pain that she thought she was in labor. At thirty-five weeks the nurse who came to her house to check on her mistakenly listened to Kerrin's heartbeat instead of her baby's and interpreted the normal but slower adult heartbeat to mean that the baby was in distress. "We live an hour from Beth Israel Hospital [in Boston]. My poor mother was going crazy," Kerrin said. "They met me at the door with a portable ultrasound machine. They threw me up on a gurney right there in the ER lobby. When my doctor came down, he could tell right away that everything was fine," Kerrin said. "He was so upset about the false alarm and the unnecessary stress it caused me and my family that he was throwing things. He took it personally. I felt like he was another member of our family. I went home that afternoon."

At thirty-seven weeks Kerrin celebrated the end of her long streak of dashed hopes with the birth by scheduled C-section of her daughter, Haylee, who was born weighing a healthy 7 pounds 7 ounces.

❧

TIP: Become familiar with your family's obstetric history. If you're pregnant or plan to get pregnant, ask your mother whether she took DES, and if she did, be sure to let your doctor know. Early notification can sensitize your doctor to any potential warning signs.

surgery, or the extra weight placed on the cervix during a multiple pregnancy. Although the cause of incompetent cervix remains a mystery in many cases, today's treatments have improved sufficiently.

TREATMENT. If cervical incompetence has been previously diagnosed and a woman is again pregnant with a normal pregnancy, a surgical procedure called a *cerclage* can be performed, usually early in the second trimester. In a cerclage, the physician places a suture (a ligature) around the cervix, physically holding the cervix shut in a manner similar to that of a purse string. You may have heard of the term *purse-string sutures*. Usually performed on an inpatient basis, this simple procedure can be carried out under local anesthesia. The physician will generally recommend bed rest for the next day, and in many cases you will be able to

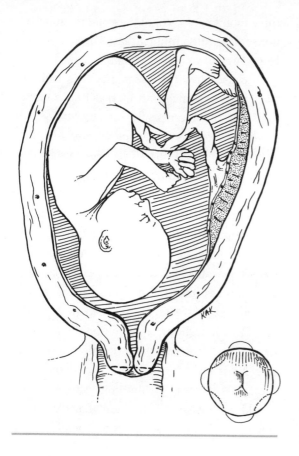

and, absent any other complications of your or your baby's health, will usually be removed within about a week of your baby's due date.

PREMATURE LABOR

Of all the mysteries of human life, those surrounding pregnancy and childbirth are perhaps the most profound. Among the mysteries of pregnancy and its complications, none is more perplexing than preterm labor. Approximately one-third of the 10 to 11 percent of all babies who are born prematurely arrive as a result of preterm labor that was unable to be stopped. Most of the remaining premature deliveries occur in connection with a known high-risk condition such as those discussed elsewhere in this chapter. Deliveries brought on by preterm labor are usually urgent in nature and are either induced or cesarean deliveries. Despite this prevalence, the medical profession today is only marginally better informed about preterm labor's root causes than it was when the discipline of neonatology was in its own infancy during the early seventies.

resume normal activities after that. (A more complete discussion of cerclage follows in chapter 2.)

Your physician will probably recommend frequent follow-up appointments to ensure the continued effectiveness of the procedure. Additionally, your physician may recommend abstaining from sexual intercourse for the remainder of your pregnancy or restrict you from certain physical activities. Bed rest beyond the initial healing period may not be necessary. However, be sure to follow your physician's advice closely. Doing so will only increase your chances for a successful pregnancy. The sutures will remain in place throughout the pregnancy

As we've noted, premature or preterm labor is any labor that begins before the full-term threshold of thirty-seven weeks' gestation is reached. Yet something so simple to define remains stubbornly difficult to explain. Though infection and dehydration have both been found to lead to premature labor, the majority of cases of premature labor remain without definitive cause. Therefore in the absence of a condition to treat, we just have to treat the symptoms of preterm labor with bed rest, close monitoring, and in certain cases medication.

Following are some signs and symptoms of premature labor.

Symptoms of Premature Labor (Regular, Sustained Contractions Occurring between Twenty and Thirty-seven Weeks of Gestation)

- Uterine contractions or tightening of the abdomen that occur every five to twenty minutes and are thirty to sixty seconds in duration
- Menstrual-like cramping in the lower abdomen that may be constant or come and go
- Dull backache felt in the lower back
- Pelvic pressure that feels as though the baby is pressing down
- Sensation of needing to urinate or have a bowel movement, especially if it is without results
- Abdominal cramping
- Increase or change in vaginal discharge
- Indigestion
- Cervical dilation (may not always be present)

As straightforward as it may seem, it can be extraordinarily hard to determine when actual labor begins. The obstetric literature defines labor as "painful uterine contractions associated with the thinning and dilation of the cervix of the uterus." Unfortunately, as we'll describe in the next chapter, these symptoms are not always easy to recognize. In fact, sometimes you can't recognize them at all without electronic assistance. If genuine preterm contractions are the first "bump" in your otherwise smooth ride through a seemingly uncomplicated pregnancy, you might ignore or make light of these signs and symptoms. "It must be something I ate. . . ." "It must be the position I slept in. . . ." "These can't be contractions; I'm not due for three months. . . ." All of these are natural reactions to your first inkling that contractions may be occurring.

Because a multiple pregnancy causes the abdomen to become so stretched out, contractions are often especially difficult to feel for mothers like Jody. Pregnant with quadruplets and on home bed rest since week twenty, she began using a home monitoring service at twenty-four weeks so that her contractions could be detected more dependably. (Jody's story appears earlier in this chapter.) The device used to monitor contractions is a recording transceiver attached to a belt that is fastened around the stomach. Twice a day, before eleven A.M. and eleven P.M., Jody would turn on the recorder for an hour, transmitting the information on her contractions to the monitoring service via telephone modem. "They would call me and say I was having contractions, and I would say, 'I was?' If I had more than three contractions in a one-hour period, I would take a Brethine [to slow the contractions]."

The uterus contracts throughout the course of a normal pregnancy. Irregular in frequency and strength, these contractions are usually painless. In the third trimester of pregnancy, however, the contractions become more frequent, more coordinated, and more consistent in intensity. Until then, however, you may not know labor is actually occurring.

Sandy's contractions first manifested themselves as a tight feeling in her stomach at around thirty weeks' gestation. The feeling was especially acute at night. Over time, the tightness evolved into sharp pain. At an appointment the day after the contractions had begun, her physician confirmed the presence of contractions. Examination of the cervix revealed that Sandy wasn't dilated. "She said I had to go home and stay in bed for a couple of days," Sandy remembers. "She told me to drink a lot of fluids, and then we would reassess. She kept saying, 'You just have to make it through the next two weeks. Thirty weeks is good, but thirty-two weeks is better.' When I got to thirty-two weeks she said, 'Okay, that's good, but thirty-four weeks is better.' I remember thinking that she was probably just trying not to scare me. But I had a feeling it was bad news." Far too often, we feel, expectant mothers experiencing preterm contractions say things like "Oh, I don't want to bother my obstetrician. I'm sure it's nothing." It is better to err on the side of caution now than to discover later on that you missed a telltale early warning sign that preterm labor was about to throw your pregnancy off the rails.

Close monitoring by your physician, strict devotion to your bed rest regimen (see chapter 2), and a hair-trigger readiness on your part to report the slightest symptoms of preterm labor are the best ways to forestall an unexpectedly early delivery and ensure the happiest outcome for you and your baby.

In her twentieth week Candace Hurley, the founder of Sidelines, the national volunteer support network for mothers with high-risk pregnancies, felt a subtle stretching in her abdomen. She decided to call her perinatologist—who discovered that her cervix was 80 percent *effaced* (or thinned) and that her contractions were coming every five minutes, lasting more than a minute and a half.

She said, "When you're pregnant, people tend to say, 'Oh, don't worry, just enjoy your pregnancy.' I got a lot of bad advice like that, but I decided to call. Had I waited, I would've lost the baby." Her perinatologist told her that she would have delivered within twenty-four hours if she hadn't called him.

PLACENTAL DISORDERS ASSOCIATED WITH PREGNANCY

The placenta is an amazing organ that forms in your uterus once you become pregnant. It transforms the uterus into a rich, nurturing environment for your infant, functioning as your baby's lungs, liver, and kidneys, producing several hormones needed to support your pregnancy, and providing your baby with vital oxygen and nutrients from your bloodstream. The placenta is fully formed and functional by week ten and reaches its final form at around twenty weeks, weighing about 1 pound. When the placenta has done its job and your baby is delivered, it is expelled by the body and becomes known as *afterbirth*.

Because of the placenta's critical role in maintaining your pregnancy, and owing to its blood-rich composition, disorders involving the placenta pose the risk of bleeding and thus are to be taken very seriously.

Placental Abruption

When the placenta *abrupts,* or becomes detached from the wall of the uterus, painful and potentially dangerous vaginal bleeding can result. Placental abruption can happen to anyone, though it most commonly occurs in women who have had several children. Its severity varies depending on the degree of the placenta's separation from the uterine wall. Mild separation involves slight blood loss and may require labor to be induced if you are in the late third trimester of pregnancy. In moderate separation you may lose enough blood to require a blood transfusion and, if you are at or near term, a cesarean delivery. Severe separation occurs when the placenta is torn from the wall of the uterus, resulting in the loss of a great deal of blood, renal failure, shock, and an emergency cesarean delivery. If a severe placental abruption takes place before the baby is viable, she will not survive.

Note: The accumulated blood lost from placental abruption may be trapped inside the uterus. So visible bleeding does not always result.

CAUSE. While the cause of placental abruption is not known, in some cases it has been linked to high blood pressure and smoking. Fewer than one in one hundred women have placental abruption. It occurs more frequently in mothers who have hypertension or PIH, or in mothers who have had this complication in a previous pregnancy.

TREATMENT. If you are found to have had a severe placental abruption, you may be scheduled for an immediate cesarean delivery. It will be performed as soon as your doctor has ascertained that your blood volume is stable. Less severe tears in the placenta that result in light bleeding or spotting can be managed with bed rest. A severe placental abruption that takes place before the baby is viable, before twenty-four weeks, will probably result in loss of the fetus.

🌿 *Placenta Previa*

Placenta previa is a potentially serious condition in which the placenta is implanted in the lower part of the uterus, thereby either par-

tially or totally blocking the cervical opening of the birth canal. The cause of this condition is unknown. It poses significant risks for both mother and fetus, for any part of the placenta that is near the cervix is exposed to the threat of rupture or damage. If labor is allowed to begin with the placenta in position to block the cervix, the baby will pass into the birth canal and tear the placenta, thus causing bleeding and potentially jeopardizing his or her supply of blood flow and oxygen. Placenta previa is rare—it affects about one in two hundred pregnancies that reach the twenty-eighth week. The good news is that about nine in ten cases of placenta previa self-correct and the placenta moves away from the cervical opening.

Placenta previa is more common in women who have had several children or who are pregnant with multiples. Often the placenta is situated near the cervix early in pregnancy but will

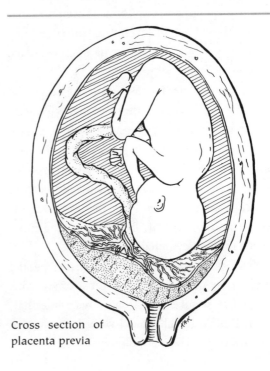

Cross section of placenta previa

move up the wall of the uterus as the pregnancy progresses, causing no problems. Otherwise an emergency cesarean section is usually called for if the condition persists.

If your obstetrician suspects placenta previa but does not detect the condition ahead of time via ultrasound (which is typically a very effective way of locating the position of the placenta), this condition may reveal itself through painless light bleeding from the vagina, typically in the later stages of the pregnancy.

TREATMENT. Placenta previa is not treatable per se. The degree of the condition will dictate the next steps. In any event, as soon as placenta previa is detected, your pregnancy is considered high-risk. You may require hospitalization, monitoring by ultrasound, or bed rest. Or, if bleeding is heavy, you may need a blood transfusion and an immediate cesarean section. For your own and your baby's well-being, vaginal delivery is ruled out; the position of the placenta creates a dangerous risk of heavy bleeding.

Other Placental Disorders

Placenta accreta is a rare condition where the placenta makes an unusually strong connection to the uterine wall. When the placenta is healthy, the delivery of the placenta triggers the uterus to start to contract. With accreta, however, this failure or partial failure of the placenta to separate from the uterine wall can lead to profuse maternal hemorrhaging. This is caused by the placenta's growth into the wall of the uterus, which causes major vessels to open up as delivery of the placenta is attempted. Without proper care, dangerous bleeding can occur when your body tries to expel the placenta after delivery. This condition may require a hysterectomy to stop the bleeding from the accreta.

Two other types of placental adherence are *placenta increta,* where the lining of the uterus, or *myometrium,* is invaded by the placental blood vessels, posing a serious threat of bleeding; and *placenta percreta,* whereby the myometrium is penetrated by the blood vessels. Effectively, the placenta grows into the lining of the uterus. The invasion or penetration may vary in strength depending on the amount of placental involvement. The major complication with all three of these placental disorders is the potential for excessive bleeding and maternal hemorrhage at delivery. The more firmly attached the placenta becomes, the more vascular the surface becomes and thus the more complicated it can be to stop bleeding at delivery. In severe cases of increta or percreta, a hysterectomy may be necessary to prevent dangerous bleeding to the mother.

MANAGEMENT OF PLACENTAL BLEEDING DISORDERS. The diagnosis of placenta accreta may not be made until delivery, when the placenta fails to properly separate from the uterine wall after delivery. A woman may need blood transfusions to replenish the lost blood volume.

Depending on the extent of the placenta's attachment or penetration into the myometrium of the uterus, a hysterectomy may be the only way to stop the profuse bleeding, which if left untreated can lead to death.

KELLY'S STORY (CONTINUED)

Kelly, the thirty-year-old former emergency room nurse, was diagnosed with gestational diabetes at twenty-eight weeks. When she was admitted to the hospital, her blood pressure was 160/110. She was started on Labetalol and didn't respond. Five days later she had had the maximum dose, and the doctor made the difficult decision to deliver that day. Kelly was given steroid injections that day to speed her baby's lung development. "I felt so terrible. I called my girlfriend and said, 'I think I'm going to be delivering soon.' My doctor told me I need to come right down to the hospital. I said, 'Let me take a shower so I can feel good about myself.' But then I did my blood pressure; it was only 120/80. My husband double-checked it: 120/80. Then a few minutes later we got 160/110. I have no idea why it fluctuated so wildly. All I know is, on the way to the hospital, I went into labor. They typed my admissions paperwork in a hurry and sent me back to Labor and Delivery."

Kelly was 2 centimeters dilated at this point, and her cervix was getting soft. Since her blood pressure was high, she was put on magnesium sulfate. And that's when the going got rough. "I felt liquid, like I was passing big, big clots. I thought at first that my water had broken. But I had abrupted. All of a sudden there were four nurses and doctors around

me, staring at the monitor. They didn't seem to be paying attention to my blood pressure anymore. Being a nurse, I knew the situation was serious when a resident put a nonrebreather [a full oxygen mask] on me instead of a nasal canula. Someone said I might have to have a C-section. I said if that was the case, I wanted to be put to sleep. My doctor said that wouldn't be good for me.

"They said my baby was having [heart rate] decelerations. We needed to deliver right now. They asked me if I was ready. I said, 'Not by C-section.' They said, 'That's not a choice now.' "

Kelly remembers a chaotic swirl of activity as the doctors raced to insert an IV, begin anesthesia, and start the cesarean. "My baby's heart rate was 40. I don't think I was supposed to know that, but I heard them talking. I was paying attention. They were about to cut, and I said, 'Look, I can still move'; I lifted my legs and said, 'you're not cutting me open. More meds, I can still feel things.' " They gave Kelly more anesthesia.

"I was starting to feel warm and sleepy. In my own mind, I thought, If I go to sleep, I'm not going to wake up. They said that they had gotten the baby out, but I didn't hear any crying. Why isn't he crying? I started hollering, 'Why isn't my baby crying?' Nobody answered. They did respiratory resuscitation [on the baby] for two minutes.

"They told my husband, 'You need to leave.' I was getting spacey. I felt like I was having an out-of-body experience. I could hear my doctor and anesthesiologist talking about a woman who needed a hysterectomy. 'Wow,' I said to them, 'it's sad to be so young and to have a hysterectomy.' My doctor said, 'Kelly, we're talking about you.' I could bleed to death if I didn't have one. I thought to myself, I'm dying. Somebody pushed my head to the left and said, 'We need to put in a central line.' I said I didn't want one. They said I had no choice.

"I was afraid that I was dying, and I just kept visualizing myself in recovery looking back and thinking, This was terrible; thank God it is over. Later I was told that it must have been my will, because even with the good medical team that I had, it was really close and I really shouldn't be here. That's weird to have someone tell me that. I had so many people tell me that I almost died. I remember waking up and not being able to breathe. I realized what was going on; I was intubated and was choking on the ET tube. I pounded my chest, and then they soon pulled it out.

"When I looked at the clock I saw that it was eleven at night. The last time I had seen the clock it was five. I thought to myself, I don't have time to die. I have two boys and many things I want to do in life. But I was so groggy that I just wasn't thinking straight.

"I was in recovery for twenty-four hours. I remember when a nurse came in, I told her that I wanted to have a breast pump and that I wanted to nurse this baby. She wouldn't let me nurse in recovery, but I persisted. They finally let me pump that night. It was hard to sit up, but it was nice to be able to do something for him."

Premature Rupture of Membranes (PROM)

The amniotic sac is a very tough membrane designed to protect the baby by cushioning her in fluid and to keep the uterus and birth canal free from infection. It is extremely strong and durable early in pregnancy, but as term approaches it becomes progressively weakened by a variety of factors: uterine contractions, fetal movements, and uterine growth that causes stretching of the membrane. Biochemical changes can affect the membrane's strength, too, including the lowering in content of a chemical called *collagen* that adds strength to the membrane.

If the membrane ruptures prematurely (your "water breaks"), a straw-colored, pale yellow fluid leaks out of your vagina. This can happen in a strong burst or a slow trickle. Unlike your urine, which smells of ammonia, the

The Mystery of PROM

Premature rupture of membranes is considered to be the cause of 30 percent of all premature deliveries. What causes it is still unknown. It is thought that the membranes, even at early gestations, are still quite strong but that local weakness caused by infection can cause the loss of amniotic fluid. Women with a history of multiple pregnancies, placental abruption, previous premature rupture of membranes, and previous cervical operations or lacerations are at heightened risk for PROM. There is no proven relationship between PROM and the mother's age, the number of times a woman has been pregnant, or maternal weight.

If you suspect that your water has broken, call your doctor immediately.

amniotic fluid has a more neutral, sometimes even sweet odor. When this happens, the sterile uterine environment is at risk of infection from bacteria in the vagina.

CAUSE. Ultimately the causes of premature rupture of membranes is not well understood. (See box on page 45.)

TREATMENT. If your membrane ruptures prematurely, your doctor will make a decision based on your individual situation whether to induce labor or adopt a wait-and-see strategy. Primarily two factors influence this decision: the risk of infection both to you and your baby on one hand, and the risk of prematurity on the other. Your doctor will want to buy as much time as possible to minimize the latter risk, while watching closely for infection. Your doctor will also be concerned about immaturity of the lungs as a result of low levels of amniotic fluid and malformities in the limbs. You may need steroids to accelerate maturation of the baby's lungs, and your labor will be induced if infection becomes apparent. If you show no signs of infection and the leaking of fluid abates, you may be sent home with instructions to avoid intercourse and bathing, either of which could encourage infection.

HYPEREMESIS GRAVIDARUM

Hyperemesis is morning sickness carried to an extreme. The cause of its characteristic excessive vomiting is unknown but appears to be more common in first-time pregnancies. If it occurs at all, it is usually most prevalent in early pregnancy. However, it can also last throughout the pregnancy. If left untreated, it can lead to dehydration, malnourishment, excessive weight loss, and harm to you as well as your unborn baby.

In her first pregnancy, Gretchen, twenty-eight, began experiencing nausea in the eighth week. "I didn't like the taste of water; I couldn't keep it down," she said. "Any motion on my bed—my husband sitting down on it, anything—would make me vomit." Going into her pregnancy, she weighed 152 pounds. By week sixteen she was down to 125. A nurse noticed that Gretchen's vomiting was mostly bile. Her dehydration was so severe that her gallbladder had to be removed via a thirty-minute laser surgery. Though she worked in a hospital office, Gretchen had never been a patient before. "I was scared to death," she said.

"After the procedure, they took me up, hydrated me, then sent me home. The second time I was in, they kept me for two days. The third time I was in the hospital for three days. The fourth time they had to carry me in because I was so dehydrated that I had no energy. My fingers would be shriveled up. You could pinch them and they would stay pinched. That's how I checked my hydration level. My lips would chap, the skin under my eyes would become dark."

Treatment for hyperemesis will depend on how severe it is. In some milder cases it can be treated with dietary measures, such as planning small but frequent meals, eating bland foods, getting plenty of rest, and taking doctor-recommended antacids or antivomiting medications. In other, more severe cases, you may need to be hospitalized for rehydration and a medical workup to rule out another cause for the vomiting. You will be given intravenous fluids to assist with rehydration and weight gain.

"How can I tell the difference between 'morning sickness' and hyperemesis gravidarum?"

First, remember that some nausea and vomiting in pregnancy is normal. In fact, some will say this is a healthy sign of a pregnancy, even though it feels like anything but healthy at the time you are experiencing it.

Now that you know it's normal to "feel sick" when you're pregnant, how do you know when it's too much? Hyperemesis, like regular morning sickness, usually starts in the first trimester but can last throughout, and you may experience them both several times a day. The difference with hyperemesis is its severity and persistence, which may result in dehydration, malnutrition, and fluid and electrolyte imbalance. The weight loss can become significant enough to interfere with your growing fetus's nutritional needs as well as your own. If you feel you have hyperemesis or are concerned about your condition, discuss your signs and symptoms with your physician.

AVOIDING NAUSEA THROUGH DIET

- Eat small quantities of food every few hours.
- Avoid heavily seasoned foods.
- Eat soups and liquids between rather than during meals.
- Avoid fried foods—they are hard to digest.
- Eat low-fat, protein-rich foods, such as skinless chicken, eggs, lean beef or pork, broiled or canned fish, and legumes.
- Sit upright after eating to minimize acid reflux.
- Have a midnight snack.
- Eat some unsalted crackers or bread in the morning or whenever nausea strikes.
- Avoid brushing your teeth immediately after meals.

Additionally you may receive stronger antivomiting medications. Once rehydrated, you will be started on a diet of clear liquids and progress toward solid food as you are able to tolerate it. To make sure you are receiving adequate nutrients for yourself as well as your growing fetus, your IV fluid may be supplemented with special nutrients as well.

Other Causes of High-Risk Pregnancy

YOUR AGE AT PREGNANCY

Extremes of age, at both ends of the spectrum, have been linked to higher incidents of preterm birth. Although there is no scientifically proven link between age and premature delivery, a number of circumstantial reasons shed light on the statistically higher rate of prematurity among mothers at both poles of the age curve. Among the youngest mothers (those in their early to mid-teens), lifestyle issues such as alcohol or drug consumption, smoking, poor diet, lack of maturity, and failure to obtain regular prenatal care may contribute to the higher frequency of prematurity. It is also possible that teenage mothers' own rapidly growing bodies may actually compete with the fetus for nutrients. While none of these individual factors alone can be linked directly to a specific instance of prematurity, the cumulative effect of one or more of these factors can increase the risk of something going wrong.

Likewise, women over the age of thirty-four face a higher risk of prematurity, but for a different set of reasons. They may be vulnerable to medical conditions that can interfere with a normal pregnancy, such as diabetes, high blood pressure, heart disease, and kidney disease. Like their younger counterparts, some of whom may be just starting to experiment with alcohol or nicotine, older women are more likely to have a history of smoking or alcohol consumption, which can harm their fetuses (see following).

YOUR OBSTETRIC HISTORY

If you've already had one preemie, are you likely to have the same problem with your next baby? Frankly, we're not sure. The biological connection between past and future pregnancies isn't well established. Nonetheless, statistics show that your obstetric history is a factor in predicting your risk for premature delivery.

According to the March of Dimes, about 10 to 11 percent of all pregnancies result in premature delivery. The rate of preterm delivery in second pregnancies where the first pregnancy was normal is less than 5 percent. Among women whose first baby was premature, about 20 percent have a second preterm delivery. For women who have had two preterm deliveries in a row, the chances of having a third preemie rise to 30 percent.

Statistics also show that for reasons unknown, women who have had more than one abortion are at substantially increased risk of premature delivery. There is no indication that the amount of time that passes between your pregnancies has any effect on the rate of prematurity.

INADEQUATE PRENATAL CARE

At least one risk factor for prematurity you have substantial control over. Failing to get sound, regular medical care during your pregnancy is itself considered a risk factor. We cannot overemphasize the importance of availing yourself of regular medical attention throughout pregnancy. While this holds true for all pregnant women, it is especially crucial for those who live with any of the other risk factors mentioned in this chapter.

Getting reliable information as you move through the stages of pregnancy, adopting sound nutritional and lifestyle habits, and making intelligent, informed decisions on the choices available to you as you progress toward your due date all can help in preventing or delaying premature delivery as long as possible. Not surprisingly, statistics reveal the costs of the failure to see a doctor regularly. Rates of prematurity are significantly higher in lower-income populations, where mothers tend to have less access to good prenatal care.

ALCOHOL, TOBACCO, AND DRUG USE

Women who smoke cigarettes transmit to their babies toxins that pass through the placenta. The frequency of placental abruption and placenta previa is decidedly higher among women who smoke, and the more they smoke, the greater are their chances of experiencing premature labor. If you are a heavy smoker and are still asking, "What's happening to me?" you now may have part of your answer. The best advice is to abstain altogether from smoking during pregnancy. The same holds true for drinking alcohol. Heavy drinking has been linked to fetal alcohol syndrome, which has been shown to cause serious physical and mental developmental difficulties in later life.

You must likewise avoid drug use of any kind during pregnancy. While cocaine is the only drug scientifically proven to be associated with preterm labor, opiates and amphetamines have been linked to low birth weight in infants. These drugs can pass to the baby during pregnancy and cause a variety of problems (see boxed list on this page). Even if preterm delivery is not conclusively caused by drug use, drugs can lead to respiratory problems, fetal addiction, and congenital abnormalities.

We strongly recommend that you consult your doctor before taking any medicine—including over-the-counter and alternative remedies. Regular aspirin can have hazardous effects on a baby. Even benign-seeming herbs from your local health food store can actually stimulate uterine contractions. These include the following:

DRUGS AND PREGNANCY: JUST SAY "NO"	
Substance	*Side Effect in Fetus*
Amphetamines	Possible central nervous system defects
Anabolic steroids	Possible chromosomal abnormalities in female fetuses
Tetracycline	Discoloration of baby and adult teeth
Streptomycin	Hearing disorders/ deafness
Aspirin	Problems with blood clotting, possible premature closing of the ductus arteriosus
Narcotics	Addiction and withdrawal symptoms
Accutane	Birth defects
LSD	Chromosomal damage, miscarriage
Sulfonamides	Jaundice, increased risk of bilirubin ecephalopathy

- Evening of primrose
- Cohosh
- Caulophyllum
- Cimicifuga
- Red raspberry leaf (tea)

ACCIDENTS

Accidents and injury are not uncommon during pregnancy, and trauma is one of the leading causes of prenatal death for infants. Fortunately most accidents produce only minor injuries, and the pregnancy outcome is seldom affected.

During pregnancy, women have less balance and coordination and thus are more likely to fall. But while the protruding abdomen is vulnerable to a variety of minor injuries, the fetus is usually well protected and cushioned from shock by the amniotic fluid, which along with the muscle layers of the uterus and abdominal wall shelters it from the bumps and jostles of a busy mother's daily activities.

However, major trauma can happen during pregnancy, and some types of accidents are increasing in frequency, perhaps as a result of the hectic pace of modern life, even for pregnant women. With travel becoming more and more common, the risk of accident has grown steadily over recent years. Injuries from automobile accidents have become a major cause of nonobstetric maternal and fetal injury. Seat belts have been known to injure an infant's head by sudden forceful pressure to the lower part of the uterus. Despite this, lap and shoulder restraints are strongly recommended. The risk is greater without them, because without restraint the mother is more likely to be fatally injured. Significant trauma to the mother can trigger premature labor. This often occurs when the membranes are ruptured as a result of an accident. Premature labor can ensue even if the woman is not injured during an accident. Moreover, the sudden force of trauma can also cause the placenta to separate from the wall of the uterus (see "Placental Abruption," page 41).

TREATMENTS. Treatment of major injuries during pregnancy focuses first on lifesaving measures for the mother, while the fetus is also closely monitored. If the baby is near term and the uterus is damaged, a cesarean delivery is usually performed. If the fetus is immature and the uterus can be repaired, it is possible the pregnancy can continue until term.

INFECTION

The sac of amniotic fluid surrounding the baby is its best protection from the infectious dangers of the outside world. The baby in utero is generally safe from flu, the common cold, stomach viruses, strep, pneumonia, and other illnesses that may afflict the mother. However, the baby is not entirely without risk.

In this section we will discuss some of the most common types of infection that can pose a risk to the baby during pregnancy. We will also list common signs and symptoms, especially subtle ones, of which you should be aware. In many instances of fetal risk due to infection, the mother will have few or no symptoms. Therefore it is essential to maternal and fetal health that diagnosis and treatment be prompt. This list will assist you in recognizing when to seek professional assistance during your pregnancy and hopefully will aid in preventing maternal and fetal complications from infection.

✿ Urinary Tract Infections (UTI)

Urinary tract infections affect approximately 2 to 10 percent of pregnant women at one point or another during gestation. The most common type is an infection called *cystitis,* or simply a bladder infection. This is usually signaled by the onset of fever, chills, discomfort while urinating, or frequent urination. These infections are generally treated effectively with oral antibiotics, increased fluid intake, and rest.

If untreated, cystitis can cause an infection to travel to the kidneys, leading to *pyelonephritis*. In addition to the above symptoms, a woman with a kidney infection may also experience lower back or flank pain, along with nausea and vomiting. Often the woman with a kidney infection is hospitalized and started on intravenous antibiotics.

Infection is thought to play a role in some instances of premature labor. Promptly report any signs or symptoms of UTI to your health care provider, as this can prevent a common bladder infection or cystitis from becoming a more serious kidney infection that is potentially harmful to mother and baby.

Signs and Symptoms of UTI

- Fever
- Chills
- Burning on urination
- Frequency in urge to urinate
- Pain in lower abdomen, lower back, or flank area
- Nausea and vomiting
- Fatigue and weakness

Sexually Transmitted Diseases (STDs)

Sexually transmitted diseases, also known as venereal diseases, are a group of diseases or infections that are contracted primarily through sexual contact with an infected person. If left untreated, they can cause harm to the mother as well as the fetus.

Following is a list and general description of these fairly common diseases, along with their implications for mother and baby, and the treatment protocol appropriate for each one.

SYPHILIS. *Syphilis* is a disease caused by an infection that penetrates broken skin or mucous membranes. Transmission occurs most frequently by sexual contact. A pregnant woman with syphilis can infect her unborn child. The infectious agent causing syphilis crosses the placenta after sixteen to eighteen weeks of gestation. If the fetus becomes infected, it could be stillborn, miscarry, or exhibit birth defects and symptoms of syphilis. Roughly thirty thousand cases of syphilis in adults are reported each year in the United States. Congenital syphilis occurs in one in ten thousand live births.

Syphilis progresses in three stages. In the primary stage, painless sores called *chancres* appear from ten days to six weeks after exposure. They sometimes disappear without medical intervention. In the secondary stage, which can begin a week to six months after the primary stage, a skin rash or lesions (which are very infectious) are the primary symptoms. A latent, or tertiary, phase follows during which no symptoms are present; but syphilis at this stage can be diagnosed by blood tests. If the disease has not been treated effectively, it will continue to invade the body, and there will be a relapse. The tertiary phase is a widespread infection that attacks the internal organs, bones, heart, and brain.

If a woman is infected, she will usually exhibit primary symptoms such as a fever, weight loss, weakness, and a sore or chancre, generally on the cervix. These sores persist for about a month, then disappear. If no treatment is received within two to six months, secondary symptoms may appear that could include acute arthritis, enlargement of the liver or spleen, and a chronic sore throat.

Today there is a laboratory test for syphilis known as a *VDRL (venereal disease research laboratory)* test. This will be performed as part of routine prenatal testing at your first prenatal visit. Early detection is important, because the sooner the condition is diagnosed and treated, the better for mother and baby. The treatment consists of medicating with penicillin, treating the other symptoms, and frequent VDRL retesting to determine whether the infection is still present. Additionally, any sexual partners should be seen by their physician and treated. The incidence of the infection will be reported to the public health department.

GONORRHEA. *Gonorrhea* is caused by a bacterial infection that invades the cervix. The symptoms are pain in the lower abdominal area and a greenish yellow discharge. After proper diagnosis by cervical sample, the treatment consists of antibiotics. All sexual partners must also be treated with antibiotics, or the possibility of reinfection is high.

As with other infections, the risk of fetal complication arises out of the chance that the infection will spread to the amniotic fluid or placenta and infect the baby. If you have gonorrhea, your baby is at additional risk for prematurity because this infection may cause PROM and premature labor. Additionally, if the fetus is delivered through an infected birth canal, the baby will be at risk for a gonococcal eye infection, which could lead to blindness. Early treatment is the best way to prevent further spread of the disease to others as well as to your unborn baby.

CHLAMYDIA. *Chlamydia* most frequently occurs among women below the age of twenty.

Up to 70 percent of women who are infected don't know they are because they have no signs or symptoms. When signs of a chlamydia infection do occur, they include increased vaginal discharge, painful urination, unusual vaginal bleeding, bleeding after sex, and lower abdominal pain. The infection has also been found in cases of inflamed cervix and pelvic inflammatory disease. If a pregnant woman is not treated, her baby has a fifty-fifty chance of developing conjunctivitis (an inflammation of the eyes) and a 20 percent chance of pneumonia. Chlamydia can also lead to premature birth or low birth weight.

The treatment of choice is tetracycline, but since this has been found to cause staining of the baby's first and permanent teeth, an antibiotic called erythromycin is usually given instead. Women who are the sexual partners of men with this diagnosis should be treated, owing to the likelihood they have been infected by their partner.

GENITAL WARTS (CONDYLOMATA). *Condylomata accuminata (genital warts)* are caused by a viral infection known as the *human papilloma virus.* Usually transmitted through sexual contact and highly contagious, the warts may be present on the vagina, cervix, or anywhere in the genital area. The virus may rarely be transmitted to the fetus during birth and rarely may cause laryngeal papillomas. Since pregnancy involves rapid cellular growth, which can cause the warts to spread rapidly, treatment of genital warts consists of removing the warts as soon as possible. Otherwise there is an increased chance of cervical infection, which in some cases can progress to cervical cancer.

Types of Vaginal Infections

YEAST INFECTION. *Yeast infections* are caused by a fungus that is normally found in the intestinal tract but can travel and infect the vagina. The symptoms are a thick white vaginal discharge, often referred to as "cottage-cheese-like" in composition. It is very itchy and irritating to the woman and can also cause painful urination. If the infection is not treated and cured prior to birth, the baby may become infected by direct contact with the infected birth canal at birth. The result is *oral thrush,* which is signaled by white spots on the tongue. It is treated with an oral antiyeast medication. This is more serious for a premature infant than an adult.

Treatment for yeast infection consists of vaginal creams and suppositories, proper sanitary techniques in the bathroom (wiping from front to back), and frequent bathing. Additionally, the sexual partners of the infected person should be treated to avoid reinfection.

TRICHOMONAS. *Trichomonas* is a type of vaginal infection common in pregnant and nonpregnant women. Though some women are asymptomatic, others have symptoms that include foamy, foul-smelling whitish or greenish gray discharge, itching, and irritation in the genital area as well as urinary frequency and pain on urination. Treatment consists of taking a prescribed medication called Flagyl, though there is some controversy over its safety in pregnancy. Additionally, any sexual partners should be treated to avoid reinfection.

BACTERIAL VAGINOSIS. Recent studies have also identified *bacterial vaginosis* as a possible cause of premature labor. It can be treated with the prescription medication Flagyl.

TORCH Diseases

TORCH is an acronym for a group of infectious diseases that are known to cause serious harm to the fetus. These are *toxoplasmosis, rubella, cytomegalovirus,* and *herpes* virus. Following we describe these conditions, how the woman or fetus becomes infected, implications of infection, and medical management and treatment for each.

TOXOPLASMOSIS. *Toxoplasmosis* is a parasite that normally produces only flulike symptoms in the adult but can seriously harm an unborn child. The pregnant woman may contract the organism by eating raw or poorly cooked meat or by contact with the feces of infected animals. In the United States the most common carrier is the cat, which transmits the infection by way of its feces. It is strongly suggested that women should not handle cat litter at all during their pregnancy. The best treatment is preventative: avoiding contact with cats or uncooked meats during your pregnancy.

RUBELLA. *Rubella,* also known as *German measles,* once a common childhood malady, today is quite rare owing to the availability of MMR immunizations (measles, mumps, rubella). Unfortunately it still exists. Women of childbearing age should be tested for immunity and be vaccinated if susceptible. Women should be vaccinated only if they are not pregnant. If a woman who is pregnant becomes infected during the first few months of pregnancy, damage usually results in fetal death. Other serious outcomes range from heart defects to hearing loss. The best therapy for rubella is prevention. All children should be vaccinated and women should be checked for immunity.

CYTOMEGALOVIRUS. *Cytomegalovirus (CMV)* is transmitted through the placenta or via the cervical route during delivery. CMV is the most frequent viral infection in the fetus. It infects up to 2 percent of neonates. Adults can acquire it from contact with an infected individual. It is not uncommon for a toddler to pick it up at day care and bring it home to the family. Most fetuses are at risk if the mother gets her first (primary) infection during the first trimester, and then the chances of serious problems are about 30 percent. Mothers who have already had their primary infection will have low levels of the virus, and their babies will have little to no risk of developing problems. Treatment for the infant may take the form of a drug called ganciclovir, which has been shown to be somewhat effective against the virus.

Tell your doctor immediately if your baby has any of the following signs and symptoms of neonatal infection:

- Fever
- Irritability
- Lethargy
- Seizures
- Skin irritation/rash
- Noticeably reddened or swollen area
- Decreased urination (fewer wet diapers)
- Poor appetite or sucking ability

HERPES. *Herpes type 2* is a viral infection that afflicts one in five adults. It usually affects the cervix, vagina, and external genitals. It is one of the most common sexually transmitted diseases. Once infected, the virus will stay in the body, even if only in a dormant form with no signs of clinical manifestation such as lesions, pain, itching, or discharge. However, the virus can pass to the fetus. Transmission of the virus to the fetus usually occurs only after your membranes rupture and active lesions manifest themselves. Transmission can also occur during a vaginal delivery when the baby comes into direct contact with the lesions. If you have a history of genital herpes, your physician will test you for active lesions as your delivery date draws near. Medications can be given to decrease the chances of spreading the virus to your baby at birth. In the presence of active lesions, a cesarean delivery may be indicated. Discuss treatment and birth options with your physician. Since the baby may be at risk, cultures may be taken of the infant's eyelid lining at twenty-four hours after birth. Your baby will be watched closely for symptoms of infection and may be given an antiviral eye ointment.

Group B Streptococcus

Group B streptococcus is a bacterial infection that is frequently found on the skin and in the vagina or rectum. It poses no harm unless the woman becomes pregnant, in which case the baby can become infected through direct contact with the birth canal during delivery. The presence of group B strep is tested for with a swab taken from the vaginal and rectal areas. This test is usually performed around the thirty-fourth or thirty-fifth week. When premature delivery is expected, the obstetrician will perform the test as the delivery becomes imminent.

Signs and symptoms of group B strep in the baby can include fever, lethargy, irritability, and poor feeding/sucking. If this bacteria is left untreated in the infant, the infection can lead to sepsis, brain damage through meningitis, and even death.

In 1997 the American College of Gynecologists and the American Academy of Pediatrics agreed that two approaches to the problem of group B strep infection were acceptable. One involves treating the mother with penicillin during labor if certain risk factors are present: premature labor, maternal fever, rupture of membranes greater than eighteen hours, or a history of group B strep in the infant. Under the second approach, a culture is taken at thirty-four or thirty-five weeks. If it is positive for group B strep, then the mother should receive treatment with penicillin during labor if any of the above risk factors become apparent. Depending on how labor and delivery go, as well as the number of penicillin doses administered, the baby might also be cultured and then observed or treated.

ABNORMALITIES OF THE UTERUS (BICORNATE UTERUS, SEPTATE UTERUS)

An irregularity that causes the uterus to be heart or horn shaped instead of the normal pear shape is a fairly common cause of premature delivery. It is not known how common malformed uteruses are, but they are usually first picked up on an ultrasound, often before a woman even becomes pregnant. Also referred to as a *bicornate* or *septate uterus,* this condition occurs when the two tubes that come together to form the uterus do not fuse completely, leaving a structural partition in the uterus. Alternatively, a wall of tissue may separate the uterus into two chambers. This condition, known as *uterine septum,* can cause the baby's movements to be restricted or to become positioned inside the uterus in a way that may hinder growth and development or complicate delivery. These conditions are rare and are usually detected either during an infertility workup or after the onset of premature labor. A cesarean delivery is generally necessary for a mother with a uterine irregularity such as this.

ABNORMAL LEVELS OF AMNIOTIC FLUID

A low level of amniotic fluid (or *oligohydramnios*) in the womb can compromise the fetus's ability to defend against infection (the amniotic sac and its fluid provide a barrier to infection when they are functioning normally and have limited antibacterial capability as well) and increase the risk of a potentially fatal entanglement with the umbilical cord. If this condition occurs before the seventeenth week or so and persists, it may retard lung growth. Too much fluid (*polyhydramnios*) can lead to a buildup of pressure within the uterus, with PROM and premature delivery commonly the result. This happens most frequently where a multiple pregnancy is involved, where the mother experiences complications from diabetes, or where there is an abnormality in the fetus. It can also happen if your baby is having difficulty swallowing because of a blockage of the esophagus or some other condition that prevents him or her from swallowing, digesting, and metabolizing amniotic fluid.

TREATMENT. If polyhydramnios becomes severe, amniocentesis can be used to "tap" fluid out of the womb. For the most part, however, this condition requires only that the mother be monitored closely.

"I FELT SOMETHING WAS WRONG WITH ME"

Melissa's story ended happily because of good prenatal care and a willingness to seek medical assistance at the first sign of trouble.

The twenty-seven-year-old from St. Louis had a bicornate uterine condition that effectively gave her two uteruses, each with a single ovary. Because of a history of miscarriage, Melissa was on progesterone and restricted activity (but short of bed rest). She was off work, forbidden by her doctor to exercise or shop the malls during her first trimester.

The restrictions loosened up in the second trimester, as her pregnancy was moving along without complication. Going in for ultrasounds regularly, she wasn't experiencing any contractions.

At about twenty-eight weeks, however, an ultrasound revealed that Melissa had a very low level of amniotic fluid in her womb. The OB began seeing her twice a week for a biophysical profile. She was placed on strict home bed rest for three weeks, during which she was allowed to shower but otherwise couldn't go anywhere or do anything.

By thirty-one weeks, however, it was clear that the fluid level was continuing to drop. It in fact got so low that the baby was in danger of distress and of the umbilical cord becoming entangled around her neck.

Melissa was hospitalized and admitted to the labor and delivery area for a few days. Then she was moved to a special area for women on bed rest. The monitoring was constant: three times a day at first; then twenty-four hours a day. "You become addicted to the [monitor]," she said. "You watch it out of fear. You just watch it and watch it, and you're afraid to fall asleep. They don't want to see dips in the baby's heart rate; I was afraid there would be a dip. But it was frustrating. Because you're not in labor, you're not a priority. Sure, you don't need help most nights. But it's easy to feel forgotten, on the back burner."

None of this meant her condition wasn't serious. At 33½ weeks her fluid levels continued to stay low, and her daughter's heart rate was staying fairly consistent. "It wasn't that she was in distress, but the environment wasn't as good as it should have been," Melissa said.

When an amniocentesis showed that her daughter's lungs were mature at 33 weeks, her physician wasted no time in deciding his next step. He delivered Lilly, all 4 pounds 6 ounces of her, at 33½ weeks. Little Lilly's Apgars came in at 8 and 9. Though she spent eighteen days in NICU, and twelve hours on a respirator, she graduated from mechanical respiration and intensive care quickly. She just had to learn to maintain her temperature and breast-feed. Then she was sent home.

"I spent a lot of time scouring the computer and searching for books, trying to find people who had this condition," Melissa said. "I felt as if something were wrong with me. It was sure nice to find others who had had this condition, to know that a happy ending was possible. Now we have our own little success story."

2

MANAGING THE
HIGH-RISK PREGNANCY

WHAT YOU'LL FIND IN THIS CHAPTER

- High-risk pregnancy:
  A numbers game
- Determining the length of pregnancy
- Some terminology
- Identifying preterm labor
- Managing premature labor

- Homeward bound
- Bed rest
- Special procedures
- Medications to promote maturation of the fetus
- Choosing a medical facility

In chapter 1 we discussed the most common reasons a pregnancy gets cut short, resulting in preterm delivery. These causes range from chronic medical conditions to the unknown causes of premature labor to lifestyle choices that you have the power to change. If you read the first chapter from start to finish (as opposed to reading only the material that is pertinent to your particular condition), it is understandable if you came away overwhelmed. The variety and gravity of the conditions that can disrupt or complicate the intricately choreographed biological minuet that is pregnancy can be extremely difficult to absorb at one sitting.

In this chapter we aim to return you to a feeling of empowerment. As you read the following discussion of the techniques for treating the conditions mentioned in chapter 1, you will hopefully come to appreciate the extent to which your diligence can have a positive impact on your pregnancy. Being a mother starts the moment you get pregnant. If you feel, however, that you are off to a bad start because you have a high-risk pregnancy, think again. Having a high-risk pregnancy is an opportunity to consciously practice motherhood right now. As you work with your obstetrician and/or perinatologist in managing your condition, using some of the techniques described in this chapter, remember: Anything you do to improve your chances of a healthy delivery now is as much a part of being a conscientious mother as anything you will do after your baby is born. That you care enough to be reading this book and educating yourself about prematurity shows your dedication to parenthood as surely as does teaching your child to read or feeding her healthy foods.

Almost every mother anticipates a full-term baby. Perhaps you don't consider yourself lucky to have received some advance warning of a possible premature delivery and birth. You may feel that anything that stands in the way of that goal cannot possibly be good news. But as you may come to realize as your pregnancy progresses, good news is where you find it. If you discover that you have a high-risk pregnancy early enough to do something about it, there is your good news: You can help yourself and your baby. This chapter is all about taking action—with the close supervision of your medical provider—and doing what you can to realize the dream of a healthy pregnancy.

"I've had very weird pregnancies," said Christine, a thirty-three-year-old Denver mother who had six high-risk pregnancies resulting in four live births. "I'm not one of those lucky ladies." Her first two pregnancies ended in miscarriage, one at nine weeks, another at six. But she endured, learning how to manage a variety of complications and successfully delivering her four children at thirty-seven, thirty-eight, thirty-two, and thirty-seven weeks despite bouts with hormonal imbalances, preeclampsia, PROM, and placenta previa. When her hormonal imbalance

was first identified, she began seeing a reproductive endocrinologist. Administrations of progesterone, increasing from 400 mg to 600 mg, coupled with blood tests every three days, made all the difference. "If I didn't take those drugs, I don't think I would have had my children," Christine said.

With two small children already at home, she had to spend a month in the hospital (recovering from PROM) in her third pregnancy. She says she set an unofficial record by watching eighty-one videos in a month while on bed rest during her fifth pregnancy! But her sacrifices, which she was motivated to make by learning about her conditions and working closely with her physician, paid off. And Christine hasn't been content to keep what she's learned to herself. She has put her extensive experience with high-risk pregnancy into service helping other mothers. Christine (like several other women we interviewed) works as a volunteer counselor for Sidelines, a national support network for women with high-risk pregnancies. When we interviewed her, she was actively supporting two mothers via e-mail and another via telephone. She has seen mothers react in different ways to their experiences with high-risk pregnancy. "One mother I'm supporting won't even pick out a name for her baby. She's at thirty weeks but had lost an earlier pregnancy at sixteen weeks. She won't look at baby catalogs. Other mothers get excited. They look forward to their next pregnancy, to the chance to make things go right. I've seen it both ways."

By the time you've finished reading this chapter about managing the high-risk pregnancy, we hope that you feel empowered with knowledge of your condition and its treatment. It is a frightening time. But better days lie ahead. Keep your eyes on the prize, follow your obstetrician's medical advice, and take one day at a time.

High-Risk Pregnancy: A Numbers Game

The great strides that perinatal medicine has made over the past few decades mean that there is a lot you and your doctor can do to bring you as close as possible to that "full-term" goal of thirty-seven weeks. If you are at high risk for premature delivery, you need to internalize the idea that, generally, the longer you hold off labor, the longer your baby stays in utero, the healthier he or she will be. Time spent in the nurturing environment of a healthy womb is time that your baby won't have to make up in a neonatal intensive care unit. As good as the equipment and staff are in NICUs today, all of their resources and talents cannot provide a better environment for your baby than your own womb. If your health is stable, your womb is the best place for your baby. However, conditions such as PIH, infection, or diabetes can make the womb an unhealthy home for your baby. In such cases the NICU will be the best place for your baby to begin life.

High-risk pregnancy is a numbers game. Every precious day counts. You and your doctor's goal, once your high-risk pregnancy has been identified, is to buy as much time as you can before your baby is delivered. There is no shortcutting the critical processes that advance an infant's growth and maturation, which progress with an almost mathematical predictability. In order to maximize the length of your baby's stay in the womb, therefore, it is important to identify any high-risk condition as early as possible.

And there is nothing "magic" about thirty-seven weeks. Everything is relative. For example, if you develop a potentially serious complication like PROM at twenty-eight weeks, holding off delivery until thirty-two weeks would be a great triumph. Statistically speaking, a thirty-two-week newborn has a much better chance of a healthy, complication-free outcome than does a twenty-eight-week newborn. In turn, the twenty-eight-weeker has a better prognosis than a twenty-four-weeker. (Please see chapter 5 for more statistics on outcomes by gestational age.) Focusing on the fact that every day your baby stays in the womb means a better chance for a healthy start will probably help you more easily tolerate the boredom and inconvenience of bed rest and the discomfort and pain of frequent blood screenings. It's a small price to pay for increasing your infant's chances of a healthy delivery.

Joan, an obstetrical nurse living in Nova Scotia, Canada, worked for thirteen years at a hospital that handled, by her estimation, five to six thousand deliveries a year. But that vast body of professional experience didn't give her any real advantage over any other mother when it came to coping with her own high-risk pregnancy. Seventeen weeks of full bed rest beginning at fifteen weeks' gestation, necessary because of bleeding that occurred throughout her pregnancy and contractions that began almost as soon as she moved, taught her at least one thing: "The advice I'd been giving [to patients] all those years was really not as good as I thought it was."

Pregnant with twins, having miscarried one of her original triplets at six weeks, she gave herself an imaginary cerclage. "The first thing I decided was that I simply *wasn't* going to deliver early. I spent time telling my cervix that I was sewing it shut visually. I knew what the procedure looked like, I'd seen it and assisted with it dozens of times, so I sat there and just imagined it. In my mind, I would simply not allow my cervix to open until the time was right. I've read a lot of Bernie Siegel. His books have been an inspiration to me with all their information about mind and body control.

"This [mental exercise] gave me one thing each day I could focus on." Through the power of her positive thinking, and the discipline to observe the rigors of her bed rest, Joan successfully delayed delivering her twins until thirty-seven weeks. Despite the seriousness of her condition, they did not spend a day in the NICU (although one of them needed resuscitation after delivery). "There is nothing in this world more important than children," Joan said. "They are the most special thing that could possibly be here."

Back at the hospital on a part-time basis, Joan has put her personal understanding of high-risk pregnancy to work in helping her patients. "My experience hasn't changed how I nurse, but it has changed the way I speak to moms. 'Yes, I know you're frustrated, tired, and can't concentrate,' I'll say. 'What can we do to help you get through this?' I used to think, Just get a good book. Before I went through it myself, I didn't really understand why they were frustrated or how frustrated they were."

Determining the Length of Pregnancy

Before we further discuss ways to extend your baby's gestational age, let's review the terminology most commonly used in discussing the length of pregnancy and in determining and confirming your baby's due date. Accuracy is important here, since most of the decisions made in the course of a high-risk pregnancy are influenced if not determined by the baby's due date (also called the *EDC*, or *estimated date of confinement*). After your baby is born, you will hear your doctor use these same terms when discussing the maturity of your baby.

Most of us grew up accepting that a normal pregnancy is nine months long. It's one of the few "facts" about pregnancy that everybody seems to know. Although nine months is an approximation, normal gestation for the human fetus is more accurately 280 days, or 40 weeks, or 10 lunar months. Understanding the term *weeks of gestation* is important since your caregivers (physician, midwife, nurse practitioner, nurse, or other health professional) will use this number to determine the current length of the pregnancy, to refer to the baby's EDC, or to describe the growth and maturity status of the infant. As you will learn, there is a great difference between what to expect from an infant born at twenty-five weeks' gestation and one born at thirty-five weeks' gestation. These weeks, and in some cases even days, can make a difference.

The accuracy of any estimate of your baby's gestational age is based on the quality of the information you give to your caregiver. The due date or EDC is calculated based on the time of ovulation—when the egg leaves the ovary and becomes fertilized. If you do not track your cycle accurately, you may not be able to give your doctor a useful approximation of this point in time. When an exact date of ovulation cannot be determined, the EDC is calculated by using the first day of your *last menstrual period* (*LMP*), adding seven days to that date and counting back three months. This formula yields the correct month and day in the following year that you can expect to deliver.

OTHER WAYS TO DETERMINE YOUR BABY'S GESTATIONAL AGE

Since many women cannot accurately recall the date of their last menstrual period, there are other methods of determining the EDC. Ultrasound is one of them. Using ultrasound, your obstetrician can take different measurements of the fetus to determine or confirm its gestational age and your actual due date. The length of the fetus (measuring from the head to the buttocks, which is also called the *crown-rump length*) is the most accurate assessment during the first five to twelve weeks of gestation. After twelve weeks and until approximately twenty weeks, the size of your fetus's head is a useful measurement. After twenty weeks multiple measurements are made to include the head measurement, the length of the thigh bone (*femur length*), and the abdominal circumference to arrive at an estimate of fetal age. This composite measurement has been shown to be more accurate than any single parameter. Ultrasound assessment tends to be more accurate when it is performed early in the pregnancy, a time when your fetus is growing more rapidly. Significant growth can take place over a few days' time, and it is easier to get accurate rela-

tive measurements then. High tech aside, your menstrual history remains the most accurate assessment of your fetus's age and due date, the "gold standard" if you will.

Also, your doctor may be able to determine this date by measuring the *fundal height,* the height of your uterus while you are lying down on the examination table (that's what he or she is measuring when your doctor stretches that tape measure from your pubic bone to the top of your protruding belly). Another benchmark is the first day that your baby's heartbeat can be heard. Your baby's heartbeat will be audible between the tenth and twelfth week of pregnancy using a Doppler (sound detection) device, and between the seventeenth and eighteenth week using a fetoscope. Your doctor will also note the date you can first feel the movement of your fetus in the womb, or *quickening.* These last two physical indicators are "guideposts" that can be integrated with the other pieces of information such as the LMP and ultrasound information to accurately fix your due date in the absence of a reliable date of fertilization or ovulation. These estimates don't always yield the most accurate results. For this reason, your menstrual history remains quite important. However, ultrasound has become increasingly accurate in assessing fetal age when it is performed by a properly trained physician during the first twenty weeks of gestation.

HOW DOES THIS ULTRASOUND WORK?

Ultrasound technology is based on the generation of a sound wave emitted by a transducer at a certain known frequency. The emitted sound strikes an object (such as a bone or an organ) and is echoed back to the transducer (that's the pad that your obstetrician moves over your belly). The strength of the echoes returning to the transducer depends on the density of the object it strikes. High-density structures, such as the fetus's bones, are strong reflectors of the echoes. Fat tissues are weak reflectors of the echoes. The different quality of echoes is electronically portrayed as different shades of gray. In this way an image of the object being examined by the ultrasound machine is produced. (In a more sophisticated variation of this technology, the movement of an object, such as a pulsating artery in the fetus's head or the aorta in the fetus's chest, can be detected by altering the frequency of the returning echoes.) These shifting frequencies are converted into a waveform that provides information about the blood flow in the fetus and the placenta. Thus the physician can determine whether blood flow between the fetus and the placenta, in the heart, in the brain, or in other parts of the body is taking place normally or is being restricted. These assessments may be quite helpful in determining whether the placenta is functioning adequately or if a congenital heart condition exists.

ALL ULTRASOUNDS AREN'T CREATED EQUAL

Ultrasound is something of a technological marvel in its ability to distinguish detail. Three-dimensional ultrasound images should be commonplace in the first decade of the twenty-first century. Scanning equipment has become ubiquitous in obstetrical offices today. Be aware, however, that the quality of the equipment will vary widely from one doctor's office to another. Some physicians may expend substantial capi-

tal to buy the latest equipment, machines that are able to see exquisite detail and motion. Other doctors may be content to use basic equipment that provides the information they deem important. Of course, while good equipment is important, the most crucial consideration is the expertise of the operator relative to the specific information required. State-of-the-art equipment may not always be necessary for gaining simple pieces of information about the fetus, placenta, or volume of amniotic fluid. But when detailed information is needed, for example, about the size and structure of the fetus's heart, then consulting with an expert ultrasonographer in cardiac anatomy using high-resolution equipment is imperative.

Some Terminology

Because of the importance of accurate gestational age assessment, there are several important terms that you should know and understand. A *term pregnancy* is one that is completed between the thirty-eighth and forty-second gestational week. After the forty-second gestational week (294 days), the pregnancy is considered *post-term*. A pregnancy loss that occurs spontaneously before a baby is viable is considered a *miscarriage*. A successful delivery that occurs before thirty-seven weeks (259 days) is considered *preterm*.

In the past, birth weight was the standard by which the maturity of infants was determined. Using birth weight as an estimation of maturity is advantageous because it is easily measured. Moreover, the information can be compared without difficulty from hospital to hospital for the purpose of keeping statistics.

However, it is now evident that many infants who are quite small by weight have the clinical profile and survival prospects of a more mature infant. Similarly, there are infants who have normal or above-normal weights for a newborn whose clinical progress and survival are that of a very immature infant, due to one or more medical complications or conditions. It is now widely recognized that many factors other than weight are important in determining a baby's maturity.

Estimating gestational age after the baby is born (using physical and neurological parameters) can be inaccurate by as much as two weeks. On the other hand, determinations of a mother's due date have become increasingly accurate with the development of improved ultrasonographic resolution. Large studies using this ultrasound information have generated standards to compare and more accurately determine gestational age. The importance of accurate estimation of gestational age using LMP, ultrasound, and physical examination cannot be overemphasized. Eventually all comparison of therapies for newborns and mothers, as well as survival and mortality rates of the preterm infants, will be based on the gestational age of the infant.

Identifying Preterm Labor

Our ability to manage and facilitate labor when it begins at the right time, or to stop it when it begins at the wrong time, is significantly hampered by the problem of identifying it in the first place. Therapy to stop premature labor treats the symptoms at best, although we are beginning to do a better job as we better understand more bits and pieces of the complex puzzle.

"Am I in premature labor?"

The following signs and symptoms may indicate that you are experiencing preterm contractions. Learn to identify the unique feeling of your own contractions. They differ from woman to woman and from pregnancy to pregnancy.

- Uterine contractions or tightening of the abdomen that occur approximately every five to twenty minutes and last thirty to sixty seconds
- Menstrual-like cramping in the lower abdomen that may be constant or come and go
- Dull ache in the lower back area
- Pelvic pressure that feels as though the baby is pressing down
- Sensation of needing to urinate or have a bowel movement, especially without results
- Abdominal cramping
- Increase or change in vaginal discharge
- Indigestion
- Cervical dilation (may or may not be present)

Your EDC will determine whether your labor is preterm or normal. But how will you know if you're in labor in the first place? You might assume it's easy to tell when you're in labor. If only things could be that simple. But if you've never been pregnant before, you might not recognize the signs. Even if you have experienced labor pains before, the nature of labor will vary from pregnancy to pregnancy, so experience isn't always a reliable guide to help you tell if you're in premature labor.

The onset of premature labor often reveals itself with subtle symptoms such as the ones listed here. Even in the absence of signs such as these, if you have an intuitive sense about your body, you may just notice that something doesn't feel right. Learn to trust your instincts, and do not hesitate to seek out your obstetrician any time your instincts tell you something is wrong.

Kathy said, "During my twenty-second week, I kept waking up in the morning feeling like I had to go to the bathroom. I would experience this overwhelming pressure, but when I would try to go, nothing would happen. The sensation, the pressure, didn't go away. Lo and behold, much to my surprise, I was in labor. I was admitted to the hospital and put on IV medication to stop my contractions. The doctor also gave me steroids and vitamins just in case my twins did deliver prematurely.

"What I learned was that anytime you have any unusual symptoms or signs, anything out of the ordinary, no matter how insignificant it seems at the time, seek medical advice."

Cheryl was in her twenty-ninth week of pregnancy when she started feeling pressure and pain in her lower back. "I was walking across campus one day and I got this nagging pain in my lower back. I described the feeling to a colleague and she insisted I go be checked out by my doctor. That struck me as an overreaction. I said, 'Oh no, let me just take five. I've just been overdoing it lately.' I started to sit down on a park bench. But my friend persisted, and I eventually gave in. She took me to the emergency room, and as it turned out, I was having contractions. I was given medicine to suppress them, was sent home, and went on bed rest. As a result of my colleague's caution and persistence, I succeeded in holding off delivering my baby girl until week thirty-two."

The Onset of Labor: Different Every Time

JOE GARCIA-PRATS: "After going through ten pregnancies with my wife, I can personally vouch for the many unknowns surrounding the onset of labor. Each of my wife's labors began and progressed differently. When we arrived at the hospital in labor with our first son, the doctor informed us that Cathy was only one centimeter dilated and probably not in active labor. She delivered our son just a few hours later. The amniotic sac ruptured only once in all ten pregnancies prior to admittance to the hospital. Two of our sons were induced postterm, at forty-two weeks' gestation. With our tenth son, we barely made it to the hospital in time. My wife experienced no early labor signs or mild contractions, as with her previous pregnancies. Contractions began suddenly, were intense, of long duration with short intervals in between. When we got to the hospital, the nurse told us that Cathy was 8 centimeters dilated—already in the transition phase of labor. Labor, I learned, is unique for each pregnancy."

"What should I do if I think I'm in preterm labor?"

Contractions can occur at any time. You will learn soon enough, if you haven't already, that children prefer to live by their own schedules and seldom accommodate their parents' convenience. (This is at least as true prior to birth as it is at twelve years of age.) You may be washing dishes, folding baby clothes, eating dinner, or sleeping soundly in bed when it happens. It is important that you take seriously any sign that contractions are beginning. "One thing is for sure: Trust your own instincts," Kathy said. "Many people without medical backgrounds feel intimidated and don't alert their doctors to something that may be wrong. I'm like that. I don't usually want to rock anybody's boat." As we hope to persuade you, there is nothing *more* important than rocking that boat when you detect—or even just think you detect—the first sign of labor.

The first thing to realize is that after you start experiencing contractions, you may have little time to act. If you were engaged in a particularly strenuous activity that you believe brought on the contractions, stop at once. Contact your physician as soon as possible, then get yourself to a comfortable place where you can lie down and take it easy. If your water has broken or you see any bleeding, call an ambulance.

Seeing the Doctor, Making the Diagnosis

If you are experiencing uterine contractions and your amniotic membranes have ruptured, you are definitely in premature labor. If you are having contractions but your membranes are intact, you may or may not be in premature

Describing Your Symptoms: Being Specific Can Save Your Baby's Life

Candace Hurley, the founder of Sidelines, a national support organization for women with high-risk pregnancy, told us, "It is vitally important that women define as precisely as possible what they're feeling and identify in clear terms what symptoms they may be experiencing.

"Though we can't and don't provide medical advice, many times, after hearing women with high-risk pregnancies describe what they're feeling, our counselors will tell them, 'Okay, hang up *right now* and call your doctor.' One woman who was six months along in her pregnancy complained to her doctor that she was feeling heavy. Her physician told her that it was not uncommon to feel that way. So she ignored it. As it turned out, what she should have said was, 'I'm feeling this heaviness on my cervix, as though my baby is falling out.' She lost that baby. Unfortunately, the way she explained it to her doctor made it sound like a question of overall weight, not pressure on the cervix. When you're describing symptoms like that, it is so incredibly important to be clear and precise.

"Many women say, 'I just don't want to sound paranoid.' Well, being vigilant is the best gift you can give to your baby."

labor, depending on whether there are changes in your cervix. Be alert to any trickle of fluid from your vaginal area. It may not resemble the proverbial "gush" you have probably heard about. Any kind of watery discharge may indicate the rupture of your membranes. Your doctor will make that diagnosis. It is important that you give him or her the earliest opportunity to do so.

If you are having contractions, you are most likely experiencing preterm labor if

1. You're at a gestational age between twenty and thirty-seven weeks.

2. Your cervix is 2 centimeters or more dilated (dilation is considered complete at 10 centimeters). Normally during your pregnancy, the mouth of your cervix, the channel between the uterus and vagina, is closed and sealed tight with a mucous plug. During labor the cervix begins to open to allow the baby passage into the birth canal.

3. Your cervix has thinned, or *effaced*, to 80 percent of its normal length. Usually the cervix is elongated. When labor begins, the cervix, in addition to widening, begins to thin down from its original elongated shape to let the baby out. Effacement is considered complete at 100 percent. If you're 10 centimeters dilated and 100 percent effaced, your baby is ready to be pushed out.

Your doctor will perform a sterile vaginal examination to determine cervical dilation and the status of your membranes. You'll probably be asked for a urine sample to check for infection. You will also be placed on an external fetal monitor to assess the effect of the contractions on the baby's heart rate. These assessments are most often done in the hospital's labor and delivery area, though they can also be performed in the physician's office or in the hospital's emergency department.

Monitoring Your Baby's Well-Being

There are a number of well-established and reliable ways for your obstetrician to keep tabs on the health condition of the baby inside you. As your high-risk condition develops, and as you move through your gestational cycle, the well-being of your baby is one of the crucial variables your doctor will weigh in making the judgment call about when to deliver. Following we describe the most commonly used techniques for in utero fetal assessment.

DOPPLER

This is a noninvasive, microphonelike device that is placed over your belly that enables your doctor to listen to the baby's heart rate and monitor the flow of blood in the placenta and in the umbilical arteries. It is most often used early in pregnancy.

ULTRASOUND (OR SONOGRAM)

Ultrasound technology, which is used early in pregnancy to provide an overall picture of your baby's health, produces grainy black-and-white images of the fetus on a small bedside television monitor. An experienced obstetrician or ultrasound technician can gain a lot of important information using this tool: your baby's size, the structure of his organs, the shape of his spine, the position of the placenta, the level of amniotic fluid, and the presence of uterine fibroids. The ultrasound transducer (which may remind you of a computer mouse) is typically placed over the belly, but it can also be inserted vaginally. If the transducer is left in one place, you may be able to see your baby moving his limbs.

FETAL NON-STRESS TESTS (NST)

Performed as you get closer to delivery, this commonly used external fetal monitoring test involves strapping two devices to your abdomen. One is an external ultrasound transducer that picks up the fetal heartbeat. The other is a pressure-sensitive gauge that measures your contractions. The purpose of this test is to gauge how the baby reacts to stimulation and thereby to determine whether she is better off inside or outside of your womb. The test first entails monitoring your baby's heart rate for thirty minutes to one hour to establish a baseline heart rate. If a reactive criterion has not been met by then, the fetus is acoustically stimulated and over the next twenty to thirty minutes is reassessed.

BIOPHYSICAL PROFILE (BPP SCORE)

This thirty-minute test will produce a score on a 0–10 scale that provides an overall picture of your baby's health. Using ultrasound, your doctor will scan the abdomen in order to assess fetal tone, movement, breathing, reactivity, and level of amniotic fluid. Each of these elements is scored 0 to 2 points. A BPP score of 8 to 10 is reassuring. A score of 4 to 6 is cause for concern. If the baby's lungs are mature and the cervix is effaced and dilated, the baby can be delivered. Otherwise the test will be repeated in twenty-four hours. If the test remains at 4 to 6 on the retesting, delivery is usually recommended if the lungs are mature. If the lungs are not mature, steroids will be administered and delivery will probably occur within forty-eight hours. A BPP score of 0 to 2 requires immediate delivery. Placental health is also assessed during this test. Oligohydramnios (a dangerously low level of amniotic fluid) or significant aging of the placenta constitutes an abnormal assessment, regardless of the overall score.

INTERNAL MONITORING

This is a less frequently used type of monitoring that takes place after the membranes have ruptured and the cervix is dilated and after the baby has moved into the birth canal. Typically used when more accurate results are required as a result of fetal distress, this test involves inserting an electrode into the baby's scalp to allow direct measurement of the fetal heart rate. At this stage of pregnancy, the baby is too low in the uterus to be monitored via ultrasound or Doppler. Internal monitoring can also be performed by using a *uterine catheter*. This is inserted into the uterine cavity and measures the pressure within the uterus—that is, the force of the contraction.

Kick Counting

If you are on home bed rest using a home monitoring service, this is something you will be doing to help keep track of your baby's well-being. Your home monitoring service will ask you (under the direction of your obstetrician) to count the number of times you feel your baby kick in a certain interval, usually fifteen to thirty minutes. You will press a button each time your baby kicks or moves. The data gets transmitted to the home monitoring service, and if your baby isn't kicking as frequently as he should, your doctor will have you in for a more thorough test.

Managing Premature Labor

If your doctor finds that you are in premature labor, she will then look for one of the conditions discussed in the previous chapter to determine what may be causing it. Your health and that of your fetus will then be assessed to determine whether continuing the pregnancy might be harmful to either's health. In most cases both mother and baby are fine, and the doctor can move to delaying the pregnancy with medications and bed rest. If dilation and effacement of the cervix are significant, however, delivery is imminent and no preventative actions will be taken.

The doctor will also check to see whether your amniotic membranes have ruptured (see Premature Rupture of Membranes [PROM], p. 42) and the amniotic fluid has become infected. A sample of the amniotic fluid may be taken vaginally to rule out this possibility. If the doctor suspects you have a bacterial vaginosis, a condition in which bacteria that are normally found in small amounts in the vaginal canal begin to overgrow the normal bacteria, you'll be given antibiotics.

What If Your Membranes Have Already Ruptured?

If your amniotic membranes have ruptured (for any number of reasons, including contractions associated with preterm labor, an increase in uterine pressure because of a multiple pregnancy, or polyhydramnios), then the decision making becomes more complex. Amniotic fluid is important to the growth and development of the fetus. Derived from the secretions of the amniotic membranes as well as from the fetal kidney, the amniotic fluid surrounds the fetus with a protective barrier that shields it from bacteria in the vaginal canal and cushions it from impacts. A proper amount of amniotic fluid creates a low-gravity environment in the womb that makes cord entanglements much less likely. The fluid also helps your baby maintain a constant body temperature.

Rupture of membranes can lead to several complications that your physician will have to consider and be prepared to address. These are 1) premature labor; 2) infection, both in you and in your baby; 3) asphyxia of the fetus caused by the umbilical cord entering the vaginal canal (this is called *cord prolapse*) and cutting off the fetus from its oxygen source, the placenta; and 4) fetal deformation syndrome.

The latter complication occurs when the membranes rupture and the chronic leakage of amniotic fluid shrinks the fluid buffer within which the fetus can move. This restricted space causes compression of the fetus, which can prevent the lungs from growing fully and cause compression abnormalities of the face and limbs. The baby with compression abnormalities may come out with a flattened nose, ears, hands, or feet. After delivery, these latter effects tend to resolve with time, as long as the lungs are sufficiently developed to sustain life.

When your doctor is examining your cervix

"What can be done to improve my baby's chances?"

Your doctor's options for intervention may be limited by how much time is available to implement them. If you are too close to your expected delivery, then some treatments may be ineffective. For example, steroid injections to increase your baby's lung maturity should be made at least twenty-four hours prior to delivery. On the other hand, if it is found that you have complications such as infection, fetal distress, or bleeding, you may be best served by having your delivery induced as quickly as possible.

Some of the most commonly prescribed options for postponing your delivery and thereby lengthening your baby's gestational age include the following:

1. Administration of tocolytics (labor-inhibiting drugs). These include terbutaline, magnesium sulfate, ritodrine, and Isoxsuprine. (See page 71.)

2. Bed rest. If you have high blood pressure or premature labor, you need to suppress them as best you can. Staying in bed, and in particular lying on your side, can keep your blood pressure down and decrease the frequency of contractions. (See the more extensive discussion of bed rest later in this chapter.)

3. An injection of a steroid medication such as betamethasone to try to speed up the baby's lung development. Such treatments, which are usually administered by your obstetrician when the baby is at less than thirty-four weeks' gestation, are most effective if given more than twenty-four hours before delivery.

for dilation, she'll check to see if your membranes have ruptured and collect a specimen of any vaginal contents to determine whether leaked amniotic fluid is present. As your doctor continues to assess and treat you for preterm labor, she will also investigate the possible underlying cause of your premature labor and/or rupture of the membranes. Sometimes an underlying cause can't be found. But if it can, there may be a way to treat it directly and forestall even further your progression to delivery.

If premature labor is discovered or suspected, you will probably be admitted to the hospital. If this is discovered at your doctor's office and your OB thinks you are in active labor, you will probably travel by ambulance. If your doctor's office is near the hospital, you may be transported by wheelchair. You should not drive if you're in labor. If you're at home, call an ambulance.

Upon your arrival at the hospital, you will probably stay in the labor and delivery area, given the ready availability there of monitoring equipment for mother and baby. Labor and delivery nursing staff tend to be closely attuned to the critical clinical signs to look for at this stage of assessment and are also familiar with antilabor medications. Should rapid or emergency delivery be required, you will be only steps away from a fully equipped facility that could handle your needs. The goal, as before, will be to stop your preterm labor if possible and if medically advisable. How long you will stay in the labor and delivery area before being moved to a room on a medical floor or in the labor and delivery area depends on the answers to several questions:

- Is the baby in any peril?
- Are the antilabor medications working?
- Do you have an additional medical condi-

tion that requires close watching—for example, pregnancy-induced hypertension?
- Are your amniotic membranes intact?
- Is your cervix continuing to dilate?
- Are contractions continuing?
- Are you at high risk for, or showing signs of, infection?
- Are you disciplined enough to remain on bed rest and not walk around?

If your physician is concerned about any of these issues, then most likely you will remain under the watchful eye of the labor and delivery nurse and doctors.

During this time your obstetrician or perinatologist will discuss with you the pros and cons of antilabor medications, including the risks and benefits to you and your fetus. Your obstetrician/perinatologist may also consider giving you steroids to help mature your baby's lungs and other organ systems (see following). Additionally, you may be placed on antibiotics or antihypertensive medication, as well as antilabor medicines. As time permits, you will have a consultation with a neonatologist, who will brief you on what to expect once your preterm infant has arrived.

While you are hospitalized, the equipment that will be used to take care of you and your fetus will range from everyday devices such as a thermometer to more complex devices such as a *fetal heart rate monitor* (*FHM*), which measures the fetal heart rate and the frequency of contractions. Ultrasound equipment is readily available should it be needed to assess the fetus or placenta. Automated blood pressure monitors will take your blood pressure at regular intervals. More often than not, your physician will recommend starting an intravenous line through which fluids and medications can be administered.

TOCOLYTICS: MEDICATIONS TO MANAGE PRETERM LABOR

Tocolytics are a class of medications designed to stop or reduce uterine contractions. Their effectiveness in suppressing preterm labor has been well established over the past two decades. As a result of the widespread use of these drugs, premature infants are enjoying a reduced rate of complications and higher survival rate as well as an improved outlook for long-term development. Use of these drugs can add weeks to a baby's gestational age and may even allow him or her to go to term.

Because most drug manufacturers have been reluctant to test new drugs on pregnant women—the cost, time, and potential legal exposure for doing full clinical trials are considerable—few tocolytics have gone through the lengthy and rigorous Food and Drug Administration (FDA) approval process. Thus most of the drugs described here have "off-label" uses as tocolytics. (Ritodrine was FDA approved as a tocolytic in the early 1970s.) Today, however, so many doctors prescribe drugs for their off-label uses that in 1999 the FDA decided to allow drug manufacturers to disseminate "sound and balanced" information about off-label uses for their drugs. This was a striking departure from the FDA's former policy of requiring its full approval before a drug's benefits could be advertised.

If the decision is made to use tocolytic medications and your physician discovers that your cervix is dilated more than 4 or 5 centimeters when tocolytic treatment is begun, there is only a small chance that the pregnancy can be prolonged for a significant length of time. While your physician will still be aggressive with treatments designed to stop or delay the progression of labor, you must understand that it will be difficult to delay labor for much longer if the cervix is so far dilated when the first assessment is performed. All of this underlines the importance of early intervention when you are first confronted with the signs and symptoms of preterm labor or any other indication that "something just doesn't seem right."

The most commonly used antilabor medications are ritodrine, Isoxsuprine, terbutaline, and magnesium sulfate. These tocolytic medications may be used in combination with other high-risk pregnancy treatments such as bed rest, intravenous hydration, and other medications to combat conditions such as infection. Women on tocolytics will also be placed on uterine activity monitors to assess the effectiveness of the medications and the status of the fetus.

Drug therapy alone is successful in stopping approximately half of premature labor cases where the amniotic membranes are intact and there is no maternal vaginal bleeding associated with preterm labor. When drug therapy is combined with bed rest (see the section on bed rest later in this chapter), that success rate rises to about 80 percent.

These medications, which each work in different ways, can be administered by intravenous infusion, by intramuscular injection, subcutaneously (under the skin), or in pill form. Where contractions are strong or recurring, you may be placed on a pump that continuously infuses low doses of the drug into your system. The route most often depends on how quickly your physician wants to get the medicine into your system. Usually you'll be started on the intravenous route, then switched to another method of delivery as your contractions begin to settle down.

You will remain on these medications as long as your doctor believes you are at risk of premature labor or until the side effects begin to threaten you or your baby. The most common side effects for the mother include agitation and jitteriness, headache, nausea and vomiting, fast heart rate, and an increase in blood sugar.

Serious complications (which occur no more frequently than one case in twenty) include heart rhythm problems and fluid accumulating in the mother's lungs. These medications do cross over into the circulatory system of the fetus, with some similar symptoms as in the mother, but they rarely cause problems.

TERBUTALINE (BRETHINE). *Terbutaline,* FDA-approved as a treatment for asthma, has been widely prescribed since the 1970s for its "off-label" benefit of controlling preterm labor. Also known by the trade name Brethine, the drug is a safe and effective replacement for ritodrine, which belongs to the same class of drugs. Terbutaline has several advantages over ritodrine, however: fewer side effects, lower cost, and greater effectiveness in small doses.

Most commonly administered by injection every three hours until labor ceases, and thereafter as a tablet, terbutaline can be taken right up to thirty-seven weeks' gestation. It may be given orally in pill form, via intravenous administration, or, in some situations, by a mechanical pump. Oral administration allows a woman to easily self-administer the medication while at home on bed rest. Administration by

pump allows for continuous infusion of this antilabor medication while at home on bed rest. If this is the method your doctor prescribes for you, you will be trained in the use of the pump by a home health agency. On bed rest you may be given a home uterine activity monitor that keeps track of your contractions and automatically administers terbutaline as needed.

Women with hypertension, heart disease, hyperthyroidism, or diabetes should not take terbutaline. This is because the drug is famous among high-risk mothers for some of its side effects. Sandy, who first began experiencing preterm contractions at thirty weeks, was hospitalized and had her contractions originally brought under control using magnesium sulfate. She was discharged for one day, but when the contractions started again, her doctor put her on terbutaline. "I found the drug really anxiety causing," she said. "Frankly, I felt as though I were going insane. I had contractions on the Brethine, but they were never painful and they never caused my cervix to dilate. I made it to thirty-six weeks. At that point my doctor said, 'You're clear, you're safe.' I went off Brethine and four days later delivered my baby."

Daryl remembers, "[Terbutaline] made me shake. My heart rate was 120. I couldn't hold a fork or go to the bathroom. I was really scared. It makes the baby's heart rate go up, too. You could see it on the monitor. I hadn't had any caffeine or Tylenol the whole pregnancy. Now here I am taking this major drug."

Side effects of terbutaline can include the following:

- Nervousness
- Shaking

- Rapid heart rate
- Anxiety
- Headache
- Nausea and vomiting

RITODRINE (YUTOPAR). Ritodrine is the only drug that has FDA approval for use as a tocolytic. It works directly on the muscles of the uterus, causing them to relax. Ritodrine also works to increase maternal blood flow to the uterus, which enhances the vital nutrients available to the fetus. This medication can be administered orally, intravenously, or intramuscularly. While on this medication, you will be frequently assessed for side effects and your physician will consider changing medications if they become increasingly bothersome or if stopping the medication becomes medically necessary.

Side effects of ritodrine can include the following:

- Rapid heart rate
- Nausea and vomiting
- Headaches
- Shakiness and tremors
- Nervousness
- Shortness of breath
- Hot flashes/flushed feeling

ISOXSUPRINE (VASODILAN). Isoxsuprine is another medication used for its tocolytic properties. Like other tocolytics, Isoxsuprine works to relax the smooth muscles of the uterus. Isoxsuprine is first administered intravenously, then, once preterm labor has subsided, you may be placed on a maintenance dosage administered orally. Isoxsuprine, with its vasodilating (blood-vessel-expanding) prop-

erties, can have the side effect of causing dangerously low blood pressure. When you are taking Isoxsuprine, blood pressure should be closely monitored by your physician.

Side effects of Isoxsuprine can include the following:

- Hypotension (low blood pressure)
- Rapid heart rate
- Tremors
- Anxiety
- Restlessness

MAGNESIUM SULFATE ("MAG" OR MgSO₄). Originally used to treat pregnancy-induced hypertension until its value in the management of preterm labor was discovered, magnesium sulfate functions by stopping the uterine muscle from contracting. It does this by working on the nervous system and blocking the effect of calcium, which causes muscle contraction. When used to counter preeclampsia, magnesium sulfate raises the threshold for women at risk for seizure activity, thus controlling and hopefully preventing seizures in these women. Magnesium sulfate's tocolytic properties slow, stop, and prevent further preterm labor in women with a history of that condition.

When used as a tocolytic, magnesium sulfate is administered by intravenous administration. After an adequate dosage has been established, the medicine will be given as an intravenous drip, which will allow smaller amounts of medicine to be administered in the hopes of maintaining effective blood levels while at the same time keeping the dose low enough to decrease the incidence of uncomfortable side effects. The side effects of magnesium sulfate can be pronounced, and may include the following:

- Flushing/flushed feeling
- Hot flashes
- Nausea and vomiting
- Blurred vision
- Drowsiness

- Lethargy
- Loss of muscle tone/reflexes
- Low blood pressure

"It's horrible," one mother said. "It made me feel as if I were insane. It gives you anxiety and makes you hot and sweaty. When you're in premature labor you have all this stuff to be anxious about, and here they are giving you medicine that makes you more anxious." The most serious side effect is possible fluid accumulation in your lungs. Magnesium sulfate's effects on the fetus are generally minimal, but the medication may cause decreased muscle tone in the infant, resulting in difficulty breathing for the first few hours after your baby is born. But this is unusual and is in any event not difficult to manage.

≫

The choice of tocolytic drug and its route of administration will be made by your physician after taking into account your whole health picture. You might be hospitalized for assessment after the initial signs and symptoms of preterm labor manifest themselves, but once your contractions have stopped or stabilized, you may be discharged and medically managed as an outpatient. When making this very individualized decision, your physician will evaluate your health status, your proximity to a hospital, and your home situation.

After you're stabilized, your OB may taper your dosage and route of administration from, for example, a high IV dose to a lower oral dose. This will allow for more ease in administration, and often the side effects are fewer and less severe in nature. And, significantly, this will make home management a more feasible option for you as well.

Trendelenburg Position: A Special Technique for Forestalling Labor

Pam, from Maryland, the mother of triplets Valerie, Stephanie, and Jennifer, spent three months in the hospital on bed rest. However, her persistent contractions defied management with magnesium sulfate, terbutaline, and bed rest. Any kind of activity or stress, it seemed, would send her into contractions. "They tended to get worse in the evening. But sometimes they were heavy in the morning, too," Pam said. At twenty-two weeks she went to the hospital for a terbutaline injection that stopped the contractions for two days. Then they started up again, coming at two-minute intervals. She began a five-day course of intravenous magnesium sulfate. But by the fourth day even that wasn't working. "I was very anxious," she said. "Any time anyone came into my hospital room, my contractions would get worse."

As fragile as she was with respect to contractions, by twenty-four weeks her cervix had dilated to 1.5 centimeters. At that point her physician decided to place her in the Trendelenburg position to manage the contractions. This involves placing the mother at a twenty- to thirty-degree head-down, feet-up incline. Pam could turn from side to back to side once or twice a day, to help keep her muscles from becoming stiff.

"I'd been getting increasingly nauseated, and that didn't help it. At first [being in the Trendelenburg position] was very hard. My muscles were atrophying from lack of use. Going to the bathroom was difficult. My physical therapist said there was very little I could do that wouldn't bring on contractions. About all I could do was flex my ankles.

"I remember having to watch television half the time in the reflection of a mirror because I couldn't turn and face the screen. It was kind of funny, because all of the mirror images were reversed.

"My hair was disgusting. I washed it once a month. I had my hair in three ponytails, but I could only brush them one at a time, every time I was rolled over in bed into a different position. I had to brush them in rotating order because they were afraid I would contract if I brushed my hair all at once. I put on lipstick once and my doctor said, 'Oh gosh, you're all dressed up.' There were crumbs all over my bed because I ate all my meals in it."

The difficulty of personal grooming and hygiene can cause stress. But there were much deeper causes of stress for Pam. "I kept having these visions of my babies being born really tiny. I was afraid at every minute that they were going to die. They put me on Ativan for anxiety. I tried not to read any books on prematurity while I was pregnant. I didn't want to hear one word of it. It was just too upsetting and would cause me to contract."

Pam's doctors were optimistic. But one day they took a sonogram that showed Pam's cervix had shrunk so much that her contractions risked causing it to tear. "The doctors were standing around me as though they were at a funeral," she recalled.

"My doctor said to me one day, 'If you can just make it to twenty-eight weeks, I'll be thrilled. If you make it to thirty, I'll be ecstatic. If you reach thirty-two weeks, I'll run naked down the halls.' Well, I made it to thirty-four weeks. But nudity was no big deal to me. You lose your inhibitions in these conditions. People were walking in on me naked all the time." No wonder, then, that her doctor's offer wasn't particularly exciting to Pam.

Pam's 3 thirty-four-weekers were born at 4 pounds 1 ounce, 4 pounds 10 ounces, and 4 pounds 3 ounces. They were fourteen weeks old and doing well as this was being written. "They're perfect," she says. "I look at them every day, and it's a miracle they're here. I was so lucky to have been pregnant when I was, when the technology was available to prolong my pregnancy long enough to deliver safely. It just takes my breath away."

When Should You Not Take Antilabor Medication?

The potential benefits of delaying labor with medication must always be weighed against the risks. If you are near term, or if you have certain medical conditions such as PROM or conditions involving maternal bleeding such as placenta previa or placental abruption, your doctor will probably recommend against tocolytics. In such a case it can be dangerous to allow the pregnancy to continue. If testing detects significant distress in your baby, it would likewise be dangerous to use tocolytics. Other medical conditions may or may not warrant forsaking drug treatment. For instance, some tocolytic medications could aggravate a mother's diabetic condition. In that case tocolytics would be warranted only if the doctor decided that close monitoring and control of the mother's blood sugar levels were essential and that the fetus would benefit significantly from a longer time in the uterus.

As you can see, each situation of premature labor can be quite different. You present your unique medical profile, as does your baby. The risks and benefits of treatment will have to be considered in that light.

Some physicians feel that if you have reached your thirty-fifth week of pregnancy, the risk of complication outweighs the potential benefit of using medication to further prevent premature labor. The neonatal mortality and morbidity rates among fetuses at thirty-five-week and thirty-six-week gestations are about the same as for infants delivered at term. In some situations, therefore, avoiding premature labor can present an unnecessary risk to the fetus as well as to the mother.

Should preterm labor stop, you may be allowed to move to the obstetrical unit, where you'll be monitored closely. It is usually quieter and less hectic there than in a labor and delivery area. How long you'll stay there will depend on your physician's assessment of the risk that preterm labor will recur. However, if the cause of the labor is unknown, the chance of recurrence will most likely be uncertain, too. Many doctors err on the conservative side in cases like that. Besides, if you have a medical condition that requires close observation or treatment, your OB may feel that the hospital is the best place for you. Lastly, if the condition of the fetus is tenuous, staying in the hospital keeps your baby in close reach of expert medical personnel. Discharge from the hospital is sometimes not a good idea for "baby reasons." Sometimes, of course, preterm labor may be brought under control to the point that hospitalization may no longer be necessary. In such cases home bed rest with medication and uterine monitoring may be appropriate.

Homeward Bound

If your doctor is satisfied that the threat of premature labor has passed, or if she feels it can be managed successfully at home, she may allow you to be discharged. At that point, because you will likely be placed on bed rest (discussed in detail in the next section)—the strictness of which will vary with the delicacy of your condition and other variables—you will need to plan a system to allow friends and family to help with your home responsibilities. If you are home by yourself during the day and you have other, younger children to care for, you will almost certainly need some help. Don't be afraid to ask for it. If it is true that "it takes a village" to raise a child, now is the time to call upon that village of friends, family, and neighbors for help. Most likely they will be eager and flattered.

If you were on tocolytic (antilabor) medication in the hospital, you may be required to continue taking it at home. Again, the decision to begin tocolytic medications will be based on the apparent cause of the premature labor and the condition and maturity of the fetus. You'll need to make preparations for another stay in

Friends May Surprise You

When Joan was on bed rest, she was surprised by two things: the amount of help she got from her friends and which friends turned out to be the biggest help.

"They were coming over and vacuuming without even being asked," she said. "One of my friends showed up with a hamper full of food—all of this ham, chicken, cookies . . . it was more food than I'd ever seen her prepare for her own family.

"The surprising thing was that there were probably five or six people I had assumed would be very supportive but would never come, and others I never imagined would be interested in my condition but who came over and really helped. It turned out to be very surprising to see who came and supported us."

the hospital when your doctor feels you've gone as far as you can on home bed rest and that you've stretched your baby's stay in the womb as long as possible.

Using home monitoring so that a mother can watch for her own uterine contractions has enjoyed mixed success. As we've noted, it can be extraordinarily difficult for you to determine when you are experiencing preterm labor. It is safe to say, however, that any unusual feelings of discomfort or abdominal or back pain warrant a call (day or night) to your doctor. It is crucial to investigate these signs as promptly as possible. Should you experience any signs of preterm labor, your doctor will need to intervene quickly to try to extend your pregnancy. Any rupture of the amniotic membranes can place you and your baby at increased risk of complications and continuing labor.

Preterm labor cannot always be halted. For reasons that are often unknown, many mothers simply won't be able to progress to term with their pregnancies. Nonetheless, with prompt medical care and some of the labor-preventing measures described here, it is often possible to add extra days or even weeks to the delivery date, reaping a potentially huge reward for your baby.

Bed Rest

Bed rest is one of the lowest-tech "treatments" that modern neonatal medicine has to offer. Yet it also happens to be one of the most effective. Happily, it is something concrete and positive you can do to improve your outcome. If you are on bed rest, you will be strictly limited as to your physical activities. Whether it is done in your home or in the hospital, you will be lying in bed the majority of the day. You will be able to get up to take care of only the absolute essentials of daily living: going to the bathroom and taking a quick bath or shower, and that's just about it. Your meals should be brought to you if possible. You may consider this a sacrifice, but sacrifice has its rewards.

The act of lying motionless in bed while pregnant can have a far-reaching impact on how long you are able to stretch your pregnancy and how healthy your premature infant is upon delivery. Bed rest by itself, without any pharmaceutical assistance, stops premature labor in its tracks about half of the time. In other cases, bed rest will be an "insurance policy" to support the effectiveness of other treatments, such as medications or surgical procedures such as cerclage (see page 93).

The strictness of your bed rest regimen and whether it will be done in the hospital or at home will be a function of several variables:

- The level of threat your condition poses to your health
- The level of threat your condition poses to your baby's health
- Your proximity to the hospital (preferably a level III center with an NICU)
- The number of weeks of pregnancy that your physician has set as your goal
- Your ability to perform home monitoring
- Your other responsibilities at home—for example, other young children
- How much help you have around the house

KEEP YOUR GOAL IN MIND

When your OB first informs you that you have to go on bed rest, you may experience a flood of emotions, including resolution ("I'll do whatever I can for this pregnancy"), determination ("It can't be that hard"), and fear ("Can I really do this?"). (See "Coping with Bed Rest's Daily Grind," page 85.) You will have to prepare yourself for the changes it will cause in your daily life. Your personal or family routine will be disrupted. Your level of physical fitness will decline. You will get stiff and have body aches from all the time you spend lying in the same few positions. The boredom you experience may become unbearable. The flow of time may seem to grind to a halt as you count the days re-

maining until you reach the number of gestational weeks that your obstetrician or perinatologist has set for you.

Jody, carrying quadruplets, was placed on
bed rest at around twenty weeks. She recalled,
"My doctor and I had discussed bed rest early
in my pregnancy, so I knew it was inevitable. I
mentally prepared myself for bed rest, I knew I
had to do it.

"It would have been really difficult to be depressed. We're active in our church, and we had
a lot of people praying for us. They sent cards,
called, brought us meals. My neighbors came to
visit, and I had family here and a supportive
husband who did everything he could to help
out. It really wasn't difficult," said Jody.

"The one thing that was hard, though: I
could not read while on bed rest. I guess it was
because of the hormones; anyway, I just
couldn't concentrate. I would read the same
paragraph over and over again. My concentration just wasn't there. I watched Rosie O'Don-
nell every afternoon at three. I lived for that
show."

The best way we know to make it through
these long days or weeks or months is to envision the end of your ordeal, to bear in mind the
reason you are doing this: so that you will one
day hold in your arms a healthy infant who
spent as much time as possible in the nurturing
environment of your womb. Unlike the many
other aspects of high-risk pregnancy over
which you have no control, the efficacy of your
bed rest treatment is in your hands. The more
disciplined you are, the more successfully you
resist the impulse to get up and run the dish-
washer, dust the blinds, and rearrange your living room for good measure, the better the
outcome will be for your baby. Knowing that—

focusing on that—will make the whole bed rest
experience much more tolerable.

In the meantime you may have to resign
yourself to certain inevitabilities of being im-
mobilized in this manner. "I made a conscious
decision to overlook housework, dishes, laundry, and work," said one mother. "These things
will keep. They can be done next week, next
month, whenever. Caring for your baby and
yourself, however, must be done now."

Candace Hurley, the founder of Sidelines,
the national volunteer support organization for
women with high-risk pregnancy, said, "So
many women say, 'You don't know how I feel!'
But we say, 'Yes, we do. We felt exactly that way.
Here's the prize. Here's my healthy baby. Just
make it one more day.' "

Reaping the wide variety of benefits that bed
rest offers does not come without certain costs.
And those costs may surprise you when you
first encounter them. Perhaps the most difficult
aspect of bed rest, as many bed rest veterans
have told us, is persuading yourself that you're
critically ill when you may not feel the least bit
sick. Joan, the obstetrical nurse from Canada
who lost one of her triplets at six weeks and experienced bleeding throughout her pregnancy,
wasn't able even to sit up without contracting
every two to three minutes. Since she believed
in low-intervention care, she kept her doctor's
office visits to a minimum (every two months)
and did ultrasounds only when necessary. "My
physician and I talked about my preference,
and he just laughed. 'You have the highest-risk
pregnancy I've ever seen,' he said." Joan had her
illusions about the leisurely bliss of bed rest
quickly dispelled when she found that she
didn't have the attention span to read for more
than ten minutes at a time. "I thought it would

be pretty cool to get to rest in bed and not have to do housework. I never thought I'd get bored. The idea that it would be easy to find things to do while on bed rest," she said, "takes no account of your complete inability to concentrate."

Christine, a Colorado mother whose hormonal imbalance has made her a veteran of six high-risk pregnancies, said, "They tell you to take it easy, but they don't really explain what 'taking it easy' means. A doctor will say, 'You're doing too much—take it easy.' Okay, you say, so I won't do dishes and laundry today, but I'll just sneak out to the store. Doctors see so many patients that they can lose sight of the fact that each patient doesn't always know what they're supposed to be doing or not doing [on bed rest]."

Even the most well-informed women have little idea what awaits them when they make the transition to spending virtually all of their waking hours in bed. For many women the prolonged periods of inactivity that bed rest involves make it among the hardest aspects of pregnancy for them to handle.

Mara Tesler Stein, a clinical psychologist who works with women who have high-risk pregnancy, said, "The thing about bed rest is people are waiting. They're waiting for it to be over. The thing to realize is that even with delivery, it isn't over. It's just begun.

"If you imagine high-risk pregnancy as a journey, you can tolerate a whole lot more, because you're not imagining that you're going to be stuck in this one place. You're not trapped. It's that fear that you're entering a nightmare and you're never going to get out that's so terrifying.

"Part of it has to do with how you walk into the experience: with how difficult it was to get pregnant; with how difficult your pregnancy was; with how much the pregnancy means to you."

Once you're on bed rest, everything else in your life takes its proper place—in the backseat. You will stop working. You will stop running errands. You will stop exercising. You will stop vacuuming, doing dishes, and washing clothes. You will rely on others to an extent you probably thought unimaginable. Even if your doctor permits you to get up for limited periods of time and for limited purposes, for the most part, you should adjust yourself to the fact that until you give birth, your bed is your home. It isn't easy. When you are being placed on bed rest, you are doing so because your body is suffering from pregnancy's stress. Being kept in bed, away from the productive routine of your everyday life, is not always the easiest way to relieve the psychological stress, good though it usually is for the physical stress.

Sandy, who lives in Brooklyn, went on bed rest after experiencing premature labor at thirty weeks. Three nights in the hospital brought her contractions under control. She was then sent home with orders to stay on bed rest. "I started from a weak place, emotionally and physically," she said. "To stay in bed six weeks was depressing. I mean, I did get around to reading a lot of books, but it was tough. You're stuck in this small world, your room, and it's hard to banish the bad thoughts. There are no distractions. All you can do is lie there, feeling your contractions all day long." For Sandy the difficulty was worth it in the end. She gave birth to a 6-pound-1-ounce baby girl at thirty-six weeks' gestation.

Whether the challenge you face is to extend your pregnancy as long as possible through creeping hypertension or to quiet down an un-expected run-in with premature labor, bed rest can be one of the most useful and effective tools at your disposal for lengthening the term of your pregnancy. If we have thus far emphasized the burdens of bed rest, let us be perfectly clear on the benefits: It is one of the most important ways for you to maximize the health of your unborn baby, not to mention your own. Throughout this book we emphasize that the goal in managing prematurity is to delay delivery as long as possible. The low-tech remedy of bed rest and inactivity, done under the supervision of experienced medical professionals, can achieve excellent results for women with a variety of pregnancy-related complications.

How Does Bed Rest Help?

The physiological benefits of bed rest have been well documented. Following are some of the benefits that accrue to you and your baby when you faithfully execute your doctor's bed rest orders:

- Bed rest helps reduce your overall fatigue level.
- It helps reduce your blood pressure.
- It helps suppress the effects of edema (swelling).
- It takes the weight of your uterus off your cervix.
- It reduces the amount of oxygen and blood you require and makes them available for your baby.
- It may reduce your nausea.
- It can reduce the frequency of Braxton-Hicks contractions.

Lying on your left side is often an effective way of lowering your blood pressure. This occurs primarily because lying in this position physically takes the pressure off your aorta. The aorta is the largest blood vessel in your body. If it is stressed, your entire circulatory system is stressed. Remaining in this position helps keep pressure off the aorta and thus helps keep your blood pressure down. If you have a blood pressure cuff at home, as you likely will if you have preeclampsia or PIH, you will notice the differences in your readings right away. It also facilitates your circulatory system's ability to deliver blood and nutrients to your fetus through the placenta.

If you are pregnant with multiples, or have incompetent cervix, placenta previa, pregnancy-induced hypertension, severe edema, or another high-risk condition, bed rest will very likely be prescribed by your physician. In women whose babies are at heightened risk for intrauterine growth retardation, the inactivity allows more blood and oxygen to flow to the undernourished infant. Women who have incompetent cervix or a multiple pregnancy benefit from the reduced pressure the cervix receives when their body is lying supine (on the back), a position where gravity is working for you instead of against you. Exactly when bed rest will be prescribed, and for what duration, will be determined by your physician in the context of your individual symptoms and prognosis. Going on bed rest may entail admission to the hospital. However, this is not always the case. Increasingly, technology is giving high-risk mothers some options about where and how they manage their condition.

HOME MONITORING

Technology is making life easier both for many women on bed rest and for the medical professionals who care for them. Through the simple device of a telephone modem, women on home bed rest today can have their blood pressure, urine chemistry, weight, uterine contractions, and baby's activity monitored electronically. Your doctor can receive instantaneously from the home monitoring service real-time reports of any change in your condition. This can ensure close supervision of your condition while allowing you to remain in the comfort of your own home. Although hospital monitoring is preferable for women who have especially delicate conditions, home monitoring is an advance that many women and doctors are finding helpful.

If your physician decides that home monitoring is appropriate for you (this is a function of the severity of your condition, how far you are in your pregnancy, and your proximity to a major medical center), a home health nurse will come to your house, set up the system, and instruct you in its use. Bedside computer consoles commonly in use today include the following:

- Blood pressure cuff
- Scale
- Urinalysis kit (for monitoring your urine protein, blood sugar, ketones, and specific gravity)
- Button counter you will use to record the frequency of your baby's movements at defined intervals
- Fetal monitor for measuring your baby's activity
- Monitor for measuring your uterine contractions
- Small keypad with which you can enter the number of hours you slept and the amount of time you spent on bed rest

At set times each day you will record whatever data your obstetrician requires in your bedside computer console. It will then be transmitted automatically to a home health nursing

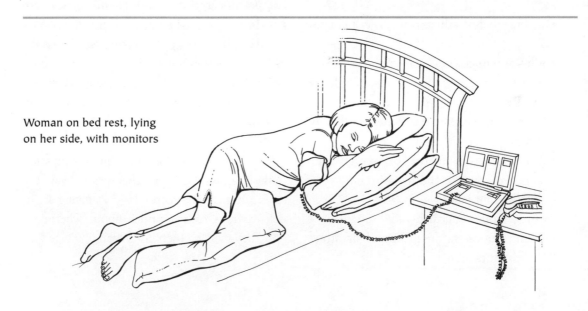

Woman on bed rest, lying
on her side, with monitors

Home Uterine Activity Monitoring (HUAM)

If you are placed on home management for preterm labor along with tocolytic therapy and bed rest, your doctor may additionally institute *home uterine activity monitoring (HUAM)*. This is a way for you to be remotely monitored while in the comfort of your own home. If HUAM is ordered, a home health agency that provides this service will be contacted by your doctor's office and an appointment will be made for delivery and equipment setup.

HUAM does not prevent preterm birth, but it can help your physician detect preterm labor in high-risk situations. Uterine monitors can pick up contractions or uterine activity that even you are unable to feel. This can be very important when close monitoring is necessary in high-risk situations.

The home health agency's representative, usually a registered nurse, will come and train you on the use of the monitor. At this time the nurse will also perform a physical assessment in order to establish a baseline of care for the home health agency, which will be acting on your behalf per your doctor's guidelines and orders. Though the nurse will check in daily and you are also free to call whenever necessary, this first meeting with the home health nurse may be your only face-to-face encounter with the agency. Though arrangements will be made for the home health agency to visit you, it will still be necessary for you to keep your doctor-prescribed appointments.

The device is commonly set up to monitor you twice a day or any time you feel contractions or a noted change in uterine or fetal activity. To perform the test, you place tranducers on your abdomen and lie still for thirty minutes to an hour. This allows time for a good, consistent tracking of any uterine activity. The doctor will be looking for consistency, length, spacing, and regularity of contractions. This vital information will be relayed via modem to your home health agency for review. Additionally, a home health worker, usually a nurse, will check in by phone every day to get the "subjective" picture on how you are feeling. All of this information will then be compiled and sent to your doctor for review.

The importance of this monitoring in a high-risk pregnancy can't be underscored enough, especially since one of its greatest benefits is its ability to pick up uterine activity that often the mother herself can't detect. This can allow for medical intervention to take place well before it would otherwise.

Note: Home monitoring is also often available for the management of hypertension, diabetes, coagulation disorders, and hyperemesis (extreme nausea and vomiting). Strides are continuing to be made in the care of the high-risk pregnancy. No one wants to need these services, but it sure is nice to know they're there. Ask your doctor whether any of these home monitoring services are available in your area.

SHARON HORNFISCHER: "When I reached my twenty-eighth week of pregnancy, I was faced with a good news/bad news scenario. On one hand, my pregnancy had reached twenty-eight weeks, the threshold where a majority of preemies not only survive, but have few complications. On the other hand was the rapidly escalating nature of my pregnancy-induced hypertension. Earlier in my pregnancy my blood pressure would sometimes reach 140/90 during a typical day at work. The pressure would quickly drop once I got home, and I could lie down and take it easy. By my twenty-eighth week, however, my high blood pressure was becoming more stubborn. Hoping to hold off delivery as long as possible, my doctor decided to pull me off work and put me on bed rest. In view of the alternative—hospitalization—I was glad about his decision to try home monitoring for my preeclampsia. He told me that it was quite common for patients with my condition to be hospitalized. But since this was my first child and I didn't have the responsibility to care for other children at home, and also because I lived within a few miles of the hospital, he felt I was a good candidate for home monitoring.

"Once the decision was made to put me on home bed rest, my obstetrician and his staff wasted no time getting me connected with a home monitoring service. That same afternoon a home health nurse was ringing my doorbell to set up and show me how to use the home monitoring kit. It was a compact, very well designed unit that turned out to be easy to use.

"Mothers will do anything for their children. For those of us who are placed on bed rest, the opportunity to go the extra yard for them begins well before birth."

service over a special telephone modem provided with your system. In this way your condition is never far from a medical professional's watchful eye. A home health nurse will call you at least once a day to see how you are doing. If any of your readings show cause for concern, a nurse from the home monitoring service or your doctor will call you to see if everything is all right and possibly recommend that you be admitted to the hospital. If you have any questions, the nurse may be able to advise you directly. In other cases an answer will have to come from your physician. While you are free to call your doctor anytime, sometimes using the home monitoring service's staff can be more convenient because of their ready accessibility twenty-four hours a day, seven days a week. If you forget to make your recordings or sleep through your alarm, the home health staff responsible for your care will contact you to see if you are okay.

For mothers who have to stay on bed rest, the convenience of home monitoring can be hard to beat. Even if you have a potentially serious medical condition, as long as your doctor has a way of monitoring your condition, you will be able to avoid the need to travel to the doctor's office as you enjoy the relative comfort of your own home. Granted, it is not the same comfort you knew when you weren't restricted to bed rest. But it beats a hospital room. Although it will never be fully comfortable as long as you are there by medical necessity, it will certainly be preferable to the cold sheets of a labor and delivery area. Pregnancy will constantly test your ability to see the bright side of things.

COPING WITH BED REST'S DAILY GRIND

Your doctor probably views bed rest primarily as a treatment regimen, as "medicine" designed to offset whatever high-risk condition is threatening your pregnancy. If you have the kind of relationship we hope you have with your obstetrician, she will also be empathetic enough to recognize the emotional and psychological dimension. Hopefully she will counsel you about what you can expect in terms of the sometimes difficult lifestyle adjustments this "life of leisure" can force you to make. Of course, there's a medical dimension as well—a good OB appreciates that your stress level is one of the most important variables in the high-risk pregnancy equation. She will understand and talk to you about the psychological and emotional strain that bed rest is likely to place upon you.

"It was the hardest job I've ever had, to lie in that position day after day, never knowing if things would be okay," said Annie, who experienced heavy contractions at twenty-six weeks and spent five weeks on bed rest before delivering her twin boy and girl. "Mood swings were a pretty big issue for me. My husband would come into the bedroom after work and ask, 'Are we having a good day or a bad day?' It took us four years to have a pregnancy last beyond eleven weeks. I was just petrified every single day. Friends would say, 'It must be nice to lie in

bed all day.' Nobody understood what I was doing, that all I wanted to do was vacuum the house or do a load of laundry. You take your child's life in your hands, there are big stakes."

Candace Hurley, the founder of Sidelines, a national support network of volunteers who help women with high-risk pregnancy, said, "I tried to be upbeat, but I felt blue and hopeless, exhausted, sore in my hips and shoulders, and speeding because of the medication I was on."

Daryl, who spent five weeks on bed rest as a result of incompetent cervix, said, "I was concerned about my mental state, about keeping myself as happy as possible. My emotions went wild. I didn't know how long I would be in this room. I was scared and angry. I thought this was all very unfair. I had been having this normal pregnancy, and all of a sudden it was gone. It was just . . . everything. For two days I sobbed all day long. So they got me a nicer room."

Fear and anger are entirely natural responses to the staggering uncertainty that surrounds so many aspects of your high-risk pregnancy. There is no shortage of uncertainty. You may notice that your doctor will seldom make concrete promises, and he will usually have more questions than answers.

Elizabeth endured successive bouts of severe preeclampsia in her two pregnancies. The writer living in Idaho delivered her daughter, Fiona, at thirty weeks, weighing 2 pounds 7 ounces. Her son, Ian, was delivered at twenty-eight weeks, weighing 2 pounds 8 ounces. Her first pregnancy had spun off the rails when at twenty-seven weeks she began to swell severely. In the space of just four hours, Elizabeth said, she gained twenty-five pounds. "I was a balloon. My feet were round all the way around. I couldn't bend my fingers or my knees, the skin was so tight. I called my husband to warn him about it, but he still couldn't believe it when he got home. He was feeling my feet; holding them up to the window, you could see through them. There was so much moisture, they were almost transparent. It was really weird."

Elizabeth spent the next three weeks at home on bed rest, with a blood pressure monitor, calling in her numbers every day and doing protein dips. She coped with bed rest by reading her entire collection of *Reader's Digest* issues—a stack about two feet high. "There were a few articles on preemies in there. I didn't think I would have one at that point. My goal was to make it to thirty-six weeks, and I was stable for a week or two on bed rest. I really didn't know what to expect. I'm usually a voracious reader. But I wasn't able to read anything much longer than a short article. I would read an article, then fall asleep. I tried to read a novel, and I couldn't get beyond one chapter."

HOW *NOT* TO HELP A MOM ON BED REST

"People need to keep it simple," said Candace Hurley. "Once, a woman came over and insisted that she would cook Cornish game hens. I kept saying, 'Oh, let's just get pizza.' She found out

---

Surviving Bed Rest

Leslie from Queens, a preemie mom and a volunteer for Sidelines, recommends the following:

- Establish a routine. Don't just sit there and watch TV. It will turn you into a zombie.
- Ask your doctor lots of questions. Consider yourself part of the team. You're paying your doctor a lot of money to take care of you. If he doesn't give you what you want, push him.
- Keep a diary of what's going on.
- If your medications make reading difficult, get a CD player for your room.
- Call a friend on the phone. I can't tell you how many times as a Sidelines volunteer people have told me, "I couldn't have gotten through this without someone to talk to."
- Think about the final outcome, not the process. Your goal is to have a healthy baby.
- Let yourself experience the emotions you need to experience.
- Don't feel you have to go back to work right away. I just entered information on 140 Sidelines moms into a database, and I can count on one hand the number who went back to work full-time. No one thinks, Okay, I've just had a preemie, now I think I'll go back to work full-time and put my baby in day care.
- Don't be scared. Be aware. Ignorance may be blissful, but it is a mistake. The truth may be offensive, but it is not a sin.

the hens were frozen, and she didn't know how to work my oven, so it was off when we thought it was on. I was so stressed out, I went into contractions."

Often people will have the best of intentions but still wind up doing more harm than good. "Medical people, friends, families—they often want to smooth things over," said clinical psychologist Mara Tesler Stein. "They have their own ideas about what parents can tolerate. It's harmful to assume what people need. What people don't often do is really listen to what people are asking them. People come to terms with what happens to them in their own way. The job of a family member or health care professional is to listen.

"I was on bed rest from twenty-four to thirty weeks. From week twenty-four to week twenty-six I asked almost no questions about my baby. My questions were all along the lines of, 'Why aren't my contractions stopping? Is this typical?' But at twenty-six weeks I finally worked up the courage to ask my nurse about my baby: 'What do twenty-six weekers look like?' I asked. She just said, 'They look small,' and then she ran off.

"This poor lady had no idea what to tell me. She was probably afraid that too much information would damage me somehow. Physicians sometimes say things like 'You know, you're just going to get upset'—probably wanting to avoid the intensity of the emotions that the parent has. Well, I would respond, 'How do you think I feel now?' What parents need is a little more information. They often just need to cry about it. Crying doesn't make things any worse."

Bed rest has its lighter moments, too. Elizabeth told us, "When you're lying there in bed, you can concentrate on the baby moving. My

SHARON HORNFISCHER: "When I was on bed rest, I passed a lot of time playing board games, a family tradition I've enjoyed since I was a small child. Yahtzee is the ultimate game of luck, so I thought it was a good omen that I was able to consistently beat my husband in our 'bed rest series.' He is so competitive that sometimes playing him wasn't the best thing for my tension level. But it was by and large a good way to burn away a few late afternoon hours on a long day of boredom. We've saved the score sheets for David's baby book. They're nice little keepsakes."

daughter moved a lot. She kept on tickling the lower side of my belly. People would come visit and think it was really funny because I would just start laughing all of a sudden.

"My husband would do most of the cooking. I would instruct him from the couch. He'd leave leftovers in the fridge, so when I got hungry later I could fix my food real fast and come back to the couch. I spent my days on the living room couch and nights in bed. I got real sore. Lying on my left side with my feet up on a pillow got kind of awkward."

GETTING THE SUPPORT YOU NEED: SIDELINES NATIONAL SUPPORT NETWORK

If you're stir-crazy from bed rest, or simply could use a sympathetic ear to tell your troubles to, you may find it helpful to join a high-risk pregnancy support group in your neighborhood, at your hospital, or on the Internet. Clinical psychologist Mara Tesler Stein said, "When parents network and talk, they feel a lot less alone and less crazy. They become more willing to say, 'This is my journey. This is who I am. This is what's happening to me.' They feel less of a need to get to a place where they can pretend it never happened."

A nonprofit organization called Sidelines has proven to be a popular way for women with high-risk pregnancy to find support from women who have been there before. A national network of support volunteers funded by donations and grants from the March of Dimes, foundations, and the health care and insurance industry, Sidelines pairs women in high-risk pregnancies with trained counselors who have themselves been through the experience of high-risk pregnancy. Working in person, by telephone, or by e-mail, Sidelines' five thousand volunteers can help you deal with your emotions and possibly even help you detect signs and symptoms of physical trouble. (Of course, the organization is not licensed to provide medical advice per se.)

According to the organization's founder, Candace Hurley, herself a veteran of two high-risk pregnancies, women sometimes feel more comfortable confiding in their volunteers—whom they consider peers—than in their doctors or nurses. When the volunteers suspect that something is wrong with the pregnancy, they encourage the women to notify their doctor.

In many ways you may find it easier to talk to another mother who has been through a high-risk pregnancy than to a medical professional. "I remember filling out my application right before Thanksgiving," said Daryl, who spent five weeks on hospital bed rest because of incompetent cervix. "The coordinator told me she didn't expect a fast response because of the holiday. But I was matched up with somebody by Monday or Tuesday. The volunteer who helped me was from Chicago and had a baby about a year old. She had lots of ideas about how to make me feel better: getting a haircut, getting dressed every day in my own clothes, showering when I could.

"Lying there in bed, I knew there were other women in the hospital in my situation. But I didn't know who they were, and I couldn't talk to them. But I had an e-mail buddy. It was great. I could completely unload on her. I didn't like unloading on my family. They were going through a hard time also. To cry to them made them feel worse."

Sometimes tough love has its place. Candace Hurley recalled one of Sidelines' very first patients, a woman who already had seven children at home to care for when pregnant once again; she was put on strict bed rest. "Her husband was losing his mind," Hurley said. "At one point she threatened, 'I'm going to go to Palm Springs. I've *got* to get out of this bed.' Had she done that, of course, she would have been at a very real risk of losing her baby. So I threatened her that I'd come out and pop her tires if she tried. I talked her down. And now her baby's fine."

BED REST AND YOUR FAMILY

❧ Maintaining Your Marriage

The disruption of the routine that bed rest creates can place strains on even the best marriage. If you were working before and suddenly had to leave, you may have money problems that cause marital stress. Many men grow deeply frustrated with their natural tendency to want to know exactly what the problem is and how to fix it. The uncertainties about high-risk pregnancy may frustrate your partner, causing you both some strain. "My husband was very frustrated," said Annie. "He wanted everything to be fixed. Of course, that's not the way high-risk pregnancy works. You just have to wait, and there's not a lot you can do."

If your husband has to take time off from his job to help out, as glad as he may be to do that, there may be strain from the added burdens of working a reduced schedule. Marie, who because of preeclampsia complicated by HELLP syndrome delivered her daughter at thirty-four weeks, said: "My husband held himself together with spit and baling wire. He lost a lot of sleep and a lot of time from work. He used to be able to work whatever overtime he needed. Suddenly, with me on bed rest, he became a clock-watcher. He would disappear from work suddenly to do a day care pickup or drop-off. At the end, when I was sickest, he disappeared from work for two full weeks. I don't think his employers understood how ill I was. Of course, they didn't have a lot of choice."

When she was on bed rest, Sandy, the Brooklyn mother who successfully held off her premature labor at thirty weeks to deliver a healthy, thirty-six-week daughter weighing 6 pounds 1 ounce, wrestled with feelings of resentment whenever her husband, Chris, would resume his normal daily life. "I would watch him go off to work, and I would be jealous that he had an escape from all of it. I'm sure it was tough for him to see me so helpless. But when the time came, he got to go away to work. He'd sometimes say to me, 'Look, I'm going through this, too.' But then he'd leave. When he went to work, it was hard to be alone. It was scary. And hard not to be mad."

Men differ from women in the way they handle stressful situations. "Men go with the flow," said Ron, whose wife, Kerry, delivered prematurely owing to preterm labor and premature rupture of membranes. "They want direction, not empathy. My mother always told me, 'You can't waste today worrying about tomorrow.' Sometimes a guy will be sitting there quiet, not thinking about anything at all, and his wife will come up and say, 'Tell me what you're thinking.' The man will say, 'Nothing.' And the woman will say, 'Nothing? You must be thinking something.' Men don't want to be pushed, and they can get mad if people try to make them talk. That's just a man thing, I guess."

"The bed rest was a real emotional ride for both of us," said Candace Hurley's husband, Brian. "Men typically sense that we have to make things seem normal even when they're not. I don't really get upset easily, but the emotional side . . . you'd get to the point that you wanted to see the light at the end of the tunnel so bad, you'd snap and start crying."

Sandy said, "Each of us reacted to my situation very differently: he wasn't trying to make light of it, but he was trying to make my situation appear to be not as bad as it was. I knew otherwise. When I was on bed rest, I was just miserable. I would be lying there and he would come in and say, 'Come on. You should walk to the park. It's only two blocks away.' He thought that my life would be better if I could just walk to that park. This was against all good medical sense. But his thinking was that if I stayed there in bed, I'd be miserable. He was right. But his solution was no help."

It is normal for even the strongest, most loving relationships to feel strain from disruption caused by bed rest. Openly acknowledging the difficulty can be a good way to bridge the gap that often forms with a spouse during the bed rest ordeal.

🌿 Handling Your Other Children

Factoring other small children into the equation further complicates the picture when you're on bed rest. If having a high-risk pregnancy makes you feel inadequate as a parent to your new baby, the feeling can be understandably magnified when another child is looking to you for love and care. "Even when you're on bed rest, you're still 'Mommy,'" said Gretchen, whose second pregnancy became complicated early on by hyperemesis and preterm labor brought on by an infection. "My daughter was still in the baby stage when I was on bed rest with my second one. It was frustrating because I couldn't pick her up. I felt like I couldn't be a loving mom. I could tell her I loved her, but I couldn't do the little things to show her." Gretchen's advice to mothers in a high-risk pregnancy who have the responsibility of caring for other young children is to recognize the limits imposed by bed rest: "Don't try to plan your child's day. Take care of yourself and that baby inside you. Someone else can help out with the children at home. Do what your doctor says."

Joan did her best to involve her other children in helping out around the house. Her eight-year-old daughter "takes everything in stride; it doesn't bother her." But when it came to her four-year-old son, she ran into the invariable frustration of trying to give a smaller child more responsibility than his years can bear. "He couldn't understand why his routine was upset. He wanted me to eat at the table with him, to be like Mom as much as possible. He just didn't get the explanation. We tried to include him in our new routine. But he would do things like put his bean bag in the microwave or enter whatever number of minutes he felt like when he tried to cook something. As much as he tried to be helpful, he couldn't be. And it wasn't fair to expect him to do better."

Candace's second high-risk pregnancy followed directly on the heels of her first. While she was on bed rest, she had a seven-month-old son to care for. It was more than she could handle. Keeping up with him always seemed to bring on contractions. Candace found that she could touch him only when the baby-sitter brought him to her bedside when he was asleep. "I felt tremendous guilt," she said. "I felt I was ignoring this baby I'd waited so long for. Anything can tip the scale; you're so precarious. Once, he chipped the front of his tooth on his bottle, right in front of me. I started crying—and went into contractions. But my mother told me to snap out of it. 'Don't sacrifice the one inside you!' she said."

One especially insightful father, Robin, whose wife, Joan, experienced preterm labor, told us, "It was rough—no joke about that. My wife and I had two kids already, and an entire family schedule that was pretty well established. It couldn't just come to a stop, yet it couldn't continue the way it was. Joan's bed rest was something the whole family went through. The challenge was to maintain stability as much as you could given the fact that one of the major people in it was so limited.

"Meanwhile, there was a question I couldn't get out of my head: 'What are the chances of coming out with any live babies after this?' I can't remember what the odds were. I don't think anybody was particularly optimistic. I'm hearing all these things—that brains can bleed, that organs can be underdeveloped—and I was really stressed out by the whole thing. Joan, being a nurse, has always been very competent. I was trying to rely on Joan's knowledge about what was happening. But in a way I was putting too much on her because she was the one who needed the support, not me. She knew more about what was going on than I did.

"I look back and say, 'Man that was really something.' You just have to realize that this isn't forever. Stay focused on the goal. It's very easy to get self-indulgent, to say, 'This is too much stress. I can't handle this.' But that makes everything harder. Every minute that something bad didn't happen was another minute closer to our goal. I felt every minute go by. It was like tick, tick, tick. . . .

"But I'd go through the whole thing again, because it was worth it. What's the old saying? 'That which doesn't kill you, makes you stronger'? I learned so much about what was really important from this experience. Until you actually face something like that, you don't realize what you're capable of."

LEAVING WORK TO GO ON BED REST

Increasingly today, women are shouldering dual responsibilities on both the home and the work fronts. If your doctor orders you to go on bed rest, however, this balance will experience a sudden shift. Ideally your supervisor and co-workers will appreciate the very real risk that a condition such as preeclampsia, incompetent cervix, or gestational diabetes presents. Sometimes, though, that is not the case.

Debra said, "I had a female boss who was not at all understanding about my need to go on bed rest. She had had perfect pregnancies. She never even had any heartburn or back pain, and she delivered on her due date. She had no comprehension of what a problem pregnancy was." Though you may not look sick to them—indeed, even a high-risk pregnancy may still have you all aglow and looking quite healthy—your boss and colleagues will have to understand the genuineness of the illness that is sidelining you from work. Like few other periods in your life, pregnancy is a time to readjust your priorities.

Whether you believe it or not, your job and all of the "important" responsibilities it entails will somehow be taken care of in your absence. Conversely, your children won't unless you take the best possible care of yourself. While many people will be able to step in and eventually perform your duties on the job, only you are capable of ensuring that your children are well cared for, whether or not they have been born yet. Learn to apply the "year from now" rule: Ask yourself, "Will my leaving work and the disruption it is supposedly going to cause truly matter in a year?" The answer to this question, as with most work-related questions, is almost certainly "No." However, the answer to any question related to your children's health is a definite "Yes."

"I used to think the world would stop if I didn't go to work or keep up the house," said Daryl, an attorney whose bout with incompetent cervix kept her on bed rest for five weeks. "But you know, it doesn't stop. I was stuck in the hospital for a month, and the world kept going. It seems like so much time. When you're in it, it seems like forever. Every day you're

Making Time Fly

THINGS TO DO WHILE YOU'RE ON BED REST

- Study your family's genealogy.
- Learn the ins and outs of mutual fund investing.
- Learn to crochet; then make a baby blanket. (Even if it doesn't turn out perfect, it will become an irreplaceable family heirloom.)
- Catch up on back issues of your favorite magazine.
- Read your favorite novel. (You sure won't have time later.)
- Listen to books on tape (especially good if you are having visual disturbances).
- Organize your photographs.
- Keep a diary or start a memory book.
- Rent and watch *The Godfather—Parts I, II,* and *III.*
- Study a foreign language.
- Persuade your husband to provide backrubs on the hour.
- Write a letter to your unborn child.
- Surprise an old friend with a phone call.
- If friends or family offer to help, let them. It will make both them and you feel better. Schedule appointments for them to come and help you.
- If you don't have cable TV, get it.
- Challenge your husband, friend, or neighbor to your favorite board game.
- Work on your baby name list.

WHAT *NOT* TO DO WHILE YOU'RE ON BED REST

- Try not to complain. It only makes the time pass more slowly. Life is 10 percent what happens to you and 90 percent how you react to it.

scared. You don't know what to prepare for. The uncertainty is what's so scary."

As we have observed earlier, technology is giving high-risk moms more and more ways to handle their bed rest experience. Daryl said, "My husband bought me a laptop so I could access the Internet from my hospital bed. I could research my condition and my medications, e-mail my friends, and do Christmas shopping on-line. As a sole-practitioner attorney, I was even able to work some from my hospital room. The nurses would sometimes come in and say, 'You should be resting!' One of them even told the doctor on me. But he told her to leave me alone. He felt it was important that I keep my mind occupied. Little did anyone know, watching soap operas for hours at a time stressed me out more than anything."

Dr. Mara Tesler Stein believes that it can be counterproductive to make "what to do" lists while you are on bed rest. It can contribute to a sense of guilt that doesn't need much contribution. The Chicago-based psychologist said, "Friends may ask you, 'So, what are you doing to keep busy?' The best answer is: When you're on bed rest, you are not *obligated* to use your time well. You don't *have* to keep a journal, knit, write letters. You don't have to do anything in the visible, concrete, tangible sense of, 'Look what I did today.' The fact is, just breathing, just getting through the day, is a momentous achievement. Every day is an unshakable gift to your baby."

Special Procedures

CERCLAGE

If the doctor's examination reveals that you have cervical incompetence—that is, premature dilation because the cervix has lost its ability to remain closed—or if you have a multiple pregnancy that is placing a lot of pressure on your cervix, she may recommend that you undergo a procedure called *cerclage*. A cerclage is a frequently performed, inpatient hospital procedure, done with local anesthesia, in which a stitch, or *suture,* is placed around the cervix, physically holding the cervix shut in a manner similar to that of a purse string. You may hear this referred to as *purse-string sutures.* Cerclage can be performed as early as the second

---

PAM'S "THINGS I CAN'T WAIT TO DO WHEN I GET OUT OF THE HOSPITAL"

- Hold my babies.
- Hold my husband.
- Take a shower.
- Shave my legs.
- Cut/color my hair.
- Eat in a restaurant.
- Go for a walk.
- Cuddle with my dogs.
- See our house.
- Look at my garden.
- Sleep—*not!*
- Have a facial.
- Have a cup of Dunkin' Donuts coffee.
- Use the bathroom.
- Get ready for babies, put away clothes.
- Build up my strength; exercise.
- Sit in my hammock.
- Drink tea.
- Never watch TV again.

And I've done all of them!

---

trimester, usually around the twelfth or thirteenth week of pregnancy in women with a known history of incompetent cervix.

The physician will usually recommend bed rest for the next day, and in most cases normal activities can be resumed after that. Your physician will probably recommend frequent follow-up appointments to insure the continued success of the procedure. Additionally, she may

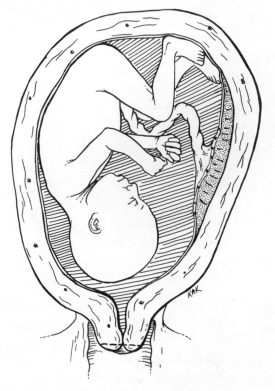

Cross section of a cerclage

nancy in utero. That success rate is upward of 70 percent when another form of management is used in addition to the cerclage, such as bed rest or medication.

Jody, the mother of healthy quadruplets, recalls an early planning session with her perinatologist. "She discussed the increased risk I was at for having conditions such as hypertension, gestational diabetes, and premature labor, and she also mentioned that multiples are at greater risk for IUGR. She said, 'Be prepared, you will be on bed rest at some point in your pregnancy. And when my patients are carrying more than triplets, I recommend a cerclage to be performed at thirteen weeks.'" Jody was undaunted by the thought of being operated on. She recalls her perinatologist declaring, "If you do what I tell you to, this *is* going to work." Sure enough, the procedure was a success. The cerclage held until her quads could be delivered safely at thirty-four weeks. "It held those babies in. I think that was key," she said.

✿ Rescue Cerclage

Susan's son, Alex, was born at 31½ weeks, at 4 pounds 4 ounces. However, this happy, healthy outcome was anything but a foregone conclusion. Susan had a difficult pregnancy. Her success was the result of a mother's being in touch with her body and the excellent medical intervention of her physician.

At twenty-two weeks Susan was going out to buy a congratulations banner for her sister-in-law, who had just had a "picture-perfect pregnancy." On the way she felt a discharge and began to have a backache. She didn't think too much of it, but something told her she should err on the side of caution. "When I

recommend abstaining from sexual intercourse for the remainder of your pregnancy. In some cases she may restrict certain physical activities. If you have had a cerclage, bed rest is usually not necessary as a long-term proposition. But whatever the restrictions, follow your physician's advice and increase your chances for a successful pregnancy. The sutures will remain in place throughout the pregnancy and will usually be removed within about a week of your baby's due date. There is a slightly higher risk of infection due to the penetration of the stitch into your cervix. But the benefits of the procedure are well established. Cerclage alone is reported to be about 50 percent successful in maintaining the preg-

called my doctor's office, they didn't offer me an appointment. But I pushed them to see me. I'm convinced if I didn't do that, I would have lost my baby. The symptoms were there, with my backaches."

Susan's backaches were in fact contractions from preterm labor. "When I have labor problems, I get backaches," she said. "It's a back spasm that comes at five-minute intervals. I'd never had a back problem before. When I went to my perinatologist she at first thought I needed a neurologist. I said, 'You don't understand: these are too regular. It's not from a pinched nerve or a sciatica.' They put me on a monitor, and sure enough, they confirmed my contractions."

Symptoms aren't the same for everybody. Contractions reveal themselves through a number of possible symptoms, not all of which signify labor in every instance. "You talk to some people," Susan said, "and they tell you to call your doctor immediately if you have any kind of discharge. Others will say, 'Oh, I had backaches and discharge all the time.' What it comes down to is, if your gut tells you something is wrong, you better follow up on it. That's what I did; and I probably saved my pregnancy because of it."

Susan was admitted to the hospital that night. Despite magnesium sulfate and terbutaline injections, her contractions did not stop. At twenty-two weeks this was a very dangerous situation—her baby would not be viable for at least two more weeks. So the next day her doctor assessed her situation—80 percent effaced, 1 centimeter dilated—and decided to do a rescue cerclage. This procedure involves, in essence, stitching the cervix shut. Susan's procedure was performed in a regular operating room, some-

thing she has second thoughts about today. "I mentioned to the recovery room nurse that I was still having contractions, and she didn't know what to do. They weren't used to dealing with maternity patients having contractions." At Susan's request she was transferred to the labor and delivery floor.

On the day after the cerclage was put in place, Susan was sent home on a uterine monitor and oral Brethine to control contractions. "Things quieted down for about a month," she said. She was on strict bed rest, lying on her left side, instructed to consume large amounts of fluid. It was tough: "I could go downstairs only once per day."

At twenty-eight weeks "all hell broke loose," she said. "My doctor said it was okay to celebrate my anniversary, and my husband and I went out to dinner. I had gotten a betamethasone shot that night [to quicken maturation of her baby's lungs]. Within forty-eight hours I was contracting heavily because of it. I woke up in the morning and I was just a mess. My heart rate was up, I was flushed, and I was having major contractions." Susan spent four days in the hospital getting stabilized, then went home again. But when her contractions started again at twenty-nine weeks, she was back in the hospital, where she was put on Procardia. "I couldn't really feel these contractions," she said. "If it weren't for the home uterine monitor I was on, I would never have known. The monitor counted thirteen contractions in an hour, but I only felt five of them." She was soon discharged yet again. A day and a half later, however, her back spasms were "incredible, coming every five minutes." She was hospitalized for the third time in less than three weeks, and a week and a half later, on the day after Thanksgiving, she

An Innovation

Most high-risk mothers are willing to explore any option to improve their babies' chances to survive and flourish. We include this story to celebrate their love and dedication. However, we wish also to remind the reader that some innovative therapies, for all their appart benefits, do not yet have clinical proof of their safety or efficacy. Any type of therapy must be undertaken under close supervision of your physician.

Because of severe hyperemesis beginning earlier in pregnancy, Gretchen had two high-risk pregnancies. The Missouri mom spent several weeks on bed rest in a Catholic hospital. It was a fairly conservative institution, but Gretchen had the good fortune to come under the care of a highly creative, progressive perinatologist. One day he came into her hospital room and told her and five other expecting moms that they had to put on swimsuits. They would all be going swimming. "There are only three places in the United States that did this," Gretchen said. "It is very unusual. My first reaction was, 'I can't go swimming. I have a terbutaline pump stuck in my leg!' But before we knew it, we were getting into our wheelchairs, with our bathing suits under our bathrobes, and heading for the pool.

"Nobody got any pictures of us, but I wish they had. All of us were carrying our babies so low that we really waddled when we got out of the wheelchairs and headed for the pool. The other patients thought it was really funny. Getting into the pool, we would put our terb pumps in waterproof Matria shower bags, set the bags on a foam kickboard, tuck Styrofoam noodles under our arms, and spend half an hour moving up and down the pool using our arms and our one free leg. The weightlessness took the stress off our muscles, which had become tense during bed rest. And the exertion helped maintain muscle tone for those of us who would go into labor and needed to push. We did this once a day right before lunch for thirty minutes—they watched us closely for contractions, of course—and we were restricted to only one wheelchair ride a day other than our trips to the pool. But the mental relief was great. It felt good to be in the water. On the days that I didn't go, my back would cramp up very badly. You get so sore and stiff lying in bed that this really enabled you to stretch out. It made the day go by, gave us something to look forward to besides breakfast, lunch, and dinner."

Another time, Gretchen and her friends on bed rest, having been hospitalized for six weeks, lobbied for the right to set up a VCR in a waiting lounge and bring in movies to watch from home. Lying on their sides in recliners and on the floor amid a pile of pillows, they would watch a movie for ninety minutes to two hours. Humor was fine, but sexy or racy films were prohibited because the perinatologist feared the aroused moms would "pop off having contractions," she said. "If we had contractions, we had to tell him or we would never get to watch the films again. I felt like we were back in school. They gave us an inch, and some of us just wanted to see how much we could get out of it. They would get up and walk to the table to get refreshments. That was a no-no."

gave birth. "I thought I'd be delivering pumpkin pie, not delivering a baby. I remember we had to battle shopping traffic to get to the hospital. When my doctor checked my cervix and pulled out his hand covered with blood, I knew there was nothing to do to stop it," Susan said. "But thanks to the cerclage, we have a birth to celebrate."

Medications to Promote Maturation of the Fetus

Steroids have had an incalculable impact on the health of premature infants. Given via intramuscular injection into the mother at least twenty-four hours prior to an expected preterm delivery, they have been shown to accelerate the maturation of the premature infant's lungs, thus reducing the likelihood of respiratory problems. Although the beneficial effects of steroids have been recognized since the mid-1970s, concern about possible complications to the mother persuaded many obstetricians not to use them. Additionally, steroids were said to be contraindicated in mothers with high blood pressure because they can increase blood pressure. There was also a concern about exposing the mother to infection by using steroids. None of these concerns have been proven. In fact, steroids are a proven way to help preemies breathe better after delivery.

In November 1994 the National Institute of Child Health and Human Development convened a panel of experts to review all the available scientific data pertaining to the use of steroids in pregnant women. It was agreed that steroids used in this manner reduced the incidence of lung immaturity and bleeding into the

SHARON HORNFISCHER: "When my pregnancy-induced hypertension reached the point where my obstetrician felt premature delivery was imminent, he wasted no time starting me on a steroid regime. This consisted of an initial injection in my hip muscle [the leg, hip, or arm is most commonly used], then a second injection twenty-four hours later. After the second injection was made, I was inside what my doctor called 'the steroid window.' This was the period of time, spanning about a week, in which the effects of the steroids would most benefit my baby's lung development. If delivery did not occur within the steroid window, I would be given a second regimen of steroids. As it happened, I delivered by C-section forty-eight hours after my second injection. My son entered the world with a gratifying scream and did not require artificial ventilation. It was truly the sweetest sound I had ever heard."

brain of the premature infant and may have beneficial effects on other fetal organ systems, such as the intestinal tract. These experts also reiterated that the risk to the mother was minimal. Since late 1994 steroids have been an accepted standard of care in the management of a mother facing possible premature delivery. Eighty percent of mothers in preterm labor are given steroids to boost their babies' lung development. Some medical experts believe that this has contributed to the reduction in infant mortality rates in the United States over the last several years.

Choosing a Medical Facility

By the late stages of your high-risk pregnancy, even if delivery appears likely to come prematurely, you may already have decided where you plan to deliver. If not, you should not delay any further in making that important decision. Knowing where your delivery will take place will give you a chance to become acquainted with the surroundings, tour the maternity ward, and visit the special care nursery. Getting to know the lay of that land will alleviate some of the fear of the unknown and give you an idea of what to expect during this time of the unexpected. Your physician and his staff can provide you with information on the various hospital settings, insurance plans, and special care nurseries in your area. If you are confined to strict bed rest, have your husband or a close family member help you out in making these plans.

For mothers with high-risk pregnancies, theselection of a medical facility can be a com-

plicated decision. If you live in a rural or outer-suburban area, you may need to travel long distances to reach a hospital that has adequate facilities to handle all of the contingencies of a high-risk delivery. You will want to find a hospital that can handle all of your pre- and post-delivery maternity needs. You may focus your choice of a hospital on the quality of its neonatal medical staff, neonatal intensive care unit (NICU), or special care nursery. Or you may be more concerned with proximity to your home and to your family members. However, if you have a multiple pregnancy coupled with a complicating condition such as PIH, it may be best to trade the convenience of delivering at the nearby community hospital for the security of delivering at an NICU-equipped major medical center in a neighboring city.

Even if your high-risk pregnancy is going well, these potential worst-case scenarios should be thought through and talked about and a fallback plan of action decided upon just in case it's needed. It's best to have the what-ifs covered, because once you find yourself in the middle of an emergency situation, it's not the best time to make such important decisions.

Your obstetrician's or perinatologist's admitting privileges may determine where you can deliver your baby. Admitting privileges are essentially what they sound like: they give a doctor the right to admit a patient to a certain hospital. If your OB/GYN does not have admitting privileges at the medical center you have chosen for its capability to handle high-risk deliveries, then he will have to consult with another physician at that facility and that other physician will take over your care for delivery. If you have a close relationship with your doctor, this may be a problem for you. If at all pos-

> "Due to my high-risk pregnancy, my husband and I made sure to tour our hospital's special care nursery during our childbirth education class. Even though it was a little overwhelming at the time, we were so glad that we did this. For one thing, we got to see what a premature baby looked like. They were so different from what babies looked like in all the magazines. It also helped to see where our baby would be spending his first days and weeks. Getting this preview made for a smoother emotional transition to becoming parents of a preemie."

sible, try to find out where your physician has admitting privileges before you settle on him for your baby's care. If you are going to be transferred into another doctor's care, it may be wise, time permitting, to meet with the new physician to further discuss your delivery and to get acquainted with one another. Of course, if your chief concerns tend more toward practical matters and less on the personal relationship you have with your doctor, this may not be an important issue for you.

When it comes to choosing a hospital, convenience to family and distance to your home are factors, as are your physician's admitting privileges, but at the end of the day the most important criterion is the type of facility a hospital is. Indeed, until you are faced with the risk of a premature delivery, the idea of choosing a hospital may seem beyond your ability to explore. Women with a normal pregnancy will probably be concerned with the comforts and amenities of the delivery suite. But when you have a high-risk condition, you have got to become more bottom-line oriented. The bottom-line question is: "What are the capabilities of this institution's staff and facilities?" You need the right kind of labor and capital: specialized neonatal professionals and a neonatal intensive care unit. More than anything else, these variables affect how well you and your baby will be cared for in an emergency situation.

Essentially there are three types of facilities.

THE LEVEL I HOSPITAL (BASIC CARE FACILITY)

Every day babies are born in community or rural hospitals all over the country, and these facilities are perfectly adequate for an uncompli-

THE PPO NETWORK

An increasing number of insurance plans are built around the concept of the preferred provider organization (PPO). A PPO is an association between an insurance company, on the one hand, and doctors, clinics, and hospitals, on the other, in a given metropolitan area. The PPO will provide for reduced rates if patients use a PPO's member facilities. If your health plan uses a PPO system, you will pay less if you use their member facilities for your care. For example, if you use a PPO's network member, most PPOs will cover 90 percent of expenses, charge you a small co-pay for doctor's office visits, and offer a reduced deductible. If you use an out-of-network health care provider, however, only 70 or 80 percent of expenses will be covered, your deductible will be higher, and your total annual out-of-pocket maximum will be higher. It can become rather complicated if your individual doctor is a member of your PPO but the hospital where he has admitting privileges is not. In that case 90 percent of your doctor's office visits may be covered, but only 70 to 80 percent of your hospital charges.

Your PPO may have procedural requirements under which you have to call the PPO to inform them of your hospitalization within a certain period of time after your admission. Be sure to sort out these details ahead of time. When the time comes to deliver your baby, the last thing on your mind will be the intricate rules of an insurance carrier.

cated labor and delivery. But when a high-risk situation arises, this isn't always the best place to be. Basic care facilities do not have advanced neonatal special care units and do not keep specialized neonatal medical personnel on staff. If you have a high-risk pregnancy and live in a rural community or smaller town, you may need to be transferred to a larger specialty or subspecialty facility in a nearby metropolitan area. The transfer can take place by ambulance, aircraft, or helicopter. Many large metropolitan facilities have their own medevac helicopters or airplanes, and this is often the fastest and most efficient way to transfer. But the means of transfer will depend on your medical status and on the capabilities of the two health care facilities. If a transfer is necessary, your physician will discuss it in detail and assist you in making these decisions. If you are transferred to an unfamiliar hospital, a staff social worker or patient coordinator will be able to assist you and your family with needs ranging from the mundane—finding food, lodging, or parking—to the complex—helping you navigate a confusing labyrinth of insurance paperwork and the like.

THE LEVEL II HOSPITAL (SPECIALTY CARE FACILITY)

These facilities, classified as level II hospitals, are able to take care of most complex problems with mother and baby. Specialty care facilities keep perinatologists and neonatologists on call and maintain a dedicated neonatal intensive care unit or special care nursery for high-risk deliveries and premature infants. If your condition requires the level of care that only a specialty care facility can provide, you will probably need to relocate to an urban area where the medical community has more resources at its disposal to offer specialty care.

THE LEVEL III HOSPITAL (SUBSPECIALTY CARE FACILITY)

These highly sophisticated medical centers offer an expanded variety of medical specialists who are able to handle almost any situation the current state of the art allows. These advanced, big-budget facilities offer doctors who specialize in perinatal ultrasound, in pediatric cardiology, or in endocrinology, just to name a few. If your baby has heart trouble, for example, she will receive the best possible care from the specialists on call here. If you require a facility with these capabilities, you may be transferred there. Depending upon the urgency of your pregnancy situation, that transfer may take place in your own vehicle, by ambulance, or by air.

If you live in a city, you need to research your options. Greater choice means greater responsibility. Talk not only to your doctor about which facilities she recommends (including which ones she has admitting privileges to), but also to friends and acquaintances who have delivered babies in your town. Their firsthand experiences can tell you a great deal about a place. If you talk to enough people, patterns will emerge and you may find one of several seemingly similar hospitals getting the lion's share of the praise. Visit a few hospitals yourself. If it's feasible, communicate your preference to your doctor. If logistics, time, or your condition doesn't allow you to visit facilities personally, have your spouse or a friend visit them for you. Together you should be able to come up with a plan that will offer you and your baby the best possible care available.

3

LABOR AND DELIVERY

WHAT YOU WILL FIND IN THIS CHAPTER

- Planning the unplannable
- Childbirth class: "Should I even have bothered?"
- It's time: when to go to the hospital
- Entering the home stretch
- Cesarean delivery

- The labor and delivery area
- Choices and childbirth
- Getting ready for delivery
- Induction medication
- Deciding about anesthesia
- The moment after birth

Even though you and your physician have made every effort to prevent or control your preterm labor, even though you have been scrupulous in adhering to the bed rest regimen prescribed by your physician in managing a condition such as PIH or incompetent cervix, it is possible that you will not be able to avoid a premature delivery. If you have been on bed rest for any length of time, or if your contractions have required you to be on medication or even to be hospitalized, you may be used to the idea that the time frame of a high-risk pregnancy is highly variable and subject to change with little or no notice. Though it is certainly a

hope, it is by no means a promise that your doctor will be able to take you to a full-term delivery of thirty-seven weeks.

There is no shame in not reaching full term with your pregnancy. It is not failure by any stretch of the imagination. As we emphasize throughout this book, even if you are able to forestall delivery by only a few weeks or even a few days, your efforts can prove to be a great success. No matter what the goal—yours or your physician's—any additional period of time you can win for your baby can greatly improve her prospects for health.

Sandy's bout with premature labor began

during her thirtieth week of pregnancy when she started feeling sharp pains in her abdomen. But thanks to an effective combination of anti-labor medication and bed rest, she succeeded in holding off delivering her baby girl until her pregnancy was at thirty-six weeks, for all practical purposes a full-term delivery. When delivery came, it came fast. Three and a half hours after her water broke, her 6-pound-1-ounce baby was born. Sandy's rapid, painless delivery was the envy of every other mother on the floor.

With most high-risk pregnancies, mother and doctor face a dual challenge: trying to lengthen the pregnancy as long as possible so that the baby will be as mature as possible at delivery, and at the same time standing ready to cut the pregnancy short in case the underlying cause of the prematurity begins to pose a health risk to the mother or the baby. The goal is to stretch out the pregnancy as long as possible, but not so long that your own health (or your baby's in the event of a condition like IUGR) is threatened. This delicate balancing act is the reason we have emphasized throughout this book the need for close supervision by a competent medical professional. Your physician will weigh all the variables and determine whether continuing to postpone delivery will be likely to put your or your baby's health in jeopardy.

This chapter focuses on the last days or weeks of your pregnancy leading up to the climactic moment of labor or delivery by C-section. We include a few last-minute tips, as well as an overview of the options you may have with respect to procedures and medication during delivery. We will discuss how you'll know when it's time and describe what you can expect in the labor and delivery area upon your arrival to the hospital. We also discuss the transfer of your baby's medical care from your obstetrician or perinatologist to the neonatologist, just minutes after your baby's arrival.

Planning the Unplannable

Planning is the first casualty of a high-risk pregnancy. Mothers with a full-term pregnancy have the benefit of a due date by which to plan these pivotal weeks and months. Armed with this information, they can make a reasonable attempt to plan their lives as their pregnancy winds down. They can pack their own suitcase, adding all the essentials and whatever luxuries they choose. They can arrange child care for their other children, if necessary, weeks or even months in advance. They can set up the nursery, pick out announcements, make a list of their first phone calls, and get the house ready for the new addition. Not so for the mother with a high-risk pregnancy. Delivery could come tomorrow, next week, next month, or in three months. There is no way of knowing. The fluidity of the time horizon is one of the main causes of stress for women with high-risk pregnancies.

"I had considered every possibility except that she would be born early," said Melissa, the mother of Erin, born at twenty-six weeks weighing 2 pounds 1 ounce, and Emma, her full-term younger sister. "I hadn't felt good for a couple of days. I was feeling nauseated, as if I had the flu. I wasn't throwing up, but I just didn't feel right. I didn't feel like eating, which was odd. So I went ahead and went to work.

"I was having a heavier discharge than normal. I put if off for the weekend. That Sunday I went into work, and I felt really bad. I had this cramping, and I thought I might have a vaginal infection. At the hospital, the nurse didn't find any dilation. The fetal monitor showed no contractions. They watched me for an hour, took some cultures, and sent me home with a prescription for a urinary tract infection.

"I was pacing the house all night. I couldn't get comfortable, couldn't sleep. At 5:00 A.M. I decided I couldn't stand it anymore. We jumped in the car and went straight to Labor and Delivery. I was going to demand they check me again. This time I was 8 centimeters dilated. They called my doctor. He got to the hospital at 6:00 A.M. I delivered at 8:22.

"She had Apgars of 5 and 7. I remember her squirming around, looking pretty blue. She wasn't breathing on her own, which was kind of scary because this was only a level II nursery. I had no knowledge that babies were even born this early. I had no clue. I asked the neonatologist point-blank: 'How bad is this?' He said she had a 70 to 80 percent chance of survival. I said, 'Please do whatever you need to do.' "

If you spent significant time on bed rest, you've had a great deal of time to ponder the uncertainty. "You're stuck in this small world, your room, and it's hard to banish the bad thoughts," said Sandy, who went into preterm labor at thirty weeks. "There are no distractions. You lie there feeling your contractions all day long."

If the end point of your pregnancy is at hand and the time to go to the hospital is fast approaching, fear will mingle with excitement as you think about finally coming to an end of your unexpected ordeal. The following information is presented to assist you during this last and most climactic phase of your pregnancy: those final tense days when you at last make the transition to parenthood of a preemie.

SHARON HORNFISCHER: "When I went in for my emergency cesarean, everything in our new nursery was halfway done. My husband went home and packed my bag after I was admitted. He did a fair job, but let's just say I never envisioned that a Boston Red Sox T-shirt and sweats would be my hospital uniform. I was very glad when my mother and sister came to my fashion rescue with a bag full of matching clothes, a gown, robe, and slippers."

Childbirth Class: "Should I even have bothered?"

Perhaps earlier in your pregnancy, or during a previous pregnancy, you and your husband were able to take childbirth education classes. That is well and good, and the techniques and helpful tips can assist you with coping with the pains and stresses of labor and delivery, even if your delivery is preterm. However, if, like many women with high-risk pregnancies, you were unable to attend childbirth education classes and instead found yourself confined to bed rest during the week of your first class, don't fret over the lost experience. You will have to take your sense of empowerment from other sources: from books like this one and from the hospital staff, who are pros with lots of experience directing women through labor and delivery, whether they attended childbirth classes or not.

If you did have the chance to take a few classes, be sure to inform your childbirth educator about your potential or actual high-risk condition. Remind her that you will be looking to her for guidance when the time comes. We don't promote any particular type of childbirth preparation class. Several good ones are available today. What we do promote is educating yourself about your and your baby's condition and being proactive in exploring your options. You are in a position to assist your health care provider in making the right decision for you. Talk to your doctor about what's available and look into the class that you feel is right for you.

"My husband and I were all excited about our childbirth education class. We had our first class just as things were starting to go wrong with my pregnancy. We attended the first class and practiced breathing. But even as I did this I felt sort of silly practicing all of those breathing exercises. I thought it was a waste of time, because somehow I knew that I was going to have a cesarean. Shortly after this class my doctor put me on home bed rest, and that was the last my husband and I saw of our classmates. My only real regret was missing the chance to tour the NICU prior to delivery. The NICU tour was scheduled for the fourth class, and I remember wishing that we had attended class a month earlier and had been able to tour the NICU prior to delivery. That way, we 'medical-necessity dropouts'—who were most likely to need the NICU—would have had a chance to see it."

—Courtney

It's Time: When to Go to the Hospital

High-risk pregnancies are just like normal pregnancies in at least one significant respect: They take on lives of their own. Even with all of the planning in the world, your pregnancy will find a way to confound your expectations. You may experience severe preterm labor in your twenty-eighth week, only to deliver a healthy baby at term after going on tocolytics and bed rest. Or you may be sailing along smoothly in your thirtieth week when all of a sudden your blood pressure becomes elevated, requiring an unexpected cesarean delivery. None of this is intended to scare you. Rather, we simply wish to point out that planning is difficult in a high-risk pregnancy. If you feel that your anxiety, lack of focus, and general inability to get and stay organized are somehow personal failings, you need to think again and appreciate the unique burden that your entire being—not just mind, but body, too—is carrying.

But believe it or not, there will come a time when the daily rituals of doctor visits, home monitoring, and frequent lab tests and those long days of bed rest and other essential elements of managing a high-risk pregnancy will be a thing of the past. There will come a day when you are no longer able to delay your delivery any further. If you haven't already been hospitalized as a result of a medical complication of pregnancy, your hospitalization will take place when you reach an end point established ahead of time by your physician. There may be any number of reasons why you have reached your end point. They vary from person to person. You may find yourself with preterm con-

When the Womb *Isn't* a Healthy Home

We have stated in this chapter and elsewhere in the book that the longer your baby can stay in utero, the better his chances to live healthily. In truth, this is not always the case. For example, the effects of pregnancy-induced hypertension (PIH; also known as preeclampsia or toxemia of pregnancy) can be seriously detrimental to your growing fetus while in the womb. The high blood pressure that is characteristic of PIH causes a restriction of the blood vessels in the placenta. This reduces the flow of nutrients to the baby. When a baby isn't getting adequate nutrition in the womb, his growth rate slows. This is called *intrauterine growth retardation* (IUGR). It is crucial to see your doctor regularly while you are pregnant. Without good obstetric care throughout pregnancy, conditions such as PIH can be difficult to detect given the variable ways in which symptoms may manifest themselves.

tractions that suddenly no longer respond to medication. Your membranes may have ruptured prematurely. Your cervical dilation may be fast approaching 10 centimeters. Or you may have been monitored as a high-risk pregnancy from the first or second trimester and have finally reached a diagnostic parameter that indicates it's time—for instance, in the case of chronic or pregnancy-induced hypertension, a urine protein reading that indicates the beginning of liver or kidney damage, or a possible progression of your condition to HELLP (see chapter 1). If this is your situation, your health or the health of your baby will be in jeopardy by prolonging the pregnancy any further.

Contractions may begin without warning, and you should take them very seriously, even if you're not positive that they have started.

"One morning I started feeling this pressure in my abdomen," said Kathy. "I felt like I needed to go to the bathroom. But nothing would come of it. It soon became apparent that the source of the pressure was contractions. My doctor admitted me to the hospital for observation and placed me on medication for premature labor. I stayed in the hospital for about two weeks. It was completely uneventful, and we felt that I was out of imminent danger. My doctor decided to reduce my dosage. But later that same day I began to have contractions—real contractions—just about every thirty minutes. By the time I was checked again, I was a full 10 centimeters dilated and delivery was imminent. I was told to push. Of course, it took only one push, and Zachary came out. He let out one small cry, then was whisked off to the NICU."

Entering the Home Stretch

You are almost there. All of your hard work is about to culminate in the experience of childbirth. Whether you will have a vaginal or cesarean delivery, being prepared mentally and physically will help you best cope with the inevitable stresses along the way. As the end point of your pregnancy nears, you will want to spoil yourself to whatever extent is possible. You can increase your chances for a smooth delivery by catching up on your rest prior to delivery. Though it's easier said than done, take every opportunity you get to take it easy. Listen to your body; it will tell you what it needs. Put your feet up. If you have the luxury of time and advance notice of your delivery, get your bag packed ahead of time (see above checklist). If you are on bed rest and unable to shop and pack, tell your husband or a family member what you need and have him or her pack it for you.

In the later stages of your pregnancy, you and your physician will review your birth plan. Your birth plan—which includes your preferred facility for delivery, type of delivery (labor or C-section), type of anesthesia, if any—may or may not still be appropriate at this point in your pregnancy. Reasons of necessity associated with the high-risk aspect of your pregnancy may pre-empt any preferences you may have. However, your physician will assess your health and the health of your baby, review your previous birth plan, and discuss what your health status means with respect to your birth plan. Even if you don't have a real choice, it's helpful to understand why. And even if you're upset that your planned "perfect pregnancy" went by the boards, take comfort in knowing that it is a considerable accomplishment to have brought your pregnancy as far as you have.

Cesarean Delivery

Conditions that call for an immediate cesarean delivery vary from person to person. Individual considerations determine whether and when the baby must be surgically delivered. The time to perform a cesarean delivery can come when either your or your baby's health begins to be compromised. As is the case with many conditions of high-risk pregnancy, the physician will monitor you and your baby very closely, and if either starts to become adversely affected by your medical condition, the physician will recommend delivery.

A cesarean delivery may be necessary in the following circumstances:

- In cases of a multiple pregnancy
- If a baby is in the breech position
- When the baby's positioning in the womb otherwise indicates that surgical intervention is necessary
- If the baby is in fetal distress
- When you are experiencing serious bleeding (placenta previa or placental abruption)
- In cases of worsening maternal or fetal condition

If you have preeclampsia, it could be possible to have either a vaginal delivery or a cesarean delivery depending on factors such as cervical dilation, weeks of gestation, or your or your baby's ability to withstand the stress of labor, induction, or a potentially slow vaginal birth. Using fetal monitoring (discussed in greater detail in chapter 2), your doctor will be vigilant to any signs of stress in the baby or other conditions (such as placenta previa or abruption) that would indicate an immediate surgical delivery. Depending upon when you last ate, this could take place within hours. In an ideal world, it is recommended that a woman fast for approximately twelve hours prior to a surgical delivery, owing

Missing Out on the "Magic" of Labor

JOE GARCIA-PRATS: "It is natural for some mothers to become upset when they discover they can't give birth naturally, 'like a real woman.' Well-meaning friends and family may say things like 'You really should try to deliver vaginally. There's nothing like it.' There are all sorts of myths about the benefit of doing things the old-fashioned way.

"Frankly, most mothers I see are so focused on their baby's well-being that they don't bat an eye when told they need a cesarean. The most important thing is your and your baby's health. Your only concern should be doing whatever it takes to get her here safely."

to the chance of aspiration of any food in the digestive system during surgery.

When Tara's water broke at twenty-three weeks, her doctor wasted no time admitting her

SHARON HORNFISCHER: "When I was at home on bed rest, my blood pressure readings and fetal kick counts were sent via modem to my physician every four hours. One night I just wasn't feeling very good. I was restless and my blood pressure wouldn't go down. A friend who worked at a movie studio had visited and brought her whole collection of videotapes, and that night I remember watching a subtitled version of *Like Water for Chocolate*. Having been on bed rest for several weeks at this point, I needed the escape. The foreign language, the beautiful imagery, the lovely romance—it was just what the doctor ordered. Although I tried hard to convince myself that I was feeling better, throughout the movie my home health nurse kept on calling me to say my blood pressure readings were elevated. I kept thinking the pressure would go back down if I could just relax, enjoy my movie, and get a good night's sleep. They kept calling me to check on things and insisted that I lie on my side to keep the pressure down. I would do so, recheck my pressure, and meet with no better results. I became convinced that the high pressure readings were just a symptom of my lack of sleep and restlessness. I had a very painful area in my neck, which I attributed to the constant need to lie in bed in an awkward position. But the nurses kept calling to check on me. When they saw what my blood pressure was doing, they started insisting that I go to the hospital.

"At two A.M. the hospital was the last place I wanted to be. I was scheduled to see my OB/GYN early in the morning. The last thing my blood pressure needed, I felt, was a late night trip to the hospital and a miserable night's sleep on a hard mattress. I finally went, mainly to humor my persistent nurse. I was convinced that I wouldn't be left alone unless I did. Though I went fully intending to turn around and come home once my pressure dropped, I was admitted and stayed the night, during which time baby and I were being closely monitored. When morning came, so did lab results that indicated we had pushed our parameters as far and as long as possible. Because of my PIH's advanced condition, my pressure was no longer controllable by bed rest and my kidney tests were showing the upper limits of safe protein buildup. It was frightening to discover, additionally, that my baby was not reacting as he should to his non-stress test. The doctor came in at ten A.M. on May 30 and gave us the news that we would be having David today. 'Are you ready to have a baby?' he asked. The rest of the day was spent with staff rushing in and out of my room, preparing me for delivery.

"It was then, thirty-two weeks and two days into my pregnancy, that I realized that my son would come into this world that very day, via an emergency cesarean."

to the hospital. She was told that she would stay there until she delivered her twin boys. "They put me on bed rest and made me lie in the Trendelenburg position. [This is a position where the head is lower than the body, thus using gravity to keep as much pressure as possible off the cervix.] My doctor figured that I would go into labor and have the babies that day. But since this was early in the pregnancy they were so concerned about the babies' viability, they decided to let the babies stay in utero as long as possible. Of course, if my health became an issue, they would deliver the babies and hope for the best. After I was admitted, I made it one more week,

then I started to go into labor. Since one of the boys was breech, I had a C-section.

"When my doctor took them out, I heard what sounded like kittens crying. I asked, 'What is that, Gary?' and my husband said, 'Those are your babies.' Kyle and Jack were born at 24½ weeks. Kyle was 1 pound 3 ounces, and Jack was 1 pound 9 ounces. They stayed in the NICU for four months. When I think back to what enabled them both to make it, I think of the steroids I was given. I think that's the one thing that helped these guys the most."

Cori, the twenty-nine-year-old mother of a twenty-four-week son, remembers her surprise, shock, and terror when the doctor came bursting into the room with a group of people wearing surgery masks. "He told me that Bo was in distress and we had to take him now. The anesthesiologist behind him was holding an epidural needle and told me it was time for my medicine. In my infinite wisdom, I started arguing with him that the epidural would hurt. He told me rather curtly that it wouldn't hurt any worse than labor would. When I said that I wasn't in labor yet, he said, 'You're about to be!' My family members were asked to leave the room as I was prepared for an emergency C-section. I found out later that all of the commotion was because my placenta had abrupted, making this an extremely urgent situation for both baby and me.

"I was crying and shaking uncontrollably, and the nurses kept telling me that I needed to calm down. As I was being wheeled down the hall to the OR, I looked at my family, and they were all so petrified but trying to keep up a brave front for me.

"As I arrived in the OR, there was a mass of people rushing around in what seemed like a panic. A man with a mask, who I later found out was the neonatologist, came by and introduced himself and told me that he would be taking care of my baby. I kept asking if my baby would be okay, knowing that the chances were not good for a good outcome. They put the sheet up at about my breastbone, and I really started to freak. I was terrified beyond belief, and then this angel, this wonderful nurse, came and sat beside me and took my hand. She told me that she was the mother of a twenty-four-weeker, too, and he was now almost sixteen and 'fixin' to drive.' Hearing that made me feel so much better. It was a ray of hope, and I grabbed on to it and held fast. She told me that my hus-

band was coming to sit with me. I told her that there had to be a mistake because my husband had told me that he wouldn't be in the room when the baby was born. This had been a pretty big argument throughout the pregnancy. He came and sat down and took my hand. When I looked into his eyes, all I could see was love and compassion and, of course, fear. I kept telling him over and over again that I was so sorry I couldn't carry his baby to term. He looked at me and told me it was okay, that he loved me regardless of what happened."

The Labor and Delivery Area

Once you arrive at the hospital, after going through the admitting procedure, you'll be taken to the labor and delivery area. This is where most deliveries, cesareans, or preoperative procedures are performed. If you've had episodes of actual or suspected premature labor earlier in your pregnancy, you've most likely been managed in the labor and delivery area

---

The Paper Chase: Take Care of It Ahead of Time

Before it's even time to go to the hospital, have your admission papers filled out and handy. Be sure and get preadmitted if there is time. Keeping your papers handy in your hospital travel bag could save you considerable time and hassle later, when you won't be as likely to have your organizational wits about you.

> "When I went into labor, I turned off my phone. It was getting so depressing with all my relatives calling: to have to keep describing the situation over and over was no fun. But it's hard to tell good people who are calling you because they're concerned, 'I don't want to talk about it.'
>
> "The nurses knew how upset I was. They hung a sign on my door saying that whoever came by had to check in with the nurses' station first. They would often tell people I was asleep."
>
> —Daryl

and thus know what to expect. However, if this is your first visit to the labor and delivery department, you will find here a sort of organized chaos: medical professionals darting into action at every turn to attend to the ever-changing needs of their patients.

You will most likely be placed in a labor room, also sometimes called an LDR (labor/delivery/recovery) room. You will be assigned a nurse who will care for you throughout your labor and delivery. (Since nurses leave after their shift ends, there is a good possibility that you will be assigned a second nurse when your admitting nurse's shift is complete.) Your nurse will start an intravenous infusion and will place a fetal monitor over your uterus to keep watch over both your contractions and the baby's heart rate. Although there is some disagreement in medical circles about the value of continuous fetal heart rate monitoring in the full-term infant who is developing normally, this type of monitoring can be useful in the observation and treatment of a mother in premature labor or one who is at risk of delivering prematurely. The data that the monitor provides gives your doctor a great deal of knowledge that enables him to decide when, if necessary, delivery should be induced or a cesarean section performed. You may also be placed on a heart monitor and an automated blood pressure machine that takes your

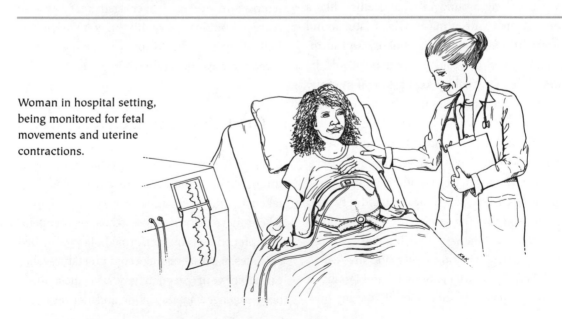

Woman in hospital setting, being monitored for fetal movements and uterine contractions.

blood pressure on a set schedule determined by your physician, based on your stage of labor and your overall medical condition.

Today many labor rooms are nicely decorated and designed to make you and your family feel right at home. There may be comfortable furniture for visitors and a television set and refrigerator in the room. But make no mistake: these are also well-equipped medical treatment rooms. If your condition warrants very close monitoring or administration of medications that have potential complications, the room can quickly transform itself into a facility capable of accommodating even complicated medical procedures.

Choices and Childbirth

Women today are fortunate to live at a time when there are so many options in childbirth. Unlike women just a few decades ago, you have at your disposal methods of modern prenatal care that can detect problems or potential high-risk situations in time for your doctor to intervene medically and give you some input into how you want to bring about a better outcome. In the following sections we discuss the options that you may be lucky enough to have during labor and delivery. Unlike women with normal pregnancies, you may find your options changing with your condition. Your physician will direct you in reassessing your options and in evaluating the different possibilities so that you can be thinking about the what-ifs that may occur. We feel it's better to have an informed idea about what's coming than to be surprised and scared when you have to change course at the time of delivery.

SHARON HORNFISCHER: "I have always been healthy, and I have always thought that I would go past term when delivering my first baby. I had imagined my water breaking while in the middle of some important meeting, being rushed to the hospital, and giving birth naturally within just a few hours of labor. If only it went that smoothly. At week twenty-seven I developed pregnancy complications. My physician informed me that we were most likely looking at a preterm birth and that a cesarean might be needed. Boy, was that a lot to digest. I can only say that I was scared but at the same time glad that I knew more of what to expect and, most important, glad that I had a physician who had earned my complete trust. I was thankful that he and his staff had the faith in me to be able to frankly let me know what was going on with my body and reeducate me by outlining my new delivery options as a high-risk pregnancy."

Getting Ready for Delivery

After your IV has been started, your medical team will consider several other therapies to prepare for your preterm delivery. You should have been given an injection of steroids as soon as your physician seriously considered you to be at risk for a preterm delivery. Ideally a forty-eight-hour lead time prior to delivery will ensure enough time for the steroids to help mature many of your baby's organ systems, foremost among them the lungs. Steroids can also help mature the brain, reduce the occurrence of bleeding into the brain (*IVH*, or *intraventricular hemorrhage*), and lower the chance of your infant suffering from *necrotizing enterocolitis* (*NEC*), an inflammatory bowel disease that primarily affects immature infants. (We'll discuss these in detail in chapter 7.) If your physician is concerned that an infection of your amniotic membranes has precipitated your premature labor, you may also have been given IV antibiotics.

Induction Medication

If your physician believes that prolonging the pregnancy could place you and/or your baby at risk, then you will be given Pitocin intravenously to augment your labor. Pitocin stimulates the uterus to contract and is considered a very potent medication that should be carefully monitored. If Pitocin is administered, your contractions will be observed very closely and the Pitocin infusion adjusted so that the rate of contractions is frequent enough to dilate the cervix but not too frequent to cause you or the baby problems. (You don't want labor to progress to the pushing stage until your cervix is fully dilated and effaced.) The goal of Pitocin when used for induction therapy is to initiate and speed labor contractions, which will hopefully lead to complete cervical dilation and effacement and eventual delivery.

Deciding about Anesthesia

Foremost among your choices is the selection of pain control. Unlike our ancestors, who had to endure the pain and pray for the best if they were at high risk or had a preterm baby, women today have several ways to manage pain. Together with your physician, you can decide which method of pain control is best for you. Some mothers feel that using any kind of artificial pain control is selling out the pureness and beauty of natural labor. Indeed, there is nothing wrong about *not* using pain control during childbirth. Just remember, though, that it can be hard to know exactly what your pain threshold will be and thus exactly what your need for pain control will be. This is especially so if this is your first pregnancy. When labor starts in earnest, you may find it necessary or desirable to take a pain medication even if you thought yourself made of stronger stuff. If this happens, don't feel like a failure. It happens, and remember: You are here for a reason. With a high-risk pregnancy coming to a close, you probably shouldn't sacrifice any degree of security or comfort in order to stand on principle.

With the realization that labor is continuing and that delivery will be a reality, you and your delivering physician must decide what type of anesthesia, if any, to use for the delivery of your baby. This decision is usually made according to the wishes of the mother. But you will be constrained by your doctor's judgment about what is the safest anesthesia for you and your baby. This is especially true if an emergency condition arises. At this stage an anesthesiologist may become involved. This is a physician with special training in the administration of different types of anesthetics. The types of anesthesia can vary from the use of a general anesthetic, where the patient is asleep during the surgical procedure, to the use of sedatives, where sensations are just dulled, to the use of an epidural for anesthesia, were the woman will have no sensations from the waist down but is awake for the experience of childbirth and new motherhood.

REGIONAL ANESTHESIA

Regional anesthesia are so called because they are designed to work by numbing certain areas or regions of the body. They may be used to block sensations or numb a relatively large area (for example, from the waist down in the event of a surgical delivery) or to block sensations to a smaller area (as in a vaginal delivery). Following are the main types of regional blocks.

CAUDAL BLOCK. This is administered via injection into your spinal area in much the same way as an epidural, but it numbs a smaller area. A caudal block has also been found to inhibit labor. It is therefore not used very frequently today.

PUDENDAL BLOCK. This is a type of regional block that is reserved for the vaginal delivery. Medication is injected into the vaginal area, blocking the pudental nerve.

EPIDURAL BLOCK. This is fast becoming the most widely used form of anesthesia for vaginal as well as cesarean birth. An epidural block is performed by injecting a numbing medication into the space around your spinal cord called the *epidural space*. This type of regional anesthesia allows for control of pain by numbing the nerves that sense pain. This medication is placed into the epidural space by using a spinal needle to introduce a very small catheter into this space and then injecting the medication through the catheter. The amount needed to keep the area anesthetized can be reinjected when needed. An epidural should remove all sensation from your waist down to your knees.

A major advantage with an epidural is the control that the anesthesiologist has in slowing and increasing the medication as needed throughout labor and delivery. The epidural acts by relaxing the muscles of the vaginal area of the mother, which potentially offers less resistance to the presenting part of the infant, usually the baby's head. Another advantage is that the epidural anesthesia can be gradually reduced so that by the time the cervix is fully dilated, the anesthesia has worn off and the mother can have a better feel for when it's time to push and can thus be a more active participant in the delivery process. Later, after delivery, the epidural's effect can be increased again as needed for delivery of the placenta or repair of an episiotomy (see next section, "Local Anesthesia"). Additionally, with the choice of an epidural you are able to remain alert for the experience of childbirth and afterward.

A disadvantage of an epidural is that it can dilate the blood vessels in the mother, causing low blood pressure. This can usually be avoided by giving the mother extra fluids by vein before the epidural anesthesia is given. But an epidural is usually contraindicated in bleeding complications such as placenta previa, severe preeclampsia, or fetal distress. Another potential disadvantage would be in the case of a fast delivery. The medicine may not be out of the system, and the mother may not have enough sensation to know when to push. In such a case, a forceps delivery may become necessary. Since epidurals are also known to lower fetal heart rate, fetal monitoring is recommended if you go this route.

LOCAL ANESTHESIA

When the baby is "crowning"—that is, when its head is pressing against the outer wall of the vagina—the obstetrician may need to perform an *episiotomy,* an incision made in the vaginal wall to allow the baby to be delivered more easily and/or to prevent tearing of the vaginal tissues. This is not necessary in all births; in some cases the stretching ability of this elasticlike skin will serve as its own anesthetic. But if it is, the doctor will generally inject a local numbing anesthetic before making an episiotomy. The episiotomy will be stitched up right after delivery and should heal in a matter of weeks.

GENERAL ANESTHESIA

Though this was once the most common form of childbirth pain relief, its use today is indicated primarily for surgical births such as an emergency cesarean when there is no time for a regional anesthetic to take effect. Occasionally it is used in vaginal birth, with a breech presentation when there is difficulty delivering the head. General anesthesia is performed by giving you a medication that puts you to sleep. When general anesthesia is given, your whole body is sedated and therefore the muscles that tell you to breathe are also asleep, and you are unable to breathe on your own. Because of this, the anesthesiologist will place a tube into your windpipe and thus be able to support your breathing during the operation and in the postoperative period until the medication wears off and you are breathing on your own again. While you are asleep an anesthetic gas is used to control your pain. The biggest drawback to general anesthesia is that the medication can cross the placenta into your baby and the baby may be sleepy when delivered. This is a particular cause for concern if the baby already is premature. Thus a neonatology team is present to deal with this as well as the other possible problems. Sedation of the baby can be minimized by administering the medication as close to the actual birth as possible. Hopefully delivery will take place before a large dose of the medication can reach the baby. Additionally, if you are given oxygen in the delivery room, it can help oxygen pass to the fetus in such an emergency situation.

Once the choice of anesthesia has been made and you are completely dilated and ready to deliver, you will be moved from an LDR room to a delivery room. This is in case an emergency cesarean section needs to be performed; LDRs are not equipped for that surgery. The move from the labor bed to a stretcher to go to the delivery area and then to the next delivery bed is often an unpleasant experience. If you're already in discomfort, it can seem almost unbearable to have to be transferred from bed to bed. However, it's necessary for the well-being of your baby.

By the time you are being readied for delivery, the neonatal team has been notified of the pending delivery and is on standby in the labor and delivery area. Though you may be in shock, you are somewhat aware of the events that will be taking place around you. You have most likely already spoken to the neonatologist, who will be supervising the team standing by to handle all eventualities for your baby. They will be readying their own version of the neonatal intensive care unit, or stabilization bay, in the labor and delivery area. Their goal will be to stabilize the baby right after birth and then transfer the baby to the NICU.

The Moment after Birth

You've no doubt imagined this moment for months; after all the work of pregnancy and childbirth, now comes the time when your newborn will be swaddled in a blanket and placed in your arms for the very first time. It can come as the cruelest of shocks instead when your preemie is taken out of your body and delivered into the hands of the neonatologist without giving you a chance even to count fingers or toes.

The neonatologist and his team will be on standby in the delivery room. If you are about to deliver multiples, there will usually be a medical team headed by a neonatologist for each baby. At delivery, the neonatologist will make a quick inspection of the infant. At one minute and five minutes, he will assess the newborn using the Apgar scoring system (see chart on page 119). If the infant is relatively mature and stable (as are most who are born at thirty-two weeks' gestation or greater), there is a good chance that she will be quickly examined, weighed, measured, bundled, and taken back to be with the mother for a few minutes of bonding. This initial bonding experience is all the more important since parents may not be allowed much actual holding contact in the NICU, at least until some time has passed and the baby is stable.

SHARON HORNFISCHER: "The neonatologist came and talked to my husband and me just hours before I was to have a cesarean. I remember his warmth and his kindness more than anything else now. He talked about all of the possible risk factors and consequences of a baby born at thirty-two weeks, and though his manner was gentle, he didn't spare us any of the details. When our son was delivered, coming out with a vigorous scream, our relief could scarcely be expressed. We had never heard a sweeter sound."

After birth, your infant will be taken to an area sometimes referred to as a *stabilization bay,* which is either in the delivery room or just adjacent to it, for assessment. This is where the neonatologist and his staff examine the newborn, the Apgar is performed and the baby's respiratory status will be stabilized if necessary. If the child is stable enough, he can go to mom's bedside for a few minutes. If the baby's condition is poor, resuscitation may be initiated and the baby transferred to the special care nursery for further treatment. Stabilization will be the goal. If the baby is very immature, then most likely your infant will stay in the resuscitation bay until she is stable. When the infant is stable, then dad and relatives may be allowed to quickly see the newborn until the neonatal team has decided what level of care she needs.

When the decision has been made as to which unit is appropriate, your baby will be placed in a transport incubator and taken directly to the special care nursery. This is necessary because the mother is usually too sedated to hold the baby or the baby's condition is fragile enough to require additional medical support. Usually dad will be asked to accompany the baby, so that he can see where the nursery is. Once dad knows where the nursery is located, he can go back to the labor and delivery area to be with mother while she recovers. Or he may stay with the baby as the special care staff receives the baby and admits her to the nursery.

4

THE FIRST TWENTY-FOUR HOURS
AFTER DELIVERY

WHAT YOU WILL FIND IN THIS CHAPTER

- The first few minutes after birth
- The first few hours after birth
- Other things to take care of when your baby is transferred to the NICU

Before your baby was born, you and your physician had at best only indirect ways to assess his health. Technology has given us wonderful tools for peering inside the womb at the miracle of life. A fetal monitor could give you information on your baby's heart rate and how he responded to stresses placed on him in the womb environment. Ultrasound could provide a grainy visual image of your baby, showing the structure of his organs, the shape of his skeleton, and his overall prenatal development. Your physician could take measurements of your baby's limbs and head in order to estimate his size at birth so as to prepare for his needs outside the womb. Specialists may have used ultrasound to zero in on particular organs at risk for complications. These tools can provide answers to many important questions about a baby's

health. All of this information was a great help to the neonatal team in preparing to assist and support your baby as he made the transition from the water-filled environment of the womb to the gas-filled environment of our world.

But now that your baby has been delivered—now that you are able to see and touch him directly—it's possible to take the full measure of his health and do something about it if necessary. This is a critical time in your preemie's hospital course, since he must now fend for himself outside the protective enclosure of the uterus. Where you once functioned as your infant's lungs and provided nutrients and warmth, now your baby must do this for himself, or rely on modern technology for assistance with these vital life processes. Lung immaturity, heart defects, and overall immaturity can make the adaptation to the outside world an especially great challenge. The neonatologist directing your baby's assessment and management will have gathered all the information available on your baby, from speaking to your obstetrician to reviewing your obstetric history. Now that your baby has been delivered, much of the estimation, probability, and guesswork can be put aside.

"Once I delivered, it was a relief finally to know: This is what I have to deal with. This is what I'm facing," one mother said.

The First Few Minutes after Birth

As soon as your baby is born, the neonatologist and her team, which will consist of at least a nurse and a respiratory therapist in addition to the doctor, will waste no time attending to your child. They will be standing by as your delivery progresses, be it vaginal or cesarean. With your baby out of the womb, the neonatologist can now perform a hands-on visual and physical assessment that is much more informative and precise than what she could do before delivery.

BREATHING: THE FIRST PRIORITY

As soon as the neonatologist receives your baby from the delivering physician, the first order of priority will be assessment of the infant—especially her respiratory system—and resuscitation and stabilization as necessary. Your baby will be attended to in a *resuscitation bay* or *pod,* which is usually located within the labor and delivery area. This area is a sort of mini-NICU where essential neonatal equipment is readily available—warmer, respirator, IV therapy, pulse oximeter, heart rate monitor, and all of the medications needed for stabilization of the infant.

Preemies who have serious medical issues at birth will undergo immediate medical intervention. This can include the administration of oxygen, intubation (the insertion of a tube down the baby's throat into the airway), and the administration of intravenous fluids to support the baby's blood glucose level. If the baby has experienced blood loss, plasma or saline may have to be infused. The goal is to stabilize the baby's vital signs as quickly as possible so that the newborn can be transferred to the NICU, where a longer-term program of care can begin. A baby may spend as little as fifteen to twenty minutes—or several hours—in the stabilization area.

THE APGAR SCORE

One minute after the baby is delivered, and again at five minutes, the neonatologist and her team will perform an *Apgar assessment.* This is a composite score measuring your baby's color, heart rate, respiration, muscle tone, and reflexes. (The neonate's team will move the baby into an incubator or radiant warmer, which are both used to keep the baby warm after delivery.) By assigning your baby a score at these intervals, the neonatologist can get a helpful thumbnail measure of your baby's need for resuscitation and how his condition progresses in these first few minutes of life outside the womb.

✤ The Apgar Scoring System

The Apgar scoring system (named for Virginia Apgar, the physician who developed it) was designed to evaluate the physical condition of the newborn at birth and the immediate need for resuscitation. The newborn receives a one-minute and five-minute score ranging from 0 to 10, based on the baby's appearance (color), pulse (heart rate), grimace (reflex irritability), activity (muscle tone), and respiration—hence the acronym Apgar. The doctor assigns a value of 0, 1, or 2 to each of these criteria. Scores between 4 and 6 often require resuscitation. This could include suctioning the airway or administering oxygen. A score below 4 means that a more dramatic kind of medical intervention is necessary as a lifesaving measure.

Sign	0 Points	1 Point	2 Points
Appearance (color)	pale blue	body pink, extremities blue	completely pink
Pulse (heart rate)	absent	slow—below 100	above 100
Grimace (reflex irritability)	none (no response to stimulation)	baby grimaces	vigorous cry
Activity (muscle tone)	flaccid	some flexion of extremities	active
Respiration	absent	slow—irregular	good (crying)

The test is administered again at five minutes after delivery. If the score is 7 or better, then the need for further support is low. Otherwise the baby will need to be observed and monitored closely until her condition stabilizes.

After your child has been assessed and placed on a radiant warmer to help stabilize her temper-

✣ FAQ:

"Will my baby be able to breathe on his or her own after delivery?"

The stability and maturity at birth of your baby's lungs and respiratory system will determine how well he or she will breathe immediately upon making the transition from the water-filled womb to our gas-filled world. Though the answer to this question won't be known until birth has actually occurred, factors such as the baby's gestational age and whether you were administered steroids (betamethasone) prior to delivery are important.

ature, varying levels of breathing support may be initiated. This may be simple suctioning of the mouth and nose, administration of oxygen, or placement of an *endotracheal tube* into the infant's windpipe so that she can be given respiratory assistance through a resuscitation bag or a respirator. If the infant is very immature (less than twenty-seven weeks), respirator support may be initiated automatically until the baby demonstrates sufficiently mature lung function. It is also at this time that special catheters may be placed into the infant's umbilical vein and/or umbilical artery. Many times catheters are placed in both blood vessels, since each serves a different purpose. The umbilical artery catheter allows arterial blood to be sampled, enabling monitoring of lung function and blood pressure, which may be very important in the first few days of life. The umbilical vein catheter serves as an avenue for administering dextrose, water, medications, blood, and blood products.

"Will I be able to bond with my baby?"

If the baby is stable, and if the doctor feels it is medically appropriate—if the baby's temperature doesn't drop after he or she is removed from the incubator—your newborn may be brought to your bedside for some bonding. Whether your baby can bond cannot be determined ahead of time. Many variables factor into this assessment—including your own health status postpartum. Some mothers of preemies will have to wait until their baby has been transferred to the NICU before they will be able to bond with their baby. Not every mother will have the opportunity to bond right away. How much bonding is allowed to take place depends on the mother's and baby's medical status after delivery. The neonatologist makes the ultimate decision about whether your baby is stable enough to handle physical contact. All other factors being equal, the chances that you will be able to bond after delivery increase in proportion to your baby's gestational age at birth.

If lung immaturity (*hyaline membrane disease,* or *HMD*) is suspected, then your baby may be given artificial surfactant (the chemical that is missing if the baby's lungs are immature) once she is stable, to facilitate the expansion of the lungs, maintain the millions of tiny air sacs in the lungs, keep airways open, and thereby promote regular breathing. The surfactant will be delivered through an *endotracheal tube* (a

tube placed down the baby's throat into the windpipe) so that the liquid can pass directly into the lungs where it is most needed. If the child has HMD, she will usually receive four doses of surfactant in the first twenty-four hours. If she doesn't have HMD, then the infant will probably need only one or two doses.

This approach is a prophylactic method, as opposed to a rescue method (administer the treatment only when one is sure the infant has HMD). The data supporting a prophylactic approach shows clearly better results.

THE ABC ASSESSMENT

During your baby's assessment, you may hear your doctor and staff referring to something called "ABCs." This is shorthand for *a*irway, *b*reathing, and *c*irculation. While assessing the airway, the neonatologist will make sure the

---

What Happens in the First Few Minutes after Birth

- Baby's respiratory status is assessed (check the ABCs—*a*irway, *b*reathing, *c*irculation).
- Stabilization and support begin.
- Apgar score is assigned (at one minute).
- Apgar score is taken again (at five minutes).
- If the baby and mother are stable, the mother may hold the baby for bonding before the baby is transferred to the special care nursery.
- If the baby requires continued medical intervention, there will be immediate transfer to the NICU.

JOE GARCIA-PRATS: "Bonding is a process that all parents will go through. In fact, it begins early in pregnancy, well before delivery. It continues from the moment of birth. But sometimes that continuation is delayed because of a medical condition that mother or baby has. The exact time that the bonding begins does not reduce its value, nor does it change the ultimate result.

"In some cultures babies are taken from their mothers after birth and cared for by other women. They feel that a newborn's needs can't be completely met by the exhausted mother. In our culture, however, there's a certain absolutism that you have to bond right after birth or it won't be okay.

"What I tell people is that bonding with an infant is like love and friendship. The really close, heart-to-heart attachment that all mothers want to form with their babies takes time. But it does happen. Although the immediacy of dealing with the medical situation can change the timing a bit, I think the bonding still happens as it would anyway. We're an adaptable species. We manage to succeed whenever obstacles are put in our way."

SHARON HORNFISCHER: "I felt that I began gradually bonding with my baby since that first positive home pregnancy test. To me, bonding is an inner feeling that grows over time. It's not like if you miss this 'window of opportunity' to bond at the time of delivery, then your relationship is doomed. I personally feel that there is a time and place for everything, and when my son was taken to the NICU soon after his birth, I knew that he was in the good hands of the neonatologist and his staff, exactly where he needed to be."

baby's mouth and throat aren't blocked by any form of obstruction. Obstructions can include mucus, the tongue, meconium (the baby's first stool in utero; this is much more common in full-term babies), swelling, or some kind of structural abnormality.

Even though the airway is clear, the baby may not be breathing properly. The "B" part of the ABC assessment involves the look-listen-feel process that may be familiar to you from CPR. The neonatologist will watch to be sure the baby's chest is rising and falling, listen for the sound of the baby's breathing, and feel for breath.

The "C" part of the ABC assessment involves evaluating the baby's circulation—the efficiency of the baby's heart in pumping blood throughout the body. If the airway is open and respiration is taking place, circulation will do the job of carrying the oxygen throughout the body. The baby's color will indicate this; a pink hue in the extremities or lips/tongue indicates good circulation. The strength of your baby's pulse will also be evaluated in assessing the quality of his circulation.

When the baby is ready for transfer to the NICU, he will be placed in a *transport incubator*—a clear plastic bed that will allow you to see and touch your infant.

The first bonding experience may last for five to ten minutes before the baby will be transported via incubator to the NICU. It could

"Where will my baby be taken immediately after delivery?"

Immediately after the delivery of your baby, he or she will be handed to the neonatologist for assessment and treatment, as necessary. The neonatologist and his team will take your baby into a "mini-NICU," or stabilization bay, adjacent to your delivery room for assessment and stabilization. Once stabilized, your baby's neonatologist will make the decision about bonding. Stability of the baby will determine whether you may hold your baby for a few minutes or not, before he or she is taken to the special care nursery. Whenever possible, your neonatologist will try to give you a chance to hold your baby, if it's medically appropriate, before the transfer to the NICU takes place. But if it would pose any danger to the baby, your child will be transferred to the NICU for stabilization.

Why are there so many different types of beds in the special care nursery?"

The preemie's bed is specially designed to furnish the kind of support dictated by the baby's health status. Generally, there are three types of beds your baby will occupy during the course of his or her special care nursery stay.

RADIANT WARMER

When you first see your preemie, she will probably be in one of these. A radiant warmer is open to air. Warmth for the baby comes from an overhead heating unit. The virtue of this setup is that the medical staff can easily access your baby in the event of an emergency.

INCUBATOR

This is a covered, transparent plastic unit heated from below. Once your preemie has stabilized, he will be moved here. Temperature is a primary concern for a preemie occupying an incubator. The medical staff can reach your baby through "portholes" in the side of the unit. This arrangement allows warmth to be preserved within the unit. The fewer calories your baby burns trying to stay warm, the faster his growth will be and the sooner your child can come home. This equipment, though used primarily to stabilize your baby's body temperature, also shelters him from the noises of a busy NICU, thus allowing him to sleep without frequent interruption.

take place in the labor and delivery room (vaginal delivery) or in the surgical suite (cesarean delivery). The doctor will be right there as you bond with your child. Neonatologists and their staff appreciate the value of mother-infant bonding and will make every effort to let you bond with your newborn if it is medically advisable. Even so, at this early stage the bonding won't last longer than a precious few minutes before your baby is taken to the NICU.

"I could hardly believe my eyes when my baby was brought to me after my cesarean," said one mother. "I didn't expect to see my thirty-two-week preemie so soon. I was so happy to see his perfect but miniature little features. They laid him on my chest; he was so light, I could barely tell he was there. He weighed just 3 pounds 4 ounces. I remember counting his fingers and toes and thanking my lucky stars."

IF YOU HAVE BEEN MEDICATED

It all happens so quickly. If you've been given medication that makes you groggy, your delivery might very well take on a surreal quality. You may regain full awareness minutes or hours after your baby has been taken to the neonatal intensive care unit or special care nursery. Your first visit with your baby in such an event will be postponed until you are well enough to make the trip to the NICU yourself. Many mothers recovering from an anesthetized or otherwise difficult delivery report a strange sense of unreality about the whole experience.

Having fended off premature labor at twenty-seven weeks, Debra underwent an emergency cesarean delivery at thirty-four weeks due to her baby's intrauterine growth retardation. When her one chance at a spinal block didn't take—time was urgent—she was given general anesthesia.

"When I woke up all I knew was my baby was gone and I hurt. My husband was gone, too. He'd gone to see the baby. Someone came over and told me that I'd had a boy. I said, 'Oh, I had a boy.' It took a while to sink in. I had no clue.

"When my husband came down, he said that our son was 3 pounds 6 ounces and was 16¾ inches long. He said Connor was breathing on his own at first, but then went downhill a bit and had to go on oxygen. It was probably two days before it clicked with me that I had had a baby. I was out when the whole thing happened. It wasn't very real to me.

"I asked Dale, 'So, do you feel like a daddy yet?' He said, 'Yeah.' I said, 'I don't.' He said,

'You don't what?' I said, 'I don't feel like a daddy yet.' I laughed so hard that my body couldn't take it. It hurt so bad to laugh. I told Dale if he made me laugh again, I would just kill him. As if it were his fault. Poor guy.

"It took a long time before it all felt real to me."

The First Few Hours after Birth

It may be after your baby's transfer to the NICU that your initial "neo consult" takes place. Your first consultation with the neonatologist is often done under less than ideal circumstances. Expediency will usually determine when and where it happens. It may very well (and indeed should, if at all possible) take place before you go into delivery. On the other hand, many times

JOE GARCIA-PRATS: "I tell parents that our job as neonatologists is to perform the role of the womb for three to sixteen weeks. In a simplistic sort of way, we're trying to do the job of the placenta and the uterus. Think about it: Millions of dollars of equipment and years of special medical training, all to replicate a system that functions inside of you that, when things go without complication, you may not spend a lot of time even thinking about. We are good—neonatal medicine has come a long way over the past few decades. But I don't think we'll ever quite match the elegance and efficiency of the placenta and uterus."

the sudden, emergency nature of what causes premature labor or delivery (for example, placental abruption) requires immediate action and allows no time for talk. As a result, your introduction to your baby's neonatologist may take place right in the labor and delivery area, just as your delivery is beginning.

This is often a difficult time for you to absorb and understand all of the information the neonatologist will provide. You and your spouse are already dealing with the unexpected issue of prematurity, with all of its implications for both your and your baby's health. With labor pains, surgical delivery, and the effects of medication thrown into the mix, that's enough anxiety for anybody. Now an unfamiliar face is outlining for you in great detail all of the health risks that go with your baby's premature birth, the treatment options that you will have, and the plans you may have to make for an extended NICU stay. It is thus understandable if everything the neonatologist says doesn't stick. There will be plenty of time to ask questions later, once you have regained your own equilibrium.

Tara, the mother of natural identical twins who had complications due to twin-to-twin transfusion syndrome, delivered Kyle and Jack via cesarean delivery at 24½ weeks, when she was twenty-six years old. It took her a long time to get adjusted to motherhood. "To tell you the truth, I probably distanced myself from the whole situation at first. They were so small, they didn't look like normal babies. It was hard for me to feel the same way about them.

"The doctor would come up and give me a status report, and I would sit there and listen to him. But if I didn't understand something, I wouldn't ask him to elaborate because I didn't know if I really wanted to understand. That's the way I dealt with everything. Whatever you want to tell me is fine. But when you ask me if I have any questions, I'm going to say no."

Owing to the twins' small size and delicate health status, contact with her babies was nonexistent. "For seven weeks I didn't get to hold them or really get to interact with them at all. I would go up there for twenty or thirty minutes at a time several times a day. But I really felt helpless."

TRANSFER TO THE
SPECIAL CARE NURSERY

Once the neonatal medical team has made its assessment and stabilized your baby, he or she will be taken to an appropriate neonatal nursery for care and observation. Although we've used the term *neonatal intensive care unit,* or *NICU,* the nomenclature is a little more nuanced than that. Most hospitals use the term *special care nursery* to indicate any level of care that differs from what a healthy full-term newborn will receive. Both critical/intensive care nurseries and intermediate care nurseries (also called *step-down units*) fall under this rubric.

JOE GARCIA-PRATS: "When I first speak to the parents, three-quarters of the time the conversation takes place in a delivery suite, with the mother in labor. In the other quarter of the time, there will be a calmer setting. So usually there's so much going on, you know that the mothers won't hear everything. Sometimes they're anxious, in the pain of labor, or already under sedation and will be nodding off while dad is trying to listen. Some parents just want to know about the big things—Will my baby survive?—and everything else is just details. Others want the details: rates of hemorrhage, chances for blindness or cerebral palsy. Often they won't even hear the answers. But I think most parents feel comforted in having a sympathetic professional ear to hear their concerns."

The special care nursery may be a single area where both intensive and intermediate care is provided (infants move from the intensive care area to the intermediate care area when their

🌿 FAQ:
"Who will take care of my baby once he or she is safely delivered?"

A neonatologist (a physician specially trained in the care of the premature newborn) will be the physician in charge of your baby's care from the time of delivery and through the end of the NICU or special care nursery stay. Additional members of the neonatology team caring for your baby can include registered nurses, nurse practitioners, clinical nurse assistants, respiratory therapists, and any of a number of other medical specialists.

After your baby is discharged, his or her medical care will be in the hands of a pediatrician. The neonatologist is charged with getting your baby to that stage.

condition becomes more stable). Alternatively, separate areas may provide these services.

Preemies with contagious infections might visit the *isolation area.* These private rooms have their own air circulation systems to minimize the chance that other newborns will catch the infection. Parents and staff will have to observe special precautions such as wearing gowns, masks, and gloves at all times. Babies requiring isolation may come from either the intensive or the intermediate care areas.

YOUR FIRST VISIT TO THE SPECIAL CARE NURSERY

Premature birth may be something that you have anticipated throughout your pregnancy. You may have known it was likely to occur since your second or early third trimester. Alternatively, it may have come on suddenly, the result of a complication at the very end of your pregnancy, resulting in emergency delivery and an unexpected special care nursery stay for your newborn. No matter how you got here, no matter how well prepared you thought you were to accept your baby's stay in the special care nursery, nothing can perfectly prepare you for the experience. For most parents, everything is a blank slate from delivery forward. Every parent has a different learning curve, but they all start in the same place. Even parents with professional medical training (including one coauthor of this book) can find themselves feeling like proverbial babes in the woods when their son or daughter has to spend time in the special care nursery.

First impressions are powerful. One father recalled, "She looked like a baby bird pinned to the bed. The nurse took a few minutes explaining the various wires, notes, and such. My only real memory of that first encounter was shock. Shock at her appearance, shock at her size [670 grams, or 1 pound 7 ounces, and 12 inches long], and shock that this was happening to me. Pretty selfish thoughts in retrospect. I figured it was only a matter of time before she died. I went back upstairs to my wife to tell her how okay everything was."

Jody, who delivered quadruplets at thirty-four weeks, said, "Trevor, my husband, was strong and fine with everything right off the bat. I, however, didn't get to go there until a day later. And when I did I was all hooked up to an IV receiving Demerol. I remember crying all over Jared. *I can't believe I have a baby this small,* I thought. *How am I going to take care of him?* On one hand it was such a relief that they were safely here in the NICU, but things were going off and beeping, it was very upsetting. The girls had an IV in their heads, they had little bruises and shaved spots where the IVs were started, and that really set me off. That hurts you as a mother.

I was there two hours, and I was just wiped out. They'll let you hold them, but then an alarm goes off, and you think, What did I do? You hold them and you feel they could break."

Dr. Mara Tesler Stein, a Chicago-based clinical psychologist and coauthor of *The Emotional Journey of Parenting Your Premature Baby,* said that while the safe delivery of a premature infant may be an occasion for some relief, the "emotional journey" of preemiedom has really just begun. "Parents actually mourn the birth of a preemie," she said. "There's a whole list of things that they've lost: the end of a pregnancy, having a choice about how and when they deliver, early time spent bonding with their baby, the joy of feeling a baby move inside them, the breast-feeding relationship, the thrill of taking your baby home. Because the infant is born early, the pregnancy never gets to the point where those things happen naturally and without a lot of stress."

"It was frustrating," Gini said. "I had formed certain expectations about how my baby should look. All the parenting magazines were full of these pictures of big, fat, healthy babies. When my baby was born, I was shocked. It wasn't at all what I expected. She was so skinny that you could see her ribs and her veins through her skin. Her ears were folded over and bent, because there was no cartilage. She was so small and there were tubes everywhere: the ventilator tubes, the intravenous lines, and the pulse oximeter attached to her foot. I just couldn't believe it. She looked like a little old man."

When you first learned that your baby would spend his or her first days, weeks, or months in the special care nursery, your first reaction may have been one of confusion and anxiety. When you were told that rather than coming home to sleep in a newly appointed nursery (already decorated and adorned with teddy bears and other stuffed friends), your baby would live in a small incubator amid beeping high-tech machinery, you might not have immediately appreciated what the development of the NICU has meant to the survival chances of premature infants. This is probably true even if you did know that prematurity was a likelihood for your baby and even if your obstetrician was able to arrange a tour of the unit beforehand. Until you became a parent of a premature infant, you probably saw the NICU as a place where *other* people's babies went. Way back when you first discovered you were pregnant, the last thing you expected was that your own baby would call an NICU home.

Tara said, "I knew there was a place where premature babies went, but I didn't know what the NICU was. I didn't visit it beforehand. I didn't get that far in my pregnancy. I thought I had time."

Melissa's daughter wasn't breathing when she was born at twenty-six weeks, weighing 2 pounds 1 ounce. She was immediately intubated for respiratory support in the NICU. The twenty-four-year-old mother from Alabama said, "I barely even saw her. There was a neonatologist on call in the delivery room, but I had no knowledge that babies were even born this early, or that if they were that they could survive. I had no clue. I asked the doctor point-blank, 'How bad is this?' He said, 'Considering her gestational age, she has about a 70 to 80 percent chance of survival.' I thought those were pretty great odds. I had no idea they were that high. I said, 'Please do whatever you need to do to help my baby.' "

Debra, a mother from Colorado, recalled a similar feeling of shock and disorientation when she delivered her thirty-four-week preemie one April. "It was just a blur. It had never occurred to me that it was possible that I could have a baby before June. It literally never crossed my mind, not even during preterm labor. This was very naive, but that's the way it was."

THE EMOTIONAL TRANSITION TO NEONATAL INTENSIVE CARE

A preemie's transfer to the NICU is a big moment for a parent. Seeing the unit in all its high-tech glory tends to crystallize the gravity of the baby's situation.

SHARON HORNFISCHER: "The whole team of neonatal nurses who took care of David was wonderful, but I remember one frustrating experience. The nurses had been telling me that the more time I spent doing skin-to-skin care with my son, the better. It is thought that the skin-to-skin contact would reduce the length of his stay in the special care nursery, and my husband and I would schedule this with the staff for every evening after the eight P.M. feeding.

"But one day another nurse suggested to me that I was keeping my baby out of the incubator too long. She said keeping him out like this was causing him to burn a lot of energy to stay warm and hindering his growth and development. I was only trying to do what was best for my baby. And to hear that I might be doing him some harm was awfully upsetting. I realize now that all they were trying to do was say that my son needed a balance between his skin-to-skin time and his incubator time, but at the time I found the inconsistency in nursing care frustrating. Parents feel anxious and helpless enough in the NICU without being accused of not doing what is best for their babies. I would love to see the staff coordinate their efforts better by being more consistent with teaching or cut down on the confusion by instituting primary care nursing whenever possible."

"My NICU experience was very positive, but also very scary," said Jackie, a Wisconsin mom who turned thirty-eight years old two days after delivering her 4-pound-11-ounce son at thirty-three weeks because of a bout with premature rupture of membranes at twenty-four weeks that miraculously sealed over. Her little boy was breathing on his own, owing in part to the betamethasone shots his mother had received. "I felt like I was holding my breath the whole time. The doctors had said the first twenty-four hours would be the most important."

If you're like most parents of preemies, you probably consider the NICU a mixed blessing. It offers your baby the best possible care and the greatest opportunity for a healthy outcome, and your rational side probably appreciates that. Yet in order to serve its function, it requires that you endure days and nights that the parenting magazines probably never told you about: Strict sanitary protocols and visitor policies that can make you feel like a stranger in your baby's own "home." Equipment and procedures that limit your freedom to touch and hold your baby. Midnight pilgrimages to replenish your baby's supply of breast milk. Unsettling images of your infant hooked up to machines and connected to tubes. Medical personnel who are so good at what they do, who take such conscientious, expert care of their little charges, that you may feel unneeded or even like a trespasser in this precisely calibrated and meticulously controlled high-tech world.

People can say the wrong thing. Even nurses and doctors, who are specially trained not just to care for premature infants, but to counsel parents, too, have their bad days. "My husband tried to get involved by helping to change a diaper," Kerry said. "Tyler was in an incubator, and Ron was holding the diaper, fanning Tyler with it, trying to dry off his wet little body. A nurse saw this and came over and said this was just 'out of line.' It would cause the baby to get cold, cause his temperature to drop. She said that was a really mean thing to do."

To become upset in situations like these is entirely normal. It's the way any loving parent would respond when faced with the thought that he or she was hurting their child, that someone else knew best when it came to deciding what the baby needed. Even for the most confident among us, the transition to life in the NICU can be a humbling time.

A few days into her premature son's NICU stay, Kerry went to her preemie support group meeting that night, a gathering comprising parents and health care professionals alike, and burst into tears. "How do you make it through this?" she asked them. The responses she got to such a raw, emotional question were telling to her. "The social worker didn't say anything. The family care coordinator didn't say anything. Finally, one of the other parents said quietly, 'We've been here six weeks. It gets easier. You just keep going. Take pictures. Be here as often as you can. Just keep going.' " Kerry said that for the rest of that night the parents did almost all of the talking. Sometimes it takes the empathy of someone who's "been there" to help you through a tough time.

Some of the women we have spoken with have described the almost unimaginable stress that can be caused by having your life transferred to an intensive care ward. "I would go in every day to see the baby," said Wendy, whose son was born at thirty weeks as a result of preeclampsia and premature rupture of membranes. "I was there by myself most of the time. My husband

JOE GARCIA-PRATS: "In the NICU, you're already scared when you see your baby for the first time. Fear of the unknown is hard to shake. Some parents think that those little pads on their baby's skin are attached with needles or stitches. (Of course, they're just pasted to the skin.) Alarms are going off, the baby is surrounded by all these medical accoutrements, and parents are usually totally surprised. Most people don't get the time to visit the NICU before their child is admitted there. Usually it's 'Boom—you've got PIH. You're in the hospital. You're on magnesium sulfate.' So you don't have the time to prepare. By my experience, in maybe 10 to 20 percent of cases we have the luxury of time, and a preadmission visit is a good idea. But whether that's possible or not, I always try to tell mom and dad, 'Here's what you're going to see in the NICU.' I try to paint a picture prior to coming in. It makes everything easier when a parent can focus on the baby instead of the equipment."

would be working in Toronto, so I had to keep my other son at the Ronald McDonald House. This was stressful for an eighteen-month-old. He actually had an accident one day. He fell out of a high chair and fractured his skull. My husband, having heard this news, had an anxiety attack. At the emergency room, they thought it was a heart attack. So here I was, in the hospital with my son in the special care nursery, my other son seeing a pediatrician with a fractured skull, and my husband in an emergency room being looked at for a possible coronary. I almost collapsed in the nursery when I got that call saying he was having a heart attack."

Eventually your appreciation of the NICU will grow and your anxiety will diminish. You will become more comfortable with the unit's rhythms and procedures. The ritual of scrubbing in with an antibacterial sponge prior to handling your baby may contribute to your own sense of the discipline that parenting requires in any setting. The high standard of cleanliness that governs every aspect of an NICU's program of care may help you in maintaining a sanitary environment throughout your baby's early years.

How Premature Is Your Baby?: "It's no red badge of courage"

Leslie is a thirty-four-year-old mother of two from Queens, New York. Her first pregnancy was a complication-free full-term delivery. Her second one was high-risk from the start, the result of placental abruption. She now volunteers for Sidelines.com, an on-line organization that supports women in high-risk pregnancies with e-mail correspondence and chat rooms. Leslie said, "Nobody should think that they have a red badge of courage because their baby was in the NICU for nine weeks and someone else's was in for only six days. Any NICU stay is a major life event for that family and shouldn't be treated with any less significance. It's their baby, and it shouldn't matter if their baby is in for two months or two days."

Believe it or not, you may eventually become so comfortable with life in the NICU that the thought of taking your baby home may become tinged with anxiety and fear. Your feelings about the NICU may have moved from "How will I live with this?" to "How will I live *without* it?" We will discuss those issues in chapter 9, "Bringing Your Preemie Home." For now we would like to acquaint you with the technology, procedures, and personnel of the NICU, to help you gain some perspective on just what this tremendous resource means for you and your baby.

Recognizing that it is impossible to prepare you fully for your experience in the NICU, we offer in the pages that follow a description of the equipment and personnel you will meet there. It can be comforting to become even passingly familiar with the equipment and its uses, with procedures and how they will benefit your baby (or babies), and with the people who implement the continuing medical breakthroughs in neonatal medicine. In the next chapter we'll give you more of a sense of the individual procedures your baby might need and a general timeline for treatment depending on his or her stage of prematurity. You'll also hear from the most qualified experts around on the "NICU experience": veteran parents who have been there. The best advice often comes from those who have walked a mile in your shoes.

GESTATIONAL AGE: YOUR BABY'S HEALTH BAROMETER

Both the length of your baby's stay in the special care nursery and the extent of care he will require there will be substantially determined by his gestational age. This one number (which may range from twenty-four weeks on the early

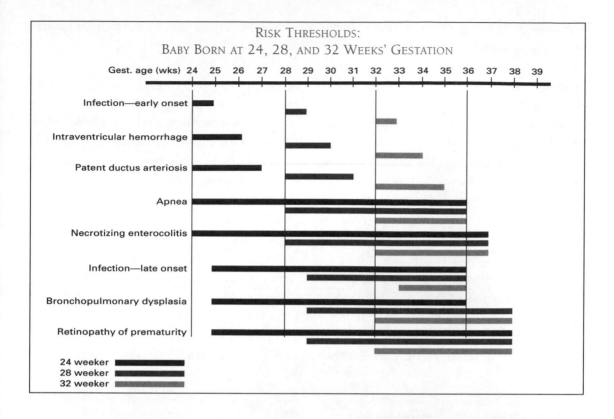

Risk Thresholds:
Baby Born at 24, 28, and 32 Weeks' Gestation

| Gest. age (wks) | 24 | 25 | 26 | 27 | 28 | 29 | 30 | 31 | 32 | 33 | 34 | 35 | 36 | 37 | 38 | 39 |

Infection—early onset
Intraventricular hemorrhage
Patent ductus arteriosis
Apnea
Necrotizing enterocolitis
Infection—late onset
Bronchopulmonary dysplasia
Retinopathy of prematurity

24 weeker
28 weeker
32 weeker

side of survivability to thirty-seven weeks at the edge of full-term) is the single most useful predictor of your baby's health and medical needs. We can't stress it enough: The longer you are able to keep your baby in a healthy womb, the better the chances of a healthy outcome will be.

The following chart gives you a visual picture of this reality. The chart graphically depicts the "risk thresholds" faced by babies of different gestational ages for eight of the most common medical complications associated with prematurity. The three sets of bars on the chart—black, gray, and white, show the periods during which preemies born at twenty-four weeks, twenty-eight weeks, and thirty-two weeks are generally exposed to risk for a certain condition. The degree of risk is highest during the earlier weeks and decreases with time, as the bars extend to the right.

However, as with any attempt to create an all-encompassing picture, it is important to note that there will be exceptions to the general trends shown on this chart, on both ends of the spectrum. Though the chart shows that the risk of a twenty-eight-weeker developing necrotizing enterocolitis ends at 37 weeks, it is possible owing to varying circumstances that this condition could manifest itself later than that. (This chart and the eight medical conditions it illustrates are discussed in greater detail in chapter 7, "Special Concerns in the NICU.")

There is simply so much variability in the health status of individual preemies of a certain gestational age at birth that attempting to forecast the future on the basis of this chart, or trying to design a program of care based on it, is not practical. A thirty-week preemie who has significant respiratory difficulty due to immature lungs will tend to fare worse than a twenty-eight-weeker whose mother received prior to delivery, two doses of betamethasone, which hastens lung maturation.

At the end of the day, we intend to use the risk thresholds chart only to illustrate a simple but essential proposition: The longer your child is able to spend in utero, the less her exposure to any number of potentially serious threats to her health. If you are still on bed rest while you are reading this chapter, use it for motivation to combat the dreadful boredom. If you have delivered already, the chart will give a rough estimation of the length of time your baby will be at risk for the conditions illustrated on it. Please know, however, that only your baby's neonatologist will have developed a truly accurate picture of the degree of risk faced by your particular child.

THE NICU'S EQUIPMENT

As the aforementioned risk thresholds chart shows, during the first twenty-four hours of your infant's life, he is exposed to the full range of possible conditions as a result of his prematurity. Most special care nurseries at major hospitals will have a broad assortment of special equipment to support your premature infant through these early days and weeks. The majority of this equipment is designed to be non-invasive and painless to your child and provide him as much comfort as possible.

Though the equipment is impressive looking with its many lights and monitors and

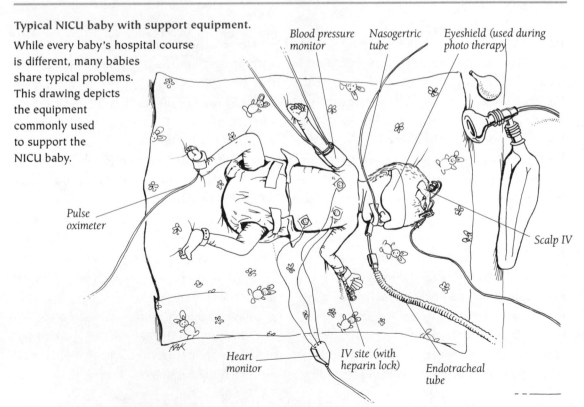

Typical NICU baby with support equipment.

While every baby's hospital course is different, many babies share typical problems. This drawing depicts the equipment commonly used to support the NICU baby.

Blood pressure monitor

Nasogertric tube

Eyeshield (used during photo therapy)

Pulse oximeter

Scalp IV

Heart monitor

IV site (with heparin lock)

Endotracheal tube

alarms, the most valuable asset in the NICU is the skill of the professionals who operate it. The skill and compassion of the doctors, nurses, technicians, therapists, and aides dedicated to neonatal special care work tend to be extraordinarily high, and their humanity tends to make the experience of being surrounded by all this high-tech paraphernalia much easier to endure.

🌿 Monitors

You may eventually find something vaguely hypnotic and comforting about watching a precisely calibrated readout of your infant's vital signs flow across a little bedside screen. You might see it as your only sure proof that your baby really is okay. As your baby gets ready for discharge, however, it is important to "wean" yourself off the monitor, to focus your attention on your infant and become familiar with her normal breathing pattern, coloration, and overall health profile without high-technology assistance.

Of course, monitors need to be properly attached to your baby to give you a correct reading. Additionally, as all medical professionals know, the medical technology at our fingertips today is wonderful in aiding in the care of patients, but the hands-on visual and physical assessments by their human caregivers will never be replaced.

CARDIORESPIRATORY MONITOR. This machine (also known as a *heart monitor* or a *C-R monitor*) keeps continuous track of your baby's heart rate and rhythm, and respiration rate and pattern, in a noninvasive, painless way. The information flows from adhesive patches attached to your baby's chest or stomach and is displayed on a small screen right at the bedside. Many machines are able to capture a history of your baby's readouts for the nursing and medical staff to evaluate later on if necessary. Of the two readouts—respiratory and cardiac—the far less reliable one is the respiratory. The accuracy of the reading depends greatly on the placement of the adhesive patches. As your baby moves about, the patches can shift or detach and you may notice sudden fluctuations in the respiration monitor or the sounding of an alarm. Unsettling as they are, these fluctuations most often are picking up artifacts that are not indicative of your baby's health status. (Check with the nursing staff if you need reassurance.) Though you shouldn't get overly alarmed about these sudden changes, it is important to have your baby physically reassessed and replace any leads or patches that are detached or tangled. The heart rate is tracked much more reliably than respiration, but these monitor patches too should be checked occasionally for correct placement so that they can accurately portray your baby's heart rhythm.

PULSE OXIMETER. Known as a "pulse ox" in the lingo of the NICU, this machine continuously monitors your infant's blood oxygen saturation. It is a noninvasive, painless device. It is sometimes a stand-alone unit and other times will be integrated with the C-R monitor (see previous). Using a small sensor light that is taped to your baby's toe, foot, finger, or palm— any place where the sensor can get an accurate reading of your baby's pulse—this machine displays the amount of oxygen being carried by your baby's red blood cells. This machine monitors the color changes that take place in the blood as its oxygen content changes. It is therefore an important element in managing your baby's respiratory health.

APNEA MONITOR. Apnea is a temporary pause in breathing that lasts longer than fifteen seconds and is accompanied by a drop in pulse rate and a decrease in the baby's oxygen saturation level. It is common in preemies, given their immature respiratory systems. This monitor flags any pause in breathing that lasts longer than fifteen seconds and is accompanied by a pulse rate drop—a sign that the baby's respiratory control center isn't fully mature yet or possibly that the baby has an obstructed airway. NICUs often have a rule that in order to be discharged, a baby must go seven days without a spell of apnea accompanied by a pulse rate drop. In that sense, you may view this monitor as your worst enemy—with but one sounding of its alarm, it can keep your baby from a long-awaited homecoming. Depending on your baby's respiratory health and maturity, your neonatologist may decide that you need to take one of these monitors home with you and keep it attached to your baby until his breathing stabilizes. Bringing the equipment home represents a major commitment on the part of parents, because its operation requires special training and constant attention. You won't be running off to the store while the neighbor watches your baby if you have one of these machines at home. (See chapter 9, "Bringing Your Preemie Home.")

TRANSCUTANEOUS OXYGEN AND CARBON DIOXIDE SENSOR. This is a small sensor that's placed on your baby's skin for the purpose of measuring oxygen and carbon dioxide in the blood. This machine is useful to your baby's physician in monitoring trends in these important blood gases. However, it may not be completely accurate. The sensor must be moved every four hours, or it may burn the skin. (It's common to find a small "sunburned" spot on your baby's skin where this sensor was placed.) Use of this device may reduce the number of blood gas assessments needed to manage your baby's lung problems.

TEMPERATURE PROBE. Because a stable body temperature is of paramount importance to your preemie, a noninvasive probe will be connected to a thermostat in the warmer or incubator and attached to your baby's skin with an adhesive strip to measure his temperature and thus determine how much warmth he will need from the incubator/warmer. It is also quite common for your infant's temperature to be checked with an ordinary mercury thermometer or electronic thermometer under the armpit (axillary) or (rarely) rectally. During routine NICU care, your newborn's temperature will be taken at least every eight hours and charted in his medical records. Once you are a veteran NICU parent, you will be quite accustomed to taking your baby's temperature yourself.

BLOOD PRESSURE MONITOR. Your baby's blood pressure will be routinely measured with a noninvasive, painless miniature blood pressure cuff fit around her arm or leg (or by an arterial catheter—see page 135). This is like a smaller version of a standard adult blood pressure cuff that you may be familiar with from your corner drugstore.

Other Equipment

INTRAVENOUS (IV) LINES. The IV is an efficient way for your baby to receive necessary medication, fluids, sugar, and other vital nutrients. The placement of an IV can be temporarily uncomfortable for your baby when the needle or special plastic catheter is first introduced.

The IV needle or a special plastic catheter will be inserted into your infant's vein, thus creating an easily accessible means for giving your baby fluids. The placement of the IV line can be disconcerting—it is quite common to place an IV in a premature infant's scalp, where the veins are more prominent and where your baby will be less likely to pull it out. A small patch of hair may need to be shaved (it will grow back) to make way for the IV. The hands and feet are also common places to insert an IV, but the IV may not last as long there. The NICU staff will frequently evaluate the IV lines for proper functioning. The insertion of an intravenous line is often an uncomfortable procedure for your baby, and you may be asked to leave the NICU while it is being performed. Don't take this personally, but it often goes more smoothly for all concerned when these types of procedures are performed without parents looking over the shoulders of the medical and nursing staff.

There are two basic types of IVs. One is a *superficial IV*, where the needle or catheter is inserted into a superficial vein near the surface of the skin. Because these smaller veins are so delicate, they cannot handle high concentrations of nutrients, medications, or sugar. Superficial IV lines usually last only two to four days and thus require frequent replacement. After your baby is finished with a round of intravenous medication, a *heparin lock* may be left in your baby's arm. This is a port that enables an infusion of fluids or of medication to be quickly reestablished if needed. If your preemie needs higher concentrations of nutrients, sugar, or medications over a period of several weeks, a

FAQ:
"Will any of this hurt my baby?"

JOE GARCIA-PRATS: "Preemies, like all babies, are fully able to feel pain. As caregivers, we are faced with the dilemma that many of the necessary things we do to help an infant also cause pain and discomfort. We try to minimize it whenever possible. Indeed it is our responsibility to comfort our patients when they feel pain. The trend in neonatal care has been to use increasing amounts of pain medication in any potentially painful procedure. This decision to use pain medication is not taken lightly because its use can have complications. It may lower blood pressure, slow bowel movements, and suppress the respiratory center. Thus most doctors and nurses will be conservative in their use of pain medication, watching out for the baby's comfort while performing necessary medical procedures."

second type of IV called a *central line* may be inserted. A central line is a thin intravenous tube made of special materials that is placed directly into one of the large veins in the scalp, neck, leg, or arm. In order to dilute the high concentration of medication or nutrients, the tip of the catheter is placed as close as possible to the baby's heart, where rapid mixing with the blood occurs. Since the catheter reaches deeply into your baby's body, this type of IV involves a greater degree of risk of infection (about 10 percent), and blood clots and must be monitored closely.

UMBILICAL ARTERY AND VEIN CATHETERS. Although an IV line is a convenient way to give your baby nutrients, medications, and fluids—including blood—it cannot be used to draw blood or monitor blood pressure. For that purpose, in the first day or two of life an umbilical catheter can be inserted via the umbilical artery into the aorta. The placement of a catheter in the umbilical vein allows for the infusion of multiple types of solutions simultaneously, since these catheters can have two or three ports (channels). In this way your baby can receive antibiotics, blood transfusions, and insulin solutions at the same time. However, both these catheters have an important limitation: they can increase the risk of infection and blood clots. Umbilical vein catheters are usually left in for one week before that risk becomes significant. Umbilical arterial catheters can be left in slightly longer before infection becomes an issue. In critically ill infants, however, it may be the decision of the neonatologist to leave both catheters in longer since in such cases the risk involved in the removal of these lines is often greater than the risk involved in keeping them in place. Other less frequent complications of catheters include the formation of large blood clots in the blood vessels in which they are placed as well as perforation of the blood vessel.

BILIRUBIN LIGHT. Bilirubin is a yellow pigment in the bloodstream created by the natural breakdown and recycling of red blood cells. Your baby's immature liver may not be ready to efficiently dispose of bilirubin. This can lead to potentially serious complications. A sign of the buildup of bilirubin in your baby's bloodstream is a yellowish tinge to your baby's skin. Fortunately *phototherapy*—light therapy—is a proven way to reduce the level of bilirubin in the blood. It involves nothing more than shining a special blue or green fluorescent lamp on the baby. The light chemically alters the bilirubin in the blood so that it can be more easily eliminated from the blood without taxing the liver. These *bili-lights* are quite effective at preventing the consequences of *hyperbilirubinemia,* an excess of bilirubin, which in its most severe form (called *kernicterus*) may cause mental retardation, cerebral palsy, or hearing loss. When the bilirubin light is on, it will be necessary for your child to wear eye coverings that will protect her delicate eyes from the intense light.

MECHANICAL RESPIRATOR (VENTILATOR). Premature infants' lungs may not function properly as a result of infection or immaturity. Preemies may be unable to maintain adequate oxygen levels in the blood. Or they may accumulate excessive concentrations of carbon dioxide in the blood. Thus it may be temporarily necessary to use mechanical respiration (also called *ventilation*) to assist in your baby's breathing. An endotracheal tube will be placed in your baby's trachea through his mouth, allowing the respirator to transport air or an oxygen mixture directly into the lungs. Some respirators require a small circular patch called a *synchronizer* to be attached to your baby's abdomen. It senses when your baby starts to take a breath so that the respirator's timing can be synchronized with your baby's inhalations. Other ventilators have this sensing device as part of the tubing of the respirator. Assisted ventilation may help your baby to better tolerate the rigors of mechanical respiration. On this type of equipment, pressure level and rate of respiration can be set to match your baby's unique needs.

NASAL PRONGS. Even after your baby's respiration has stabilized to the point that she no longer needs artificial ventilation, sometimes the infant's blood oxygen level will remain a concern due to very soft ribs and/or very weak muscles in the throat (*hypopharynx*) that may allow the upper airway to collapse. In that instance, small tubes may be placed just inside her nostrils to deliver an oxygen mixture at a constant pressure. A technique called *nasal continuous positive airway pressure* (NCPAP) keeps the air at a steady pressure in the back of the throat and thus keeps this portion of the upper airway (deep throat) from collapsing. This technique also stabilizes the flexible rib cage.

MEETING THE SPECIAL CARE NURSERY STAFF

The modern neonatal special care nursery features an assortment of professional medical personnel to care for your preemie. So that you can have a better idea of who is responsible for what, in this section we provide brief descriptions of their roles.

THE NEONATOLOGIST. Your baby's primary caregiver in the NICU will be his or her admitting neonatologist. The discipline of neonatology did not exist until the American Board of Pediatrics recognized it in 1975 as a result of the rapid advances being made in the care of newborns and the special training it required to oversee not only specialized procedures, but also a new array of medical equipment. The training regimen for neonatologists is intensive: four years of medical school followed by three years in pediatric residency and then three more years' training in neonatol-

ogy. A rigorous examination is the final step. Together with their neonatology team, including the neonatal staff nurses, neonatologists will have the most contact with your child and be primarily responsible for reporting your baby's daily progress to you.

THE NEONATOLOGY FELLOW. Neonatology fellows are pediatricians who are in the final stages of their training to become neonatologists. Though they have responsibilities for teaching, research, and supervision, fellows typically spend the bulk of their time in the NICU caring for their tiny patients. A neonatology fellow usually spends three years in concentrated, specialized study of intensive care for newborns.

THE RESIDENT OR INTERN. An intern is a doctor in the first year of specialized training. A resident is in the second or third year. As part of their pediatric curriculum, pediatric residents or interns must spend a one- or two-month rotation in the neonatal intensive care unit.

THE PHYSICIAN'S ASSISTANT. This is a graduate of either a bachelor's or master's degree program who has specialized training in neonatology or pediatrics and who may provide certain elements of your baby's medical care under the guidelines determined by the physician.

THE NEONATAL NURSE PRACTITIONER. This is a registered nurse who has received additional neonatal training through a master's degree program and who is thereby qualified to provide elements of the baby's medical care that were once the exclusive domain of a physician. The nurse practitioner may perform certain procedures and write orders under delineated guidelines decided upon by the medical staff.

THE REGISTERED NURSE (RN). An RN is a nurse who has graduated from an accredited school of nursing after two to four years of study and who has passed a state board examination licensing her or him to practice nursing in that state. The specially trained RNs in the neonatal intensive care unit are responsible for a major portion of the care given to the babies in the unit. They perform a wide variety of procedures for your child twenty-four hours a day. Of all the personnel in the NICU, you will in all likelihood come to know the staff nurses best. As the caregivers closest to your baby's daily life, they are often active advocates for the special needs of their charges. You may be surprised at the close bond that can develop between parents and nurses.

THE CLINICAL NURSE SPECIALIST. This is an RN who has received additional neonatal training in patient and nurse education.

THE NURSE'S ASSISTANT. With special training, nurse assistants help the staff nurses and are responsible for much of the basic yet very important care for your child, including monitoring daily vital signs, tracking weight, changing dressings, diapering, and feeding. Their role is especially prominent in the "step-down" unit (see chapter 8), which is where your baby may go after he or she no longer requires the critical care of the NICU.

THE RESPIRATORY THERAPIST. This specialist is primarily responsible for setting up, calibrating, and maintaining the respiratory equipment in the NICU in accordance with the instructions of your baby's doctor. Respiratory therapists play the crucial role of ensuring that the physician's instructions as to breathing rate, oxygen content, air pressure, and humidity are properly implemented on the respiratory support equipment. They also have the responsibility of recording your baby's data on a chart for review by the physician. Respiratory therapists may also perform arterial blood draws, suctioning, and other procedures under a doctor's supervision.

THE SOCIAL WORKER. Social workers may be available to consult with you on nonmedical aspects of your baby's care, including insurance coverage, transportation, lifestyle issues after discharge, and emotional support and counseling. They can be excellent resources due to their knowledge of the inner workings of the health care system.

THE AUDIOLOGIST. Audiologists specialize in the evaluation and treatment of hearing problems. They may perform hearing tests on your baby. They work under the supervision of an otolaryngologist, a physician specializing in the ear, nose, and throat.

THE LACTATION CONSULTANT. Lactation consultants assist new mothers with difficulties associated with breast-feeding.

THE VOLUNTEER. Some hospitals have community service programs that allow volunteers (often senior citizens) to assist in some aspects of hospital care. They can offer valuable extra personal attention to NICU families and will often be found changing, swaddling, holding, and rocking the babies. They take their responsibilities seriously and are a significant part of the neonatal team.

PHYSICIAN SPECIALISTS. If your baby has a particular problem, your neonatologist may choose to call in a doctor with further specialized training. Common subspecialists include

- *cardiologist*—heart specialist
- *pulmonologist*—lung specialist
- *endocrinologist*—glands and hormone specialist
- *gastroenterologist*—intestine, liver, and nutrition specialist
- *hematologist*—blood specialist
- *nephrologist*—kidney specialist
- *neurologist*—brain and nervous system specialist
- *orthopedist*—skeletal, joint, and muscle specialist
- *ophthalmologist*—eye specialist

In the event that surgery is necessary, a surgeon and an anesthesiologist (preferably one with pediatric training) may be called in to assist as well.

Other Things to Take Care of When Your Baby Is Transferred to the NICU

TAKE A DEEP BREATH—THEN TAKE CARE OF YOURSELF

The first twenty-four to seventy-two hours after the birth of a premature baby can be an overwhelming experience. Childbirth is exhausting.

SHARON HORNFISCHER: "The day after my son's evening birth, my husband was out taking care of some details, and my mother, who was visiting, helped me get dressed and wheeled me into the NICU to see my baby. It was good to see him up close for the first time. Once there, I recognized he was being very well cared for. The neonatal nurses, who are usually briefed on the mother's postpartum condition, knew about my preeclampsia and continuing postdelivery problems with labile blood pressure, vision disturbances, and overall pain and fatigue from my surgical delivery. I recall a nurse saying to me, 'Your son is in good hands, but remember: You're also still a patient. If you don't take care of yourself, you're not going to be able to take care of your baby.'

"It didn't take long to get their message. I decided to follow the doctor's and nurses' advice and try to get myself healthy before spending every spare moment in the NICU. I simply wasn't ready to be Supermom. There was plenty of time for that later."

Becoming parents, especially if it's your first time, is a major life passage. Now you're being asked to face the prospect of coping with a preemie and navigating the foreign, high-tech terrain of the special care nursery. It's easy to lose sight of your own needs in this situation. But taking care of yourself is essential if you want to take the best care of your baby.

Mothers who have just completed a high-risk delivery should continue taking their pain medication and catch up on their sleep. Caring for yourself is the most important preparation you can take at this stage.

REMEMBER THAT YOU ARE A PATIENT

If you have been on extended bed rest, it may take you some time to recover due to the loss of muscle tone and reduced cardiovascular fitness you have undergone during this period of inactivity. You may have difficulty walking, or you may experience dizziness, fatigue, depression, and other symptoms. Full recovery will be a slow, steady process before you can return to the active life you led before you got pregnant.

Allow yourself a certain period of time to heal, both physically and mentally. If it is medically advisable, physical therapy may provide a structured way for you to regain your strength. Ask your physician whether he might refer you to a physical therapist. (A referral from your physician might make your insurance company more willing to pay this expense.) While you're recovering, you might want to use a wheelchair to navigate the hospital corridors if your baby is in the NICU. That way you can conserve your strength and won't arrive too exhausted to enjoy your visit. Your mental health may be helped by taking advantage of a support group or enjoying the company of friends or family.

Cori remembered the flood of emotions from frustration to anger during her postpartum recovery period. "During the first few days of my son's life, I was still bedridden and wasn't able to go up to the NICU and see him. I vaguely remember being furious with my mother and stepfather because they could go and see Bo as much as they wanted, while I had to lie in bed and wait for their reports. I felt as if they knew more about my son than I did. I resented their visits with Bo. Eventually we worked it out, but there were some very deep feelings those first few days. I wanted to see for myself that Bo was doing okay, but all I had was their word. Finally, on the second or third day I was able to go up and see him. What a relief! I could see with my own eyes how my precious, tiny baby was doing."

HIGH-RISK MOTHER: MANAGING AFTER BIRTH

If your baby's prematurity was due to any kind of health problem that also affected you, you may need to continue to be closely medically managed. This may require continued hospitalization. Sometimes mom's health is so fragile that she becomes the one who needs intensive care. If that's the case for you, you'll be fighting two battles: one to get your health back to where it was and another to come to terms with your baby's being under the care of the special care nursery. Even if you're comfortable with that intellectually, emotionally it can take a toll. Get rest while you can. Remember that no matter what your post-operative situation is, you have been through a high-risk pregnancy. You need to focus on getting yourself well again.

The following high-risk conditions can persist well after your baby has been delivered.

HYPERTENSION. Though the cure for pregnancy-induced hypertension often comes with the delivery of the baby, PIH can persist long after delivery, for days, weeks, and even months. Sometimes PIH can even lead to chronic high blood pressure. In any event, your blood pressure must be stabilized before you can be safely discharged. If you have persistent hypertension, you may be able to be treated in a regular hospital room. Rest, diet, and oral antihypertensive medications such as Procardia or Zestril are the main tools for managing hypertension.

If you were a chronic hypertensive before your pregnancy began, it may take a while to stabilize you and return you to your prepregnancy equilibrium.

Owing to PIH, Gini spent forty-eight hours in the hospital following delivery of her daughter at thirty-one weeks. She believes she should have been there longer. "I was not ready to go home. I was so sore and so unstable, I was surprised they were going to let me go. Because my daughter was in the NICU, I was going to be going back and forth to the hospital regularly. Another two days in the hospital getting my blood pressure under control could really have made a difference in terms of getting back on my feet again. When I got out it took me a while to get my vision back. I couldn't really drive. I was too sore even to sit in the car, really. I would definitely push for another day in the hospital if I had to do it over again."

ECLAMPSIA (SEIZURES). If you are a severe hypertensive, have already experienced seizure activity, or are thought to have a low seizure threshold and are close to being eclamptic (having seizures), you will need to be closely managed in an intensive care unit after delivery. You will need to be observed for at least forty-eight to seventy-two hours postpartum or until the physicians feel the risk of seizure activity or other complications has passed.

✒ FAQ:
"When will my blood pressure go back to normal?"

For most women with PIH, blood pressure will stabilize within hours of delivery. Delivery is the only cure for PIH. However, it doesn't always work. For other new mothers with elevated blood pressure, it may take weeks or even months for blood pressure to return to normal prepregnancy levels. And some women, luckily only a minority, will develop chronic hypertension. Women who remain hypertensive after delivery will continue to need medical management by their physician. This can include a restricted diet, carefully monitored exercise, and antihypertensive medications.

Management of eclampsia involves seizure precautions, which can include close observation, safety precautions such as padded bed rails and elevated rails at all times, full bed rest with no bathroom privileges (or at least assistance with these activities), heart monitoring, oxygen administration, a heparin lock IV site to offer a quick route for medication if needed, and IV lines for administration of magnesium sulfate or other medications necessary to stabilize your blood pressure and help lower your seizure threshold. The risk for seizures and preeclampsia, though normally cured by delivery, can continue for several days postpartum.

Cheryl was thirty-five when she was pregnant with her first baby. She fought high blood pressure for the last eight weeks of her preg-

HELLP Syndrome

Severe cases of preeclampsia can combine with other conditions to bring on HELLP syndrome. The name of this potentially very serious condition derives from its diagnostic elements: *h*emolyic anemia (characterized by breakdown of red blood cells), *e*levated *l*iver transminases (liver compromise or failure), and *l*ow *p*latelet count (inability of the blood to clot).

Normally, delivery of the baby is the "cure" for HELLP syndrome. However, as with some rare cases of preeclampsia, HELLP can persist after delivery, requiring continued hospitalization of the mother to be sure the blood pressure returns to manageable levels.

For more information, see p. 27.

nancy. When her blood pressure hit 200/110, she was admitted with a diagnosis of severe PIH. On the night before she delivered, she was feeling awful. "I was anxious, irritable, and showing significant swelling in the extremities. When he was assessing me, the resident pressed down on my liver to check its size. I screamed in pain. The doctor told me that if I didn't deliver, and fast, my health could be in grave danger." She was induced the next day, delivering her 4-pound-4-ounce preemie daughter at thirty-five weeks. "I didn't see her for three days. It was upsetting. I had this all planned out. I had waited years for this baby.

"I wanted to see this baby so bad. When the nurse asked me if I was having headaches, I knew that answering truthfully with a 'Yes' would mean a further delay in seeing my daughter. I said that I wasn't having any headaches. At this point I was allowed to go to the NICU in a wheelchair. I had barely gotten to my baby's bedside when I began to feel worse. It's sort of a blur, but I remember that I couldn't breathe. I was hyperventilating. I couldn't move my arms, couldn't talk, but my eyes were open. I vaguely remember hearing the nurse say, 'Oh, my God . . . code blue!' and I remember seeing her push the panic button. The next thing I knew I'm waking up in the intensive care unit, and the doctor is telling me that I had had a seizure."

Cheryl spent the next few days recovering in the NICU. Her story is an effective reminder of the importance of following your doctor's orders.

DIABETES. Gestational diabetes usually resolves with the delivery of the placenta. This causes blood sugars to normalize almost immediately, in most cases. However, a women with chronic diabetes will need to have her blood sugar tested and adjusted and her prepregnancy diabetes management resumed. This can consist of diet, oral medication, or insulin administration.

Kelly was twenty-seven when she became pregnant with her first child, a thirty-week preemie. At twenty-eight weeks she badly flunked her glucose tolerance test. "When your doctor calls you at home on a Sunday night and tells you to come in, you know something's really not right," she said. Her blood sugar was so elevated that her doctor immediately placed her on insulin. To control her blood sugar, she had to take two insulin shots a day. She was also placed on a diabetic diet. Upon admission to the hospital, she was placed on an intravenous insulin drip, providing her with a steady flow of insulin. Her baby looked great on ultrasound, but her blood pressure was 160/110.

Immediately after delivering her 3-pound-15-ounce boy, the IV insulin was stopped, since blood sugar problems typically resolve after the baby and placenta are delivered. Kelly remembers the joy of returning to a regular diet during her four-day stay in the hospital after delivery. "They gave me a Rice Krispies treat with chocolate chips. I was so excited to see those chocolate chips. I wanted to savor each and every one of them." After the pregnancy, her sugar continued to remain slightly elevated, but she was able to control it with diet and exercise, which included—on the advice of her doctor—walking several times a week and continuing to practice tae kwon do exercises.

INTRAUTERINE BLEEDING. Conditions that cause excessive bleeding such as placental abruptions, uterine rupture, and various forms of placenta previa can lead to serious postdelivery concerns for a woman's health. These conditions can cause a woman to lose moderate to large volumes of blood, leaving her weak, dehydrated, hypotensive (low blood pressure), and anemic. In its most serious form, large sudden blood loss can lead to shock and even death if not treated promptly and aggressively.

Management of bleeding requires nothing less than stopping the bleeding (which can be a challenge because of the intensively vascular nature of the uterus) and replenishing fluid volume. When immediate fluid replacement is necessary, the physician will estimate the amount of blood loss to determine the amount of blood product or fluid replenishment needed. Additionally, a laboratory test known as a *complete blood count,* or *CBC,* will be performed on your blood sample to determine more accurately just how anemic you are. Using this lab result, your doctor can normalize your fluid volume by administering the right number of blood transfusions. Sometimes these transfusions take place in the delivery room. In other cases they will be given once you have been transferred to your postpartum room.

As your doctor continues your postpartum management, your blood counts will be taken frequently, you will remain on IV hydration, and your diet will be high in iron. In addition, you may be placed on iron supplements.

HYSTERECTOMY. A *hysterectomy* is the surgical removal of the uterus. In their most severe forms, many of the previously discussed bleeding tendencies can lead to emergency hysterectomies. This is usually the case where the woman is in danger of losing her life because of the rapid and extremely large volume of blood loss. As we mentioned earlier, it can be difficult to stop uterine bleeding owing to the uterus's large number of blood vessels, which help maintain a pregnancy and give a fetus the nutrients needed to sustain a baby's life. However, this can in turn endanger or take a mother's life when uncontrolled bleeding occurs.

With all cesarean deliveries, full-term and preemie alike, you will be given a surgical informed consent document to sign that informs you of the risk of any complication, including hysterectomy and death. At the risk of generalization, we don't think many people today take this risk very seriously: "It won't happen to me." And granted, a decision of life or death is an easy one to make. Nonetheless, having an emergency hysterectomy can be extraordinarily difficult for a young woman or couple hoping to have other children. Emergency and emergent hysterectomies can be a mixed blessing. They save lives, but the loss of the potential to have more children can be a devastating experience for couples planning on having larger families. Once a woman has recovered physically, it might be necessary for the couple to work through the loss with professional guidance.

Kelly, the ER nurse, and her husband don't regret that a hysterectomy was necessary following her traumatic delivery brought on by a placental abruption. She has her own good health, plus two healthy sons, Aaron and Ryan, to show for it. Having gone through this difficult experience, Kelly was interviewing for positions in her hospital's obstetrics unit at the time we interviewed her.

CALL YOUR INSURANCE CARRIER

In the midst of delivering your baby, it might slip your mind that someone has to pay for all this. Insurance companies and managed care organizations have rather rigid guidelines for how long they will cover your hospitalization following delivery. It is usually necessary to prequalify for coverage. This requires contacting your carrier and informing them ahead of time of the procedure you are about to undergo. Advance, predelivery notification is often required

Designated-Donor Blood: Your Preemie's Own Blood Bank

Most hospitals today allow you to donate blood ahead of time in the event that your baby needs it. If you choose to become a designated or directed blood donor (your baby's neonatalogist may recommend it because of a particular health problem your baby has, or you may simply decide to do it as a precaution), you may be able to put compatible blood at ready access to your baby's physician in the event a transfusion becomes necessary. If you meet the screening requirements—blood of the right type and Rh factor (hospitals require additional screening for viruses such as CMV, HIV, and hepatitis)—your blood will be taken and stored for your baby. The blood requires processing that may take an additional twenty-four to forty-eight hours. Please be aware that in an emergency situation there may not be enough time to draw blood from a designated donor and have it ready for use on your baby. So be prepared for the possibility that not every transfusion given to your infant will come from a designated donor. It has also been shown that designated donor blood is not necessarily "safer" than that of the general population. The reason is that all of us are just as susceptible to viruses such as CMV or hepatitis as any family member.

for coverage of your health needs. Your OB may have to get involved in order to make sure any necessary treatment is covered by the policy.

Generally, in today's HMO-dominated, cost-conscious time, medical justification is required for a hospital stay lasting beyond what is traditionally allowed—forty-eight hours after a vaginal delivery and seventy-two hours after a cesarean delivery. For the mother who has had medical problems, such as PIH, that require further treatment *following* delivery, obtaining approval may not be difficult as long as your physician can prove to the HMO that hospitalization is medically necessary. Nonmedical reasons for a prolonged hospital stay—such as your wish to stay and bond with your infant—probably won't be approved. It is best to speak with your physician to get the details of coverage worked out. He will manage your recovery closely and will also assist you in making arrangements with your insurance provider to qualify you for an extended hospital stay if it is medically necessary.

Regarding your baby's hospitalization and care, most insurance companies or HMOs require you to contact them after your baby has been delivered in order to obtain approval. For them, the infant doesn't really exist until delivery has taken place. If you are hospitalized unexpectedly, realize that you or your spouse will need to contact your insurance carrier within a certain period of time, usually twenty-four hours. Your neonatologist and her office can provide you with the necessary backup to establish medical justification. Find out if your hospital can give you a social worker to assist you. And be sure to ask whether the hospital's billing office has any information or other valuable resources you can use.

> ### Tips and Reminders
>
> - Keep your insurance cards and policy numbers handy in your wallet or purse when you go into the hospital. It will speed all of the paperwork you'll be asked to fill out.
> - If your insurance requires it, be sure to prequalify your admission. Otherwise it may be a hassle to get these procedures paid for.
> - If you were admitted to the hospital on an emergency basis, your insurance company generally requires you to call them within a set time period after the admission. Don't forget to make that phone call or have your spouse do it.
> - Remember to add your baby to your insurance policy. Most companies give you several weeks following delivery to take care of this. Mark it off your list as soon as you can. Most insurance companies have rather strict guidelines for signing up a newborn for coverage. Call your employer's human resources department or your insurance company directly for instructions.

Preterm deliveries can be staggeringly expensive. The daily charge for a routine hospitalization runs as high as $1,000 per day in some metropolitan areas. Even a short, noncomplicated delivery or post-operative hospital stay can cost several thousand dollars. It is not uncommon for a full regime of neonatal intensive care to cost as much as $3,000 to $4,000 per day. A lot of money is at stake—thus the tight control by the insurance companies. Be sure to inform yourself about your carrier's requirements. Otherwise you could end up liable for a huge hospital bill.

If You Don't Have Insurance

If you don't have insurance coverage, the social worker at the hospital can assist you in locating social service agencies that offer financial aid for eligible new parents. Federal Medicaid, as well as county-administered assistance such as Aid to Families with Dependent Children (AFDC) and Women, Infants and Children (WIC) programs, may be available to you depending on your income and number of dependents. After you and your baby come home, you should contact your city or county clerk's office to find out whether home energy assis-

tance is available to pay for the utility consumption necessary to heat or cool your home in accordance with your baby's needs. Food stamps may be available depending on your income profile, and other governmental agencies may be able to assist you with home health services, nursing care, travel expenses, and other costs associated with your newborn. (See Appendix C for Internet resources and telephone numbers.)

Accommodating Visitors, Family, and Friends

Almost immediately after the delivery of your newborn, you're likely to have a rush of well-wishers at the hospital. They will arrive in your room with flowers, balloons, and candy. They will come alone and in groups. If you have a large family or a wide circle of friends, they may arrive with such regularity that you might feel you need a break from it all. Though you'll probably be glad to have such a show of support, you may also feel some guilt (there's always plenty of that to go around) if you feel understandably exhausted by your preemie ordeal and would just as well catch up on your sleep as invest your little remaining energy in a social visit. In the face of this rush of goodwill, it can be difficult to say enough is enough. But sometimes there's no other choice.

Your journey to this point—a long, trying pregnancy and the intense, exhausting twenty-four hours since the delivery of your baby—has probably taxed you beyond your ability to maintain social graces. If that is the case, loved ones should understand. Don't shy away from explaining to them what your needs are at the moment. After all, that's why they're there, to help take care of your needs. Immediately in the wake of a premature delivery, the best help can be no help at all. You may need a good old-fashioned three-hour nap, quiet time spent staring out the window, or time absorbing the rush of recent events with your spouse and any older children you may have. Your spouse may be the best one to deliver this message to visitors. Let him answer that knock at the hospital room door. Ask him to take visitors aside and say something along the following lines: "We really do appreciate your coming today, and your support means a lot to us right now. We would love to visit with you for a while. What my wife really needs now, though, is some time to decompress and rest and take everything in. She really needs a little quiet time. So if you could keep this visit to fifteen minutes or less, or come back in a few hours, or tomorrow, it

> ## FAQ:
> ### "How long will I stay in the hospital?"
>
> The length of your hospitalization will depend on your high-risk pregnancy condition, on the type of delivery you had, and on your overall postpartum health. Many conditions that lead to a high-risk pregnancy—for example, multiple births, incompetent cervix, and (usually) PIH—will be resolved by your baby's birth. Recovery from conditions such as chronic hypertension or uterine hemorrhage will probably require a longer hospitalization. In general today, a mother who had an uncomplicated vaginal delivery stays in the hospital for about forty-eight hours, or two days. A mother who has an uncomplicated cesarean delivery can expect to be admitted for seventy-two to ninety-six hours, or three to four days. These numbers vary somewhat but are generally used as hospital policy per insurance guidelines.

would help. You know that we'll be glad to make it up to you later on, when the baby's home and we're all feeling better."

LEAVING YOUR BABY BEHIND

At discharge from the hospital, Kelly remembers sitting in a wheelchair in the lobby, watching other mothers walk out the door with their full-term babies. "It was the hardest thing, watching them holding their babies and going home," she said. "I don't want to say that I was angry, but I felt cheated. I had a hard time with that."

Eventually—and you may have a hard time realizing this so soon after delivery—you will come to a place where the difficult challenges ahead of you take on a sense of larger meaning. We were touched by Kerrin's description of what her experience with preemiedom meant to her:

"I learned how precious children are. You can't take for granted having a baby. You see things on the news, and see people having all these children. You want to say, 'You don't know how lucky you are that nature came to-gether in just this way so you can have that child. You need to treat your child that way.'

"I hesitate to say that I love my daughter more than other people love their children. But I feel that because of what we went through, my love comes from a deep understanding of how special she really is. Women who get pregnant on the first try never really stop and think about what it really takes to get them there. Of course, just because someone got pregnant and delivered successfully the first time doesn't make her baby any less special. But it may mean she doesn't fully *realize* how special she is. I don't take my daughter for granted. She's my world."

5

YOUR PREEMIE'S GROWTH AND MATURATION

WHAT YOU'LL FIND IN THIS CHAPTER

- Very premature infants: twenty-four to twenty-eight weeks' gestation
- Premature infants: twenty-eight to thirty-two weeks' gestation
- Moderately premature infants: thirty-two to thirty-seven weeks' gestation

A premature baby is more or less characterized by his or her gestational age at birth. Mothers of preemies inevitably refer to their babies using that number. It's a sort of shorthand that anyone familiar with preemies and their needs can understand. It's a quick way of introducing yourself and what you've been through.

It's medically important as well. That single piece of information is one of the most important factors that predict the infant's potential overall health profile, his potential risks for developmental difficulties, and the potential extent of the baby's medical needs while in the NICU. A full-term baby is born between thirty-eight and forty weeks' gestation at an average weight of between 7 and 8 pounds. On the other end of the spectrum, the earliest gestational age at which survival is likely is about

twenty-four weeks. Babies at that stage usually weigh in the neighborhood of 1 pound. Between these two points lies the entire possible range of prematurity.

THE IMPORTANCE OF GESTATIONAL AGE

Gestational age is one important gauge of whether the infant's organs have developed sufficiently to permit him or her to thrive outside the womb. Your neonatologist will use this important information to make an assessment of your baby's prospects. Many factors play into this assessment. However, the importance of gestational age is such that a wide range of expectations is shaped by it.

Your baby's gestational maturity influences the level of care he will need in intensive care. It

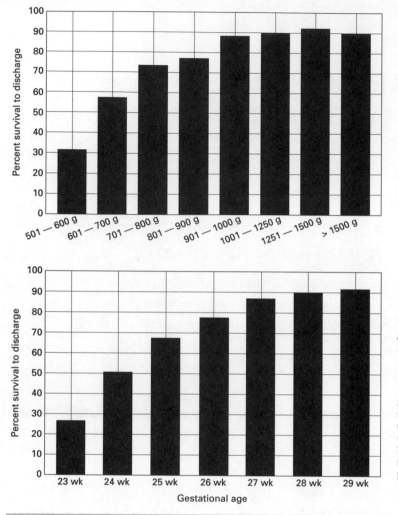

Birth-weight-specific survival from admission to discharge among all infants 23 to 29 weeks' gestation.

Gestational-age-specific survival from admission to discharge among all infants >500 g birth weight.

Source: "Actuarial Survival in the Premature Infant Less Than 30 Weeks' Gestation," by Timothy R. Cooper, Carol L. Berseth, James M. Adams, and Leonard E. Weisman, *Pediatrics* 101, no. 6 (June 1998): 975. Reprinted by permission.

also affects his ability to resist infections and deal with other problems that can arise during the NICU stay. The more mature your baby is, the more mature are his organs systems (brain, lung, skin, kidneys, and so on), so the better prepared they are to handle the outside world.

It is important to appreciate the significance of the differences between preemies of different gestational ages at birth. One good way of doing that is to actually visit the NICU, if you are able, and actually see the preemies in their incubators. This was not lost on Daryl, thirty, the mother of a thirty-week baby boy born in December 1998. "When I was hospitalized on bed rest, I learned a great deal about prematurity through reading and surfing the Internet from my hospital room. But because of my medical condition, I wasn't able to tour the NICU before my baby was admitted there. I think it would have made a *big* difference to me if I could have

Resilience, Persistence, and Individuality

JOE GARCIA-PRATS: "Just about every neonatologist I know is attracted to the calling of caring for premature infants because they are constantly amazed by preemies' resilience, persistence, and individuality. Each in his own way, preemies seem determined to complete their task of growth and development. Their individuality is almost always there to see. Sometimes you wonder how much personality a twenty-four-weeker could have. But they really do have their personal likes and dislikes. Because they work with the preemies so closely on a day-to-day basis, the neonatal nurses can always tell you: 'That one's real different, she's really strong-willed, he does this differently.' I am just constantly impressed by what even the tiniest of these little guys and gals can do, and how much they're driven to fight, and how much they can put up with."

seen, up close and personal, a twenty-six-weeker next to a twenty-eight-weeker next to a thirty-weeker. You wonder what the difference is. You think, What's the big deal? It's just a few weeks. But if I could have *seen* the physical difference between babies of different gestational ages, it might have helped me become more motivated to stay on bed rest."

Although gestational age is one of the most important determinants of how your baby will fare during the first weeks and months outside the womb, it is not the only barometer of her health. Other factors such as your medical problems, the presence of infection, congenital abnormalities, or breathing problems can have a significant effect on a preemie's health, regardless of her maturity. A twenty-eight-week preemie with a robust constitution and strong, mature lungs may do better than a thirty-weeker who is anemic and has immature lungs. But overall, gestational age (sometimes abbreviated as GA) has been statistically shown to be the most crucial element of a preemie's health equation.

The two bar charts shown here give the overall rate of survival for preemies of gestational ages from twenty-three to twenty-nine weeks and the overall rate of survival for preemies of birth weight strata, from 501 grams to greater than 1,500 grams. This study of 1,925 premature and low-birth-weight infants born at Baylor Affiliated Nurseries in Texas from 1986 to 1993 (including Texas Children's Hospital, Ben Taub General Hospital, and the Woman's Hospital of Texas) clearly illustrates the importance of gestational age and birth weight in a preemie's probability of survival.

This chapter goes into week-by-week detail about the premature baby's development, beginning approximately at twenty-four weeks' gestation and carrying through to the latest stage of maturation that can be said to be premature, less than thirty-seven completed weeks. If you are at risk for premature labor and are working with your obstetrician to postpone delivery as long as possible, it may be helpful to you to know the developmental difference between a

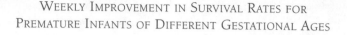

WEEKLY IMPROVEMENT IN SURVIVAL RATES FOR PREMATURE INFANTS OF DIFFERENT GESTATIONAL AGES

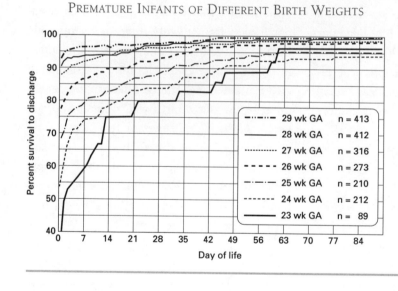

Percent survival to discharge

—·—·—	1251-1500 g n = 262
———	1001-1250 g n = 458
··········	901-1000 g n = 224
— — —	801- 900 g n = 211
—··—··—	701- 800 g n = 260
- - - -	601- 700 g n = 212
———	501- 600 g n = 147

Day of life

Effect of gestational age on actuarial survival. The survival rate to discharge, recalculated at daily intervals on the surviving cohort and stratified by gestational age, is presented for all inborn infants of 23 to 29 weeks' gestation, >500 g birth weight, and admitted from 1986 through 1993.

WEEKLY IMPROVEMENT IN SURVIVAL RATES FOR PREMATURE INFANTS OF DIFFERENT BIRTH WEIGHTS

Percent survival to discharge

—·—·—	29 wk GA n = 413
———	28 wk GA n = 412
··········	27 wk GA n = 316
— — —	26 wk GA n = 273
—··—··—	25 wk GA n = 210
- - - -	24 wk GA n = 212
———	23 wk GA n = 89

Day of life

Effect of birth weight on actuarial survival. The survival rate to discharge, recalculated at daily intervals on the surviving cohort and stratified by birth weight, is presented for all inborn infants of 23 to 29 weeks' gestation, >500 g birth weight, and admitted from 1986 through 1993.

Source: "Actuarial Survival in the Premature Infant Less Than 30 Weeks' Gestation," by Timothy R. Cooper, Carol L. Berseth, James M. Adams, and Leonard E. Weisman, *Pediatrics* 101, no. 6 (June 1998): 975. Reprinted by permission.

twenty-eight-week and a thirty-week preemie. If you have already delivered your premature baby, you will likewise want to gain a sense of how far he has come and how far he has to go.

Armed with the information in this chapter, you will be able to appreciate the important strides your baby makes with every week in the womb and understand the urgency your obstetrician, perinatologist, or neonatologist places on delivering as mature an infant as close to term as possible. Furthermore, understanding the stages of growth your baby is progressing through may help you to deepen your relationship with your baby.

Two more graphics from the Baylor study, shown opposite, illustrate the improvement in a preemie's survival chances for every week that goes by following birth. This "actuarial" analysis gives us much more useful information than the overall survival-from-birth analysis. For example, in the first chart, a preemie born at twenty-four weeks (the second line from the bottom) begins with an overall survival probability of 51 percent at birth. By day seven of life survival jumps to 74 percent. By day fourteen it is 78 percent. And by day twenty-eight survival stands at 84 percent. The improved survival rates illustrate the fact that most of the deaths in these infants occurred during the first few days after birth. The authors of the study write, "Actuarial survival data may also be useful in making health-care policy decisions concerning the use of aggressive care in extremely low birth weight infants."

Very Premature Infants: Twenty-four to Twenty-eight Weeks' Gestation Approximate Expected Birth Weight: Less Than 1 to 3½ Pounds

Suspended in and cushioned by the womb's amniotic fluid, your baby has by this time acquired many of the tools necessary for surviving outside the womb. However, babies at the earliest end of this age range are the youngest that are likely to do so. Survival rates for infants in this gestational age span a rather broad range, depending on other health factors. For twenty-four- or twenty-five-weekers, survival rates range from 40 to 80 percent. Chances of survival are higher for twenty-six- and twenty-seven-weekers: 80 to 90 percent. Many preemies born this early, especially those closest to twenty-four weeks, may have some kind of developmental difficulty or health problem. The medical literature states that the occurrence of neurological difficulties or problems (cerebral palsy, blindness, mental retardation, learning difficulties) range from 10 to 25 percent in preterm infants born less than 1,000 grams (less than twenty-eight weeks). If your baby has no major complications, she will likely spend three or four months in the neonatal ICU, where these concerns can be addressed on a continuous basis. This length of stay is derived from the length of time the baby is away from her original due date. Serious infection, illness, or congenital abnormality may require your baby to have a longer hospitalization. Likewise, rapid progress could shorten this date.

As a general working guideline, a preterm infant's chances for survival at this gestational age range increases by 2 to 3 percent for every day spent in the womb.

IF YOUR BABY IS DELIVERED NOW

Considering that your baby is born as much as four months early, he still has a good chance of survival at this stage of maturation, thanks to the great advances made in neonatology. However, the odds of some kind of developmental difficulty are higher for very premature preemies than they are for preemies born later. Your baby's gestational age, coupled with the quality of his prenatal life (which encompasses things

In utero, the fetus is in its element, where movement is easier, suspended in amniotic fluid with support all around by being in the mother's womb. At twenty weeks fetal movements are vigorous enough to be felt by the mother. From twenty-four weeks the fetus shows more movement of the extremities when turning in the womb. Hand-to-face contact and thumb sucking have been seen by ultrasound, and some fetuses have sucking blisters on their thumbs or hands. What a change once the fetus leaves the womb. The premature infant is now totally dependent on caregivers to support developing muscles, posture, and environment and is unable to get away from stimulation or interventions that overwhelm or disrupt. To support neuromotor development:

- Provide containment and security by making a nest of towel rolls or other positioning equipment.
- Assist supporting their arms and legs so that they will develop flexed and tucked posture as they would normally in the increasing confinement of the womb.
- Help posture hands to mouth for calming or comfort.
- Use their hands to provide warm touch and nurturing even if the baby is not ready to be moved from the bed into a parent's arms.
- Massage has not been performed in infants this young and may be too much stimulation, whereas just cradling your own baby in your hand may be acceptable.

Your baby will tell you just how much is enough and when the stimulation or interaction is too much.

Providing stimulation to only one sensory system at a time is usually better tolerated until your baby is more mature and shows signs of better ability to remain stable physically and calm during handling and interaction. For example, using hand containment without talking is stimulating touch without stimulating hearing. As your baby becomes more capable, both touching and talking at the same time would be appropriate and important for your baby's development.

like placental difficulties, maternal health, and the quality and administration of prenatal care), will determine the course of his prematurity.

PHYSICAL MATURITY

Befitting his gestational age, your baby at this point still resembles a fetus more than the full-term babies you're seeing in the parenting magazines. At this early stage of growth, the head receives priority and is thus going to be out of proportion in size to the rest of the body. As the body plays catch-up, your infant will more and more begin to resemble a fully proportioned baby. Though he is continuing to build up deposits of subcutaneous fat, your baby's physical stature will be quite slight right now. His skin may still be wrinkled and reddish, with a translucence that reveals veins and arteries within. His muscles have not matured yet. He is quite skinny still and does not have the strength to lie in the typical fetal position. If your baby is placed on a bed or bassinet, he will offer little to no resistance if you try to move his arms or legs and won't be able to roll over or change positions in bed. The baby's neck muscles are immature and will offer no control over his head movement. Soft *lanugo* (fine, downy hair) is all over his body, and his ears have little cartilage to give them rigidity, so they will fold over easily on themselves. The sexual organs are fully formed. However, in boys the testes have not descended yet, and in girls the vaginal area is fully exposed, as the protective skin folds (labia) are not yet their full-grown size.

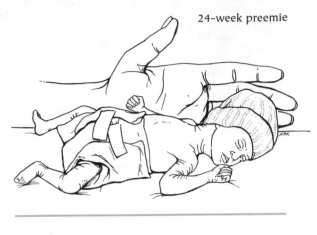

24-week preemie

NEUROLOGICAL DEVELOPMENT

Your baby is making important strides here every day. As the brain grows larger, its "circuitry" forms increasingly complex networks of neural interconnections. With each week that goes by, there will be an observable difference in your baby's capabilities. She will make more subtle and purposeful movements and have increasingly sharp perceptions of her surroundings. Sheaths of fat are beginning to insulate the spinal cord and nerve fibers, permitting faster transmission of signals within the brain. This increase in speed allows for more rapid learning and more coordinated physical movements. These movements in turn contribute to muscular and skeletal growth and to your baby's fine motor ability.

For now movements are jerky, and extremities twitch and tremor in jerky movements. These movements are quite normal owing to the infant's immaturity. You will watch this change to smooth, coordinated movement as your baby matures.

It is believed that neural connections at birth are not complete. Neurons that are specialized for survival such as breathing and circulation are functional for the term infant, and as we have observed, they are not all functioning for the prematurely born infants. It is now believed in some medical circles (although somewhat controversial) that an infant's brain is shaped not only by genetic material, but also by her experiences with the environment and by her experiences with the people in that environment. For these reasons, the typical NICU environment is often modified to provide sensory experiences more appropriate to your baby's stage of development. Dim lighting, sound awareness and reduction, comfortable bedding all support the neuromotor development. Gentle handling and opportunities for families to support their baby are a few ways to accomplish an appropriate sensory environment for the small premature infant. Just think about what the uterine environment must be like. Even though your infant is tiny and fragile, your baby can communicate through physical signs and behavior or

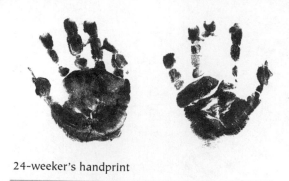

24-weeker's handprint

ways that help us to provide nurturing care that is right for your baby's age and abilities.

A head ultrasound may be performed on your baby soon after birth to check for brain bleeds, also known as *intraventricular hemorrhage* (IVH).

Temperature control is a significant concern for your baby because she has so little heat-insulating fat. To keep warm, your baby will be placed in an incubator or open warmer, where the temperature will be regulated carefully. At first it may be an open-air bed warmed from above. Medical personnel can access your baby more easily this way. If your preemie is very small, she may be wrapped in plastic, a thermal barrier designed to preserve the small quantity of heat your newborn's body is able to generate. Once your baby's vital signs are stable, she may be moved to an incubator.

Respiration is another concern. Air sacs called *alveoli* are growing at a rapid rate inside the lungs. These are the tiny sacs that must expand and contract easily for breathing to take place. Now that your baby doesn't have your placenta to breathe for her, her lungs must perform this vital work. Inside the uterus, even though the alveoli were not yet ready to do this job full-time, your baby was beginning to exercise her breathing muscles, practicing for the moment when the first breath must be taken after delivery. Prior to delivery, you may have felt your baby hiccuping, which revealed itself through sudden, gentle jerks in your abdomen.

≈

In all likelihood, a preemie born this early will need respiratory assistance. A twenty-four-weeker will almost certainly be intubated and be given respiratory assistance with the aid of a mechanical respirator. A twenty-eight-weeker might breathe without high-technology help or may require less invasive respiratory assistance such as *continuous positive airway pressure* (*CPAP*), which keeps your baby's lungs from collapsing in on themselves, or an oxygen hood or tent. The length of time the baby remains on the respirator will depend on the rate at which her respiratory system matures and how well the baby makes the transition from life in the liquid-filled womb to our gas-filled environment. Prenatal maternal injections of fetal-lung-maturing steroids such as betamethasone could have a significant favorable impact on your preemie's respiratory prognosis. Babies who require mechanical ventilation will be weaned off it gradually, moving to other types of respiratory assistance, including CPAP or oxygen delivered via an oxygen hood. Additionally, your baby may require surfactant or other medication (such as caffeine). Even after your baby is off the respirator and breathing on her own, concerns about apnea and periodic breathing will likely persist. (See page 162.)

SLEEPING AND OTHER BEHAVIOR

Your baby is still devoting most of his energy resources to growing. His growth will be fastest when he's not burning calories making eyes at his parents or engaging in other social activities. Periods of wakefulness may still be rather brief—fifteen to twenty minutes a day. Each week your baby will become more acutely aware of his surroundings. Though he may not show obvious reactions to stimuli right away, he knows when you are present and is learning to recognize your voice. Your baby is still too young to respond to stress in the usual way—with a loud cry. Instead he will show other signs and distress that you should learn to look out for: an arching back, attempting to move the arms or legs, rapidly changing heart rates or respiration rates, and a stiff or limp posture. Remember to trust what you see. Your baby's facial frowns, grimaces, and stiffly extended or limp extremities and trunk are your baby's way of saying, "I am upset." Stress often arises from exhaustion or overstimulation. Your baby will start to become more active physically over time, stretching his arms and legs, clasping his hands together, making a fist, and putting his hands to his mouth in an effort to suck. His muscles are not sufficiently developed to sustain this activity for any length of time, however. If your baby or his NICU neighbor is having many visitors, or if you are playing with him excessively, the result may be stress. Slow things down, make your baby comfortable with blankets and pillows, speak softly, and try not to overload his immature nervous system with lots of light, sounds, or touches.

FEEDINGS

In the first few hours to days after birth, the twenty-four- to twenty-eight-week preemie will not receive feedings by mouth. Rather, she will be given fluids and nutrients directly into the bloodstream via an intravenous (IV) line. Beginning anywhere from a few hours to a few days later, depending on your baby's health status, your baby will be started on breast milk or formula. The means of administration will depend on your baby's feeding maturity. Your baby will be watched closely by NICU staff to determine her ability to tolerate feedings, and the feeding quantities will be increased accordingly.

GUT PRIMING FEEDING. Prior to going on breast milk or formula as the principal means of sustenance, your preemie may undergo a technique called *gut priming*. This involves administering very small amounts of milk or formula to the baby ahead of the time when she would normally receive it. The route of administration will depend on your baby's maturity. Most likely these feedings will be given via a nasogastric (NG) tube. Infants with immature bowels may not tolerate full feedings without undergoing this preparation. Gut priming helps the intestinal system's motility, the manner in which it coordinates the movements of food and fluids through the digestive tract.

TOTAL PARENTERAL NUTRITION (TPN), OR HYPERALIMENTATION. Babies who are so small or ill that they cannot make the transition from IV feedings to oral feedings may continue to receive all of their nutritional needs, for a short period of time, via IV fluids supplemented with proteins, fats, and vitamins. Since it is so concentrated and artificially formulated, TPN is intended for short-term purposes. Possible side effects from excessive, prolonged use of TPN include fibrosis (scarring) and liver failure.

GAVAGE FEEDING. If your baby is too immature to suck from a bottle or breast—or if the sucking reflex is there, but the doctor feels that bottle- or breast-feeding would tax your preemie's limited energy reserves too heavily—gavage feeding may be used in order to ensure a sufficient quantity of formula or breast milk. This involves the insertion of a *naso-gastric tube* (also known as an *NG tube*) through the nose or mouth and into the stomach. A syringe will be attached to the tube and used to propel milk or formula directly into your baby's stomach. The more premature your baby, the more likely the need for gavage feedings. Though your baby may graduate within a few weeks to bottle- or breast-feeding, it may be necessary to supplement her feedings via gavage feeding until the neonatologist is confident the baby can fully manage regular bottle or breast feedings.

BOTTLE-FEEDING. It is very unlikely that your preemie is mature enough to be able to bottle-feed right away. It usually takes a few weeks. Preemies who take a bottle will begin with tiny quantities of milk or formula—as little as 4 or 5 cc (a teaspoonful). The quantity will be increased steadily as the baby is able to tolerate it. The NICU staff will closely monitor your baby's reaction to feedings, watching out for any signs of intolerance to feedings, which can include vomiting, excess gas, loose stools, or blood in the stool.

BREAST-FEEDING. Preemies almost always lack the strength to breast-feed immediately after birth. Even if they do have the strength, the coordinated tasks of sucking, swallowing, and breathing take time to develop. Thus mothers who want to breast-feed a twenty-eight- to thirty-two-week preemie will need patience. But take heart. Until your baby gains the strength to breast-feed, you have the alternative of expressing breast milk via a hand or mechanical breast pump and feeding your baby via bottle. (See chapter 6.)

HEARING

Though he is well insulated and protected from the highly variable and unpredictable conditions of the outside world, he is not entirely unaware of it. Indeed, by your baby's twenty-seventh week the ears will be functionally developed. If your baby is still inside the womb at this age, voices and other noises are audible to him, and he can hear the sounds of your bodily functions at work—heart beating, stomach growling, blood pumping. The physiology of your baby's tiny ear makes higher-frequency sounds easier for him to hear. Even in the uterus, he is beginning to distinguish one voice from another and is thus in the process of getting acquainted with the rhythms and accents of your speech. Loud noises can actually startle him and accelerate his heart rate. As his awareness and faculties develop—at this stage of maturation your baby's sensitivity and intelligence are beginning to blossom—the bond between you strengthens.

Some time during your preemie's NICU stay, an audiologist (an individual specializing in hearing evaluation) will test your child's hear-

"How will I know if my preemie has long-term developmental problems?"

Developmental problems could take years to manifest themselves. Research has shown them to be statistically correlated with extreme prematurity combined with an illness, infection, or congenital abnormality. For this reason it is important for premature infants, especially those with serious complications or conditions, to have their development monitored closely after leaving the hospital. Consistent follow-up is very important since some signs of possible problems may be present at one visit but not at the next. Single visits are not as helpful as consistent follow-up examinations. And it will take a long time (eighteen to thirty-six months) to know with any degree of accuracy whether your child will have problems and, if so, the extent and severity of those problems. Likewise, consistent follow-up may allow you to begin helping to ameliorate those problems that might be identified. Signs of possible problems can include the following.

Motor (movement) problems:

- Slow to crawl, stand, or walk
- Moving arms or legs on one side more than the other
- Frequent arching of the back (not just when angry or at play)
- Seizures or convulsions

Slow cognitive development:

- Does not react to your voice (three to four months after hospital discharge)
- Does not vocalize (eight to nine months after discharge)
- Understands and speaks few words by twelve to thirteen months after discharge

Less serious problems are more difficult to detect and may not be apparent until your child reaches school age:

- Poor coordination or balance
- Specific learning disabilities (math or reading)
- Very short attention span
- Difficulty with activities that require eye-hand coordination, for example, catching a ball or copying a simple drawing

If you are worried about something that you think might be abnormal, keep your follow-up appointments or ask your physician to refer your baby to a specialist in developmental pediatrics to have your baby examined as soon as possible. (See chapter 11 for further information on later-life development.)

ing. When your baby is ready for discharge, you will be given instructions and recommendations for follow-up hearing exams.

VISION

By twenty-four weeks the external structures of your baby's eyes will be normally formed. However, the important blood vessels that supply the retina of the eye (the photoplate that receives the images) haven't yet developed. This won't be evident from looking at your baby. Your infant will be able to distinguish light, and you will notice that when the lights are on around her, she won't open her eyes readily. But because she's spent most of her life so far in the dark environment of the womb, your baby will open her eyes with greater ease and less discomfort when the room lighting is turned down.

While in the womb, a baby's eyelids normally remain fused until about week twenty-six. Thus a twenty-four- to twenty-five-week preemie may be born with fused eyelids. Though the sight of your baby with closed eyes may be upsetting, this is no cause for alarm, medically speaking. No medical intervention is necessary; the eyelids will open on their own after a few days.

At about four to six weeks of age, and weekly thereafter, for the duration of the NICU stay, your baby's vision will be checked by a pediatric ophthalmologist. Subsequent vision tests will be scheduled at regular intervals during the first year.

Cori's son, Bo—who is a beautiful, healthy boy today—was born at twenty-four weeks weighing 1 pound 3 ounces (555 grams) and was 8 inches long (21 centimeters).

"Never had I seen such a tiny, red baby with his eyes fused shut. My lasting impression was of his head, which was about the size of a tennis ball. At birth, Bo had very reddish pink and translucent skin. His eyes were still fused shut (like a newborn puppy's eyes), and they did not open for about two weeks. Bo was covered in goop because his skin was so thin and they were trying to keep it from drying out. It was explained to us that he had two or three layers of skin on his little body, as opposed to us having around forty layers. The nurses had to be very careful because if his skin was even just rubbed, it could come off and scar him badly. His bed was covered with a little tent that looked like plastic wrap, to keep in the moisture. We were told that the first forty-eight hours were critical, and they gave him a 20 percent chance to live. After he made it through that, we were told that the first week would be the honeymoon period. After that first week, things could go any which way. Well, we did the preemie two-step (one step forward and two steps back) for most of his 104 days spent in the NICU."

Premature Infants: Twenty-eight to Thirty-two Weeks' Gestation Approximate Expected Birth Weight: 2½ to 4½ Pounds

IF YOUR BABY IS DELIVERED NOW

Although a preemie born at this gestational age range does not live without risk, your physician will breathe a sigh of relief if you are able to make it to this point in your pregnancy. There is no magical threshold that is crossed when your twenty-seven-weeker becomes a twenty-eight-weeker. But by any measure, a baby who reaches twenty-eight weeks or more enjoys better survival odds and less chance of developmental problems owing to more advanced physical and neurological maturity. Survival chances for a baby who reaches this age range are in excess of 90 percent. (See chart on page 152.)

A baby with no major complications will likely spend eight to twelve weeks in the neonatal ICU/intermediate care/special care nurseries. This rather conservative estimate used by most neonatologists takes into account how far the preemie is from the original due date. Serious infection, illness, or congenital abnormality may require your baby to have a longer hospitalization. Likewise, rapid progress could shorten the stay. Temperature maintenance and respiration are two concerns that any baby born this early will have.

PHYSICAL MATURITY

Your baby will be skinny in appearance, as he lacks most of the body fat that a full-term baby would have. The good news, of course, is that his internal organs are by and large fully formed and relatively more mature (certainly more mature than the twenty-four-week infant), so his chance of better functioning is higher. However, your infant is still at risk for all of the problems that the twenty-four-week infant may suffer, although the chances are smaller and your baby will handle them more readily. Your baby's physique is generally proportioned as you would expect a newborn's to be, except that any preemie still has a great deal of weight to gain.

On the outside, the twenty-eight- to thirty-

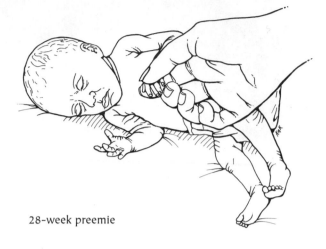

28-week preemie

two-week preemie is still playing a game of catch-up. The skin is very thin, possibly almost translucent, showing veins and arteries, and still rather reddish in color. Much of the body may still be covered with lanugo, the soft hairs that fetuses are covered with in utero. A preemie at this age lacks the muscular strength to curl up in the "fetal" position and if placed on his back will extend the limbs out to the side.

NEUROLOGICAL DEVELOPMENT

Your baby continues to make important progress here. With each week that goes by, there will be an observable difference in your baby's capabilities. She will make more coordinated and purposeful movements. These movements help muscular and skeletal growth and your baby's fine motor ability. Your baby will also have increasingly sharp perceptions of her surroundings.

Your preemie may receive a head ultrasound soon after birth to check for brain bleeds, also known as intraventricular hemorrhage (IVH). (See chapter 7.)

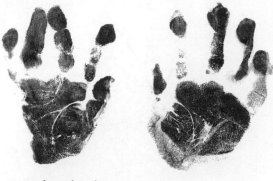

28-weeker's handprint

TEMPERATURE CONTROL

Your baby will need to be kept in an incubator for warming owing to the absence of subcutaneous fat beneath the skin, which serves as insulation. Initially an open-air warmer may be used, in order to allow the medical staff unimpeded access to your baby. Once the vital signs stabilize, he may be moved to a covered incubator. Your baby's size at birth and overall health (including the ability to maintain body temperature) will determine how long he needs to remain in the incubator.

RESPIRATION

The lungs are more fully developed and are producing increasing amounts of surfactant, the vitally important lubricating fluid that prevents the lung's tiny air sacs from collapsing on exhalation. If your premature delivery was anticipated and your obstetrician gave you a steroid injection, it is possible that your baby's lungs may be sufficiently mature for her to breathe on her own. Even if that is not the case, however, your preemie may be far enough along not to need full mechanical ventilation; rather, it is

possible that she'll need only CPAP or an oxygen hood/tent to help her breathe. You may be able to tell at delivery whether your baby can breathe by herself; a loud cry is a probable sign. If not, it is quite routine for the attending neonatologist to provide artificial respiration until the baby's lungs are mature enough not to need it.

SLEEP AND OTHER BEHAVIOR

A preemie born eight to twelve weeks prematurely will spend most of his time sleeping. Periods of wakefulness are quite brief—though usually long enough (from fifteen to thirty minutes) to make feedings and diaper changes an interactive experience. Because his range of vision is still rather short, your preemie will not be able to see you from any distance greater than a foot or so. The ability to focus is increasing, however, so you may notice the baby fixating on objects within immediate range of sight. Since his neck muscles are still weak, he won't be able to hold his head up, though it is possible he may be able to turn it from side to side while lying down. Your baby's movements will be rather uncontrolled and jerky as a result of a still immature central nervous system. For this same reason, he'll be easily fatigued by long periods of handling and interaction. Your baby may not yet be able to express that fatigue in an infant's usual manner—by crying. Instead he may show it in other ways: increases in the respiration rate or heart rate, a change in skin color, adopting a rigid or limp posture, or arching the back.

FEEDINGS

Once your twenty-eight- to thirty-two-weeker has been fully assessed and stabilized, the

Aaron Remembers

Kelly's son Aaron was born at thirty weeks, at 3 pounds 15 ounces. He was 16¾ inches long. Kelly said, "I remember when he was born, and the doctor said, 'Here he is!' He was just screaming his little lungs out. I was so surprised. I really expected him to be a little lump, not making noises. It was very exciting. After they cleaned him and gave him a little oxygen, they wheeled him over to me while the doctor was finishing suturing me. He peeked open with one eye. It was so cute. I wonder if he truly did recognize my voice. I talked to him a lot while carrying him. He looked right at me when I said, 'Hi, Aaron. It's Mommy.'

"I also remember how *red* he looked. He looked like a normal term baby—just a bit small. When I saw him, he was breathing independently on room air. But owing to my postpartum health concerns, that was the last time I saw him until after he was twenty-four hours old. And then I just couldn't believe how small he was. But what a fighter. He was initially placed on CPAP because of his lung immaturity. But when Aaron was three days old he developed respiratory distress syndrome (RDS). He needed to be intubated and given surfactant. This resolved, and he was extubated within twenty-four hours. He also had to have an umbilical artery line for his frequent blood gases, which were necessary to monitor the respiratory distress.

"He also had elevated bilirubin levels so he was put under the bili-lights and had a little tiny mask protecting his eyes from the light. And he also had a partial exchange transfusion and a grade II brain bleed, which resolved on its own. These conditions along with his overall prematurity required him to spend six days in the NICU, then twenty-two more in the step-down unit. It was scary the first week he was there. We had many ups and downs. He came home on an apnea monitor.

"Just a week or so ago, at age two, while I was getting ready for work, he came into the bathroom and said, 'Remember, Mom? Do you remember?' I said, 'Remember what, Aaron?' He said, 'Mommy, do you remember when I was born?' 'Yes, I do,' I said, then added just for fun, 'Do you?' He said, 'Yes—I came out and cried and cried and then I peeked at you!' You could have knocked me over with a feather."

neonatologist will establish a very individualized feeding routine for her. The routine will depend on the child's level of maturity and tolerance to feedings. The means of feeding may involve a few different techniques. It is possible your preemie will make use of some or all of these feeding techniques. A baby at this twenty-eight- to thirty-two-week range will make faster progress to bottle- or breast feeding than will a twenty-four- to twenty-eight-weeker.

GAVAGE FEEDING. If your baby is too immature to suck from a bottle or breast—or if she is capable of sucking, but the doctor feels that bottle- or breast-feeding would tax her limited energy reserves too heavily—gavage feeding may be used to administer a sufficient quantity of formula or breast milk. (Preemies are able to suck well before they can manage the more complex combined process of sucking, swallowing, and breathing.) This involves the insertion of a naso-gastric tube (also known as an NG tube) through the nose and down into the stomach. A syringe will be attached to the tube and used to move breast milk or formula directly into your baby's stomach. The more premature your baby, the more likely the need for gavage feedings. Though your baby may graduate within a few days or weeks to bottle- or breast-feeding, it may still be necessary to supplement feedings via gavage until the neonatologist is confident the baby can manage regular bottle or breast feedings on her own power.

BOTTLE-FEEDING. If your preemie is mature enough, she may be able to bottle-feed within days of delivery. Preemies who take a bottle will begin with tiny quantities of milk or formula—as little as 4 or 5 cc (a teaspoonful). The quantity will be increased steadily as the baby is able to tolerate it. The NICU staff will closely monitor your baby's reaction to feedings, watching out for any signs of intolerance to feedings, which can include vomiting, excess gas, loose stools, or blood in the stool.

BREAST-FEEDING. Preemies often lack the strength to breast-feed immediately after birth.

Even if they do have the strength, the coordinated tasks of sucking, swallowing, and breathing take time to develop. Thus mothers who want to breast-feed a twenty-eight- to thirty-two-week preemie will need patience. But take heart. Until your baby gains the strength to breast-feed, you have the alternative of expressing breast milk via a hand or mechanical breast pump and feeding your baby via bottle or tube. (See chapter 6.)

HEARING

The twenty-eight- to thirty-two-week preemie's ears will be functionally developed at birth. If the baby is still in the womb, he can hear the sounds of your bodily functions at work—heart beating, stomach growling, blood pumping. He is able to distinguish one voice from another and is thus in the process of getting acquainted with the rhythms and accents of your speech. Loud noises can actually startle him, accelerating his heart rate.

Because of the preemie's overall neurological immaturity, his hearing is highly sensitive and vulnerable to overloading. Many NICUs have instituted procedures designed to protect this vulnerability. They include such things as covering incubators to muffle sounds reaching the baby; switching off ringers on telephones; keeping conversations at low levels; and playing soft, soothing music.

An audiologist (an individual specializing in hearing evaluation) will test your child's hearing prior to discharge from the hospital. When your child is ready for discharge, you will be given instructions and recommendations for follow-up hearing exams.

VISION

Preemies have poor eyesight—vision is the last of the sensory systems to mature—and have a hard time focusing on objects beyond a foot from their face. It may frustrate you that you aren't able to make meaningful eye contact with your premature newborn. But you can help stimulate your baby's visual maturity by trying. Human faces are a baby's favorite objects to look at. As the days and weeks go by, you will notice steady improvement in your preemie's ability to focus. Try moving from side to side and see if your baby can follow you. Additionally, soft child-safe objects with black-and-white stripes, polka dots, and geometric patterns can help your baby focus on the world around her. As with sound, many NICUs are increasingly aware of the need to avoid visually overstimulating preemies, using indirect, recessed lighting, and blankets over incubators.

While in the NICU or possibly soon after discharge, your baby's vision will be checked by a pediatric ophthalmologist. Subsequent vision tests will be scheduled at regular intervals during the first year.

Moderately Premature Infants: Thirty-two to Thirty-seven Weeks' Gestation Approximate Expected Birth Weight: 4 to 6½ Pounds

Your baby has now crossed the threshold where almost all—approximately 99 percent—of premature babies survive. The incidence of developmental delay or difficulty is likewise much lower. However, this is not to say your experience parenting a preemie will necessarily be an easy one. Though your baby will probably have a shorter NICU/intermediate care/special care nursery stay than a preemie born earlier, your feelings of anxiety and concern are no less valid than those of a parent of a less mature infant. These concerns are shared by the neonatologist caring for your infant. Prematurity is a significant condition that is still associated with the potential problems of immature organ systems. Although the chances are much less of your baby experiencing these problems, the potential still exists. So you and your baby's physician will worry together.

IF YOUR BABY IS DELIVERED NOW

For the thirty-two- to thirty-seven-weeker, survival chances are close to 99 percent. However, a stay in the neonatal intensive care unit may still be necessary. Typically, babies born at this gestational age simply need some time to put on weight and stabilize their temperature and vital signs. Your baby will need to be monitored closely for a few days or weeks after birth. Once respiration, temperature, and other vitals are stable, your baby will be placed in the step-down unit, or "feeder-grower" unit. Once here, and assuming there are no intervening medical conditions or complications, your child is well on his way to being able to live on his own. As the term *feeder-grower* suggests, he is playing a game of catch-up with his full-term peers. He will likely spend an estimated two to eight weeks in the NICU/intermediate care/special care nursery.

PHYSICAL MATURITY

With organs more fully formed and functional, your baby's primary task at this stage is to gain weight. She will still be quite skinny. During the final eight weeks of gestation, infants are gaining half a pound per week. Thus she has a few pounds to put on still, which represent a significant percentage of her total weight. Internally your baby's organs are fully formed and functional (including, significantly, her lungs), and from her skin to her eyes to her hair, she looks like a full-term infant. Your baby has shed most of her lanugo, the fine hair that has covered her body for several months now. Her fingernails are fully grown. (In fact, she may have scratched herself in the womb, so her nails may need to be clipped.) And her muscle tone is sufficient to enable her to move her arms and legs with more authority. She will be able to grasp your fingers with her hands, and her arms may be strong enough to enable you to pull her to a sitting position.

NEUROLOGICAL DEVELOPMENT

Your baby continues to make important progress here. With each week that goes by, there will be an observable difference in your baby's capabilities. He will make more coordinated and purposeful movements. These movements help muscular and skeletal growth, and your baby's fine motor ability. Your baby will also have increasingly sharp perceptions of his surroundings.

Like many preemies, he may undergo a head ultrasound soon after birth to check for brain bleeds, also known as intraventricular hemorrhage (IVH). (See chapter 7.)

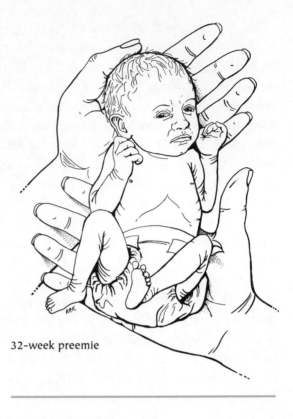

32-week preemie

TEMPERATURE CONTROL

Your baby will need to be kept in an incubator for warming owing to the absence of subcutaneous fat beneath the skin, which serves as insulation. Initially an open-air warmer may be used, in order to allow the medical staff unimpeded access to your baby. Once her vital signs stabilize, she may be moved to a covered incubator. Your baby's size at birth and overall health (including the ability to maintain body temperature) will determine how long she needs to remain in an incubator.

RESPIRATION

Whether your baby requires respiratory support after delivery or will breathe on his own at birth will depend on which end of the thirty-two- to thirty-seven-week range he occupies. Most thirty-seven-weekers can breathe on their own at delivery and require no respiratory assistance or even oxygen. Some thirty-two-weekers will; it's a function of a particular individual's lung maturity, which depends not only on gestational age, but also on whether the mother received steroid injections prior to delivery. Medications such as betamethasone are often given to mothers to aid in maturation of the baby's lungs if a premature delivery is anticipated. If your preemie does need respiratory assistance, it will most likely come in the form of supplemental oxygen delivered via nasal canula or an oxygen tent or hood. Mechanical ventilation or the less intrusive continuous positive airway pressure (CPAP) is seldom needed with preemies at this stage of maturity; this determination is made on a case-by-case basis. There is a great deal of variability in this rather broad age range. A thirty-two-weeker whose lungs aren't mature may well need CPAP or mechanical ventilation. Apnea and periodic breathing will be conditions to watch out for, even if your baby is breathing on his own.

SLEEP PATTERNS AND OTHER BEHAVIOR

A preemie at this gestational age will spend a lot of time sleeping, but periods of wakefulness are becoming longer and more frequent. Again, there is a good deal of variability among babies within this rather broad age range; every week brings progress. Your baby may become rather easily fatigued by long periods of handling and interaction. Babies on the earlier end of this age range may show stress through other ways: increases in respiration rate or heart rate, a change in skin color, adopting a rigid or limp posture, or by arching the back. But the progress made between thirty-two and thirty-seven weeks will be rapid and noticeable.

Babies born with only slight prematurity have central nervous systems that are much better developed than preemies born at an earlier gestational age. This allows them to move their limbs with more precision and purpose, to stay awake for longer periods of time, to sleep without interruption, and to be less irritable. They are able to interact with others without becoming overstimulated, exhausted, or stressed after a short time. And they respond to your voice and touch in a way that younger preemies sometimes don't.

FEEDINGS

Once your thirty-two- to thirty-seven-weeker has been fully assessed and stabilized, the neonatologist will establish a very individualized feeding routine for him. The routine will depend on level of maturity and tolerance to feedings. The means of feeding may involve a few different techniques. It is possible your preemie will make use of some or all of these feeding techniques, although a baby at this thirty-two- to thirty-seven-week range will make faster progress to bottle- or breast-feeding than his more immature NICU-mates.

GAVAGE FEEDING. If your baby is too immature to suck from a bottle or breast—or if he is capable of sucking, but the doctor feels that bottle- or breast-feeding would tax his limited energy reserves too heavily—gavage feeding may be used to administer a sufficient quantity of formula or breast milk. (Preemies

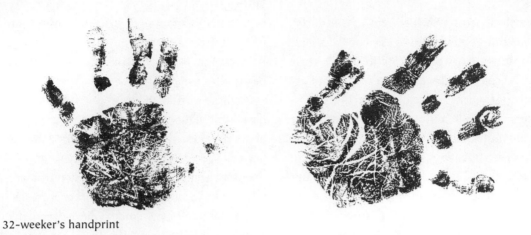

32-weeker's handprint

are able to suck well before they can manage the more complex combined process of sucking, swallowing, and breathing.) This involves the insertion of a naso-gastric tube (also known as an NG tube) through the nose and down into the stomach. A syringe will be attached to the tube and used to propel breast milk or formula directly into your baby's stomach. The more premature your baby, the more likely the need for gavage feedings. Though your baby may graduate within a few days or weeks to bottle- or breast-feeding, it may still be necessary to supplement feedings via gavage until the neonatologist is confident the baby can manage regular bottle or breast feedings on his own power.

BOTTLE-FEEDING. If your preemie is mature enough, he may be able to bottle-feed within days of delivery. Preemies who take a bottle will begin with tiny quantities of milk or formula—as little as 4 or 5 cc (a teaspoonful). The quantity will be increased steadily as the baby is able to tolerate it. The NICU staff will closely monitor your baby's reaction to feed-

ings, watching out for any signs of intolerance to feedings, which can include vomiting, excess gas, loose stools, or blood in the stool.

BREAST-FEEDING. Preemies often lack the strength to breast-feed immediately after birth. Even if they do have the strength, the coordinated tasks of sucking, swallowing, and breathing take time to develop. Thus mothers who want to breast-feed their preemie will need patience. But take heart. Until your baby gains the strength to breast-feed, you have the alternative of expressing breast milk via a hand or mechanical breast pump and feeding your baby via bottle. (See chapter 6.)

VISION

Your baby's range of vision is about 10 to 12 inches now. She will be making eye contact with you for the first time and will be intensely curious about objects and light sources placed within her field of vision. She may lift her head briefly when something catches her eye. Sources of light, movement, and sharply contrasting patterns will fascinate her. Babies born at thirty-six to thirty-seven weeks will be able to see almost as well as full-term babies.

HEARING

The thirty-two- to thirty-seven-week preemie's ears will be functionally developed at birth. If he is still in the womb, he can hear the sounds of your bodily functions at work—heart beating, stomach growling, blood pumping. He is able to distinguish one voice from another and is thus in the process of getting acquainted with the rhythms and accents of your speech. Loud noises can actually startle him, accelerating his heart rate. Because of the preemie's overall neurological immaturity, his hearing is highly sensitive and vulnerable to overloading. Many NICUs have instituted procedures designed to protect this vulnerability. They include such things as covering incubators to muffle sounds reaching the baby; switching off ringers on telephones; keeping conversations at low levels; and playing soft, soothing music. An audiologist (an individual specializing in hearing evaluation) will test your child's hearing prior to discharge from the NICU. When your child is ready for discharge, you will be given instructions and recommendations for follow-up hearing exams.

Ryan, born at thirty-two weeks, weighed 4 pounds 3 ounces, was 17½ inches long, and spent fifteen days in the NICU. According to his mother, Kelly, he had a bilateral grade II brain bleed that resolved by itself. "During the delivery, I remember them telling me, 'Your baby is out.' I listened and listened and can still hear my own voice echoing, 'Why isn't he crying?' Well, no one answered, and when I read his discharge summary the day we came home, I knew why. He didn't cry when he came out because they were assisting his ventilations."

Ryan came home on an apnea monitor and stayed on it for four months. But those days are long gone. "He's big and bad now, really getting into things." Eight months old as this is written, he weighs a solid nineteen pounds. That's a long way away from the time he and his mother conquered danger together, delivered to safety by the skill of the neonatal team, and nurtured by the compassion of the NICU's team.

SHARON HORNFISCHER: "David, born at thirty-two weeks, was 3 pounds 4 ounces. He was born early related to complications from maternal preeclampsia. Though he breathed on his own at birth—what a relief that was—David had some apnea to deal with during his six-week NICU stay. A typical feeder-grower, he had few problems, needing only some time under the bilirubin lights to counter his jaundice. He was diagnosed with IUGR related to the maternal hypertension, and this seemed to be his biggest problem. But generally he just needed time in a healthy environment in order to be nurtured and grow. At about 4 pounds 8 ounces and six weeks of age—around the Fourth of July—David was given his own independence day and was discharged home."

6

THE RHYTHMS OF THE NICU

WHAT YOU WILL FIND IN THIS CHAPTER

- Common medical procedures in the NICU
- Parenting in the NICU

- Keeping the home fires burning
- Parent support groups and other useful resources

Your introduction to life in a modern neonatal intensive care unit (NICU) will probably come at a time when you are under stress as never before in your life. This stress will likely exist whether or not you have been able to visit the unit ahead of time and no matter how much you know about neonatal medicine. You may not even notice it right away. The stress, which is usually a product of fear and exhaustion, may reveal itself through such things as general irritability, fatigue, impatience (with your spouse, other family members, or medical staff), or numbness to the reality of what's going on around you. Everyone has a different way of coping with stress. But it is one of the constants of the first days and weeks in the NICU.

There is no dress rehearsal for the actual experience of seeing your infant lying on a radiant warmer, generally helpless and dependent on high-tech equipment and busy medical professionals. After the initial fear wears off, it may be replaced by a feeling of helplessness or uselessness, driven by the feeling that with all of this machinery and highly trained medical staff caring for your child, you're little more than a passive observer. As we hope to show in this chapter (which, chronologically speaking, picks up where chapter 4, "The First Twenty-Four Hours after Delivery," left off), such impressions are far from reality. Your individual parenting skills are urgently needed by your baby in the NICU. The warmth and comfort you can offer him or her will contribute to a sense of belonging and togetherness that, it is believed, may actually shorten your baby's NICU stay.

"Begin with the End in Mind"

"Begin with the end in mind." It's the second tenet in author Stephen Covey's famous *7 Habits of Highly Effective People* (after "Be proactive"). It's worth bearing in mind as you begin your NICU experience. The "end" you should focus on looks something like this:

By the time your infant is discharged from the NICU, he will have been in the unit for roughly the number of weeks remaining until his original due date (it may be sooner than that if he does well). He will have learned to breathe, to maintain his temperature, to suck from a nipple, and to look you in the eye. Though he will be doing none of these things at the outset, every day he will make steady progress toward these goals (although he may actually lose some weight initially and will probably have setbacks along the way). On the day your preemie is discharged and you get to carry him out of the hospital's front door all swaddled and wrapped, the bond you have developed will be all the stronger for what you have been through—no matter what you may be feeling, or not feeling, right now.

If your premature infant is your first child, this is probably not what you expected—learning the parenting ropes amid the bustle and clutter of the modern NICU. Among the many expectations to be confounded by the preemie experience, this is about the most significant. If your preemie is not your first child, the experience can be all the more upsetting. Having been through pregnancy before, you may have formed certain expectations that are now all the harder to let go. You've been here before, and it was never as hard as this.

A mother ideally has nine months to prepare for parenthood, and throughout pregnancy she is with her baby every day, forming a deep bond that makes delivery the culmination of a long acquaintance. For this reason, dealing with the institutional barrier between you and your baby can be especially difficult. For fathers, parenthood arrives all of a sudden. Even the most attentive father is only an observer to his wife's pregnancy. Thus when delivery comes, the transition to parenting is all the more sudden and overwhelming. Just as sudden and overwhelming can be the way the baby is taken into this other, temporary family, the one called the neonatal intensive care unit.

In time, a transition will occur. You may not even notice exactly when it happens. But all of a sudden you will feel at home in the NICU. You'll start to know the nurses and staff by their first names. Doctors' faces will be familiar. You'll get to know the other parents looking after their babies there, and you may find them valuable sources of collegiality and support. You may also begin to feel at home with the NICU routine. Replenishing your baby's milk supply (if you are breast pumping), giving the staff a break by changing his diapers, checking his temperature, and cuddling him—all will help you feel needed by your baby. As hard as it is to imagine, you may even associate the smell of the antiseptic sponges at the scrub-in station with pleasant thoughts—the thought of seeing your baby after many hours away. These emotions will likely take hold whether or not your infant is in perfect health relative to his size.

Before we move to the challenge of parenting in the NICU, we introduce in the following pages the common procedures and protocols that generally govern most NICUs. Then we will start to explore the experience of being a parent in the unit. We hope this material helps you through the scary initial impressions and into the gradual progression toward becoming an active and involved NICU parent for whom taking care of most of your baby's daily needs is virtually second nature. Having grown into your role as an NICU parent, you will be armed with many of the tools needed to handle life after your baby's discharge, when you will be on your own at home.

In these early weeks of life in the NICU, your baby's full-time job is to grow. As we have mentioned previously, though he appears to be inactive, your baby is actually staying quite busy, working hard to breathe, maintain his temperature, grow, eat, fight off infection, and keep his vital signs stable. All of this is a pretty tall order for a being so small. But with the help of well-trained and compassionate medical professionals, advances in the field of neonatology, and loving, involved parents and families, preemies today are growing and flourishing in a way that could only be dreamed about just a few decades ago. And although not all of our babies will win the battle against their immaturity, most will beat the odds and eventually reach their full potential as healthy, active, normal children. If "it takes a village" to raise a child, the NICU is an extremely special sort of village for the 11 percent of all children today who are born prematurely.

"WHY ARE THEY SO STRICT IN THE NICU?"

One of the first things you will notice about the NICU is that it is not a visitors' gallery. As a specialized medical unit designed to meet the needs of critically ill newborns, it was not necessarily built with the comfort of visitors and parents in mind. Unlike the loved ones of full-term newborns residing briefly in the hospital's nursery, viewable on demand through large Plexiglas windows, you and your family and friends will have to abide by the restrictions most NICUs impose in order to maintain an appropriate intensive care environment. Though you will probably find the staff empathetic and helpful and willing to accommodate as many of your wishes as possible, there is a line that cannot be crossed when it comes to preserving the integrity of the unit, in terms of noise level, crowding, cleanliness, and general orderliness. This may be upsetting to you at first. Kristi, the mother of a 4-pound-11-ounce, thirty-two-week boy, said, "I was totally unprepared for the preemie experience. I was just kind of thrown into this atmosphere where the feeling coming from the staff was sort of like 'Hands off, let us do our job.' "

The idyllic image many parents have of themselves gazing upon their newborn through the large window in the newborn nursery or holding their baby beside mom's hospital bed can become deeply ingrained. It's part of the fantasy of the "perfect pregnancy" that you must find ways to dispel.

The NICU may place limits on the number of visitors your baby can have at any one time. In that case you'll have to inform your eager callers that they'll have to take turns. (The big group photo they wanted of everybody with the baby will have to wait. And certainly you should discourage anyone with an infectious ailment, even a minor cold, from visiting, lest he or she spread germs to these vulnerable infants.) The NICU will require all visitors to observe a strict sterile/sanitary protocol. Before entering the unit, all visitors—parents included—will have to "scrub in" much like a surgeon entering an operating room, scouring their hands and forearms with specially formulated hand soaps and medicated scrub bars. You may also be required to wear gowns, gloves, and surgical masks. The extent of the protocol will depend on the practices of the particular institution and on the sensitivity of your baby's condition. But over time, as we show in this chapter, you may come to feel at home here as your preemie makes her way through her program of intensive care. At the end of the day you may well find comfort in the routines and policies of the NICU and reassurance in the realization that all of these protocols are designed with your baby's health in mind.

For a number of reasons, we believe it is important for parents to become closely involved in caring for their infants amid the day-to-day rhythms of life in the NICU. For one, your baby, though small, is aware of her surroundings. Your infant will often be aware of your presence even when she shows no obvious outward sign of it. Second, participating in your baby's care will help you come to know the NICU staff and develop a level of comfort and confidence that she is being well cared for. That kind of confidence can be helpful during those nights when you wake up wondering how your baby is doing so far away from home.

Common Medical Procedures in the NICU

While in the NICU your baby will undergo a variety of diagnostic and therapeutic procedures. By "procedures" we mean everything from simple physical assessments to more invasive procedures like central lines or chest tubes performed by the unit's specially trained neonatal medical staff. Because of the self-contained nature of the NICU, the full range of medical procedures can be performed there—including surgery. Since it can be jarring to see procedures being performed in an area of the hospital that at first appearance might be a glorified nursery, we want to give you a sense of what to expect in the NICU. It will help you make a smoother transition to being an active, involved, and loving parent in this unusual medical environment. Following we survey some of the most common procedures that your baby will likely undergo while in the care of the neonatal medical staff.

ARTERIAL BLOOD GAS TESTS

Also known as ABGs, these are common laboratory tests performed on arterial blood samples that are essential to managing the effectiveness of your baby's respiratory health. The term *blood gases* refers to the oxygen and carbon dioxide levels in your infant's blood, as well as the blood's pH (acid/base) balance. A proper balance is essential to life (for adults and preemies alike). If your baby is on any kind of assisted respiration, ABG tests are an important tool the medical and nursing staff will use to assess the effectiveness of his respiratory therapy and make necessary adjustments.

BLOOD DRAWS

As the carrier of nutrients and oxygen through your baby's body, blood is one of the most important sources of information the neonatologist has on your baby's progress and health status. Blood tests are therefore frequently necessary to monitor your infant's health, regardless of his gestational age. The blood samples are usually taken from the baby's heels ("heel sticks"), which have a good blood supply. If your infant is very premature or has medical conditions that require an arterial catheter to be in place, the catheter may be used whenever blood draws are needed, thus sparing your preemie the need for frequent needle pricks, which can create exposure to infection.

PHYSICAL ASSESSMENT

Head-to-toe physical examinations of your infant are performed daily by the physicians and nurses in the NICU. The most comprehensive one, however, is given shortly after delivery. It is usually noninvasive—a painless procedure that the baby may very well sleep through. It entails an examination of the baby's lungs and heart using a stethoscope and an examination of the head (especially the soft spot, or *fontanel*), ears, palate, and eyes. Your baby's caregiver will also check for abdominal bloating (signaling problems in the intestine or other organs such as the kidneys), developed genitalia, good muscle tone, and symmetry (including overall posture and limb positions).

In addition to the physical assessment, the physician will frequently analyze and interpret lab data on your infant and review the nursing reports for the preceding twenty-four-hour period, the purpose being to make sure the infant is continuing to develop and mature without complication or undue stress.

EYE EXAMINATIONS

By the time hospital life has become a routine for you, your infant will have had several retinal examinations. The first will take place at about six weeks of age (and usually weekly thereafter) to look for abnormal development of the newly forming blood vessels in the retina. The retina is like a photographic plate that receives the light that allows the brain to form a picture. The more immature the baby, the less developed the retinal blood vessels and the higher the possibility of the blood vessels growing abnormally, leading to possible scarring of the retina. (See "Retinopathy of Prematurity [ROP]," page 220.) Because further development of the retinal blood vessels must occur after delivery, a preemie is at greater risk of having that development adversely affected by other factors (such as his overall immaturity or late-onset infections). A specially trained ophthalmologist will examine the infant's retinas with a bright light and magnifying glass after the pupils have been dilated, looking for abnormal blood vessel formation. He will try to determine how much of the retina is vascularized (contains blood vessels) and whether any abnormalities are present. Ask the ophthalmologist to explain his or her findings to you.

HEARING EXAMINATIONS

Prematurity places your baby at heightened risk for hearing impairment. Indeed, it is one of the most prevalent handicaps in the world, and people who were born prematurely constitute a disproportionately large share of the hearing-impaired population. Your baby's hearing will be tested before going home or shortly after discharge on an outpatient basis. Early detection of hearing disorders means early intervention and a better result.

A specially trained individual called an audiologist, working under the supervision of an ear, nose, and throat doctor, will perform this test in the NICU or step-down unit right before discharge. These are ideal environments for hearing tests, since they are so quiet. The test entails placing a cushioned metal receiver on your baby's head so as to detect electrical impulses that the brain gives off whenever your baby hears a sound. A large earphone, placed over one ear at a time, will emit different frequencies of sound and measure your baby's ability to hear each one.

If your baby does not pass this initial screening test, a more sophisticated test will be performed. Since impaired hearing is not a good reason to keep an infant in the hospital, this next test is usually performed later, on an outpatient basis.

NUTRITION

The difficulty that many preemies have in making the transition to the outside world reveals itself not only through respiratory trouble, but through feeding difficulties as well. The premature infant's stomach and intestines are seldom ready to begin digesting food and formula right away. Often the baby is busy fighting off small infections or other problems within the bowel, thus delaying his ability to digest food. Thus, as the neonatologist and his or her team assess your baby's health status, including his ability to tolerate feedings, your baby's nutritional needs will be met via intravenous feedings for a period that usually lasts several days—about forty-eight to seventy-two hours after birth. This is generally a simple dextrose (sugar) solution designed to be easily tolerated and sufficient to meet your infant's basic nutritional needs. It will contain additives such as sodium and potassium and calcium added as needed.

If your infant is looking good (if he is handling the IV feedings well and the neonatologist doesn't find any significant problems in the physical examination), he will graduate to an amino acid solution, which is richer in nutrients. It contains essential building blocks for protein (as well as electrolytes, trace elements, and vitamins) and is usually a yellowish clear fluid.

A fat solution may also be administered. This is a thicker, calorie-dense, white emulsion that is also administered by vein. Smaller quantities of this heavier, fat-rich substance will be needed.

This intravenous feeding program is known as *total parenteral nutrition,* or *TPN.* The term simply means that all of your baby's nutritional needs will be met intravenously until his stomach and bowel are ready for the main event—breast milk or formula feedings.

Naso-gastric (NG) Tube Feeding

A few days after birth, your baby will have matured to the point where the neonatologist can decide whether his bowel is mature enough to handle breast milk or formula for the first time. The time frame for this is highly variable and individual. Determining the baby's digestive maturity is a matter of trial and error. Very small amounts of breast milk or formula will be tried at first—as little as half a teaspoon. If the baby handles the initial small quantity—if he does not spit up, become bloated, and so on—the amount will be increased. When the neonatologist is trying your preemie with milk or formula, it's likely that your baby's ability to suck, swallow, and breathe isn't fully developed yet. Thus the neonatologist will use a

feeding technique that bypasses the immature suck-swallow-breathe mechanism: a naso-gastric (or NG) tube. Using an NG tube buys your baby the time to learn how to coordinate his sucking, swallowing, and breathing functions. It also saves the calories your baby would have burned while trying to do these things. Once that coordination has developed, the neonatologist will introduce expressed (pumped) breast milk or formula by nipple. The time frame for this progression is, again, very variable. Generally, however, by thirty-four weeks most preemies have the ability to

✤ FAQ:

"One time I was in the middle of feeding my baby and a nurse came over and told me to leave the NICU because of the shift change. Why all the secrecy?"

When the nursing staff has a shift change, comprehensive reports on the condition of each infant are given to the oncoming team. It is critical for the outgoing shift to update the incoming shift on developments on the medical status of each and every preemie in their care. To protect your and other parents' privacy (and to minimize crowding and other potential distractions for the staff), most NICUs have a no-visitors policy during these change-of-shift briefing periods so that the medical and nursing staff can freely discuss their charges' conditions and prognoses. The no-visitors periods typically last about an hour, twice a day.

coordinate sucking and swallowing. The quantities will be tiny at first, as little as a few cc's. As your baby shows the ability to tolerate these feedings, the amounts will increase. Eventually your baby will be strong enough to take from the breast or bottle on his own. He will make his way slowly and gradually into taking the nipple: at first, just one of his eight daily feedings will be delivered by nipple (breast or bottle). But as your baby succeeds with these nutritional baby steps, the number of nipple feedings will increase.

SONOGRAMS/ULTRASOUNDS

You may be familiar with the sonogram/ultrasound examination from your own visits to your obstetrician. Also performed by the hospital's radiology department, sonograms are a useful, noninvasive way for physicians to visualize what is going on inside your infant's body. The development of portable ultrasound equipment represents a major step forward in the ability of a neonatologist to evaluate a premature infant. These lightweight devices long ago took the place of bulky CAT (computerized tomography) scan equipment, the use of which required that premature infants be transferred, ventilators and all, to a hospital's radiology department. Portable ultrasound equipment has made that kind of inconvenience and risk a thing of the past. Sonograms, like CAT scans, can be performed on almost every organ of the body. For example, by passing an ultrasound transducer over the soft spot (or fontanel) in your baby's head, your physician will be able to take an early look at your baby's brain anatomy to check for any intracranial bleeding or abnormal brain anatomy or development.

ULTRASOUND OF THE HEAD. At around the same time your baby's neonatologist is thinking about beginning to wean your preemie off the respirator, he or she may also consider performing an ultrasound of her head to rule out a bleeding in the brain that can occur in premature infants. The initial ultrasound is usually done in the first seven to fourteen days of life but could be performed sooner if the neonatologist suspects a large hemorrhage into the brain. (See "Intraventricular Hemorrhage [IVH]", page 213.)

ULTRASOUND OF THE HEART. If your infant has a heart murmur (turbulent blood flow in the baby's heart caused by an abnormal blood vessel such as the ductus arteriosus or a structural problem such as an abnormal heart valve or abnormal heart anatomy), the neonatologist will usually ask a pediatric cardiologist to see the infant. The doctors will usually perform an *echocardiogram* (a noninvasive ultrasound of the heart) to confirm the diagnosis and recommend further tests and treatments such as heart medications (indomethacin) or surgery.

RESPIRATORY THERAPY

Since every premature infant's respiratory and oxygen needs are unique to his particular age, weight, and physical maturity, the respiratory team will have to monitor your baby closely in order to determine what assistance, if any, he'll need. Babies who spontaneously breathe on their own at birth will need less monitoring than infants who need artificial ventilation. Some may need only supplemental oxygen. All babies in the NICU will at least initially be monitored by one or a combination of pulse oximeters, apnea monitors, transcutaneous oxygen and carbon dioxide monitors, and a cardiopulmonary monitor (see chapter 4). A respiratory therapist specially trained in the use of this equipment will continually maintain the equipment and check on its proper use given your baby's evolving needs.

Most twenty-four-weekers, some twenty-eight-weekers, and a very few thirty-two-weekers will need mechanical respiration soon after birth. Again, this is a very individualized issue that depends heavily on a particular preemie's lung maturity. The usual course of treatment is for the preemie to progress from mechanical ventilation to a less invasive respiratory therapy such as CPAP or an oxygen tent or hood.

WEANING YOUR PREEMIE OFF THE RESPIRATOR

If your baby has been put on a respirator for any reason (the most common reasons are for treatment of hyaline membrane disease, pneumonia, infection, or severe overall immaturity), then the goal of her medical management will be the gradual reduction of respirator support so that she can slowly learn to breathe on her own. Typically the goal is to remove the baby from mechanical respiration within seven to fourteen days of birth. Of course, any attempt to give you a time frame in the NICU is subject to a great deal of variability.

Your baby's respiratory function will be closely watched as this reduction in support takes place. The primary means for measuring breathing efficiency is by monitoring the arterial blood gases from an arterial catheter. Alter-natively, pulse oximetry and transcutaneous oxygen monitors may also be helpful in measuring the efficiency of your infant's breathing. Pulse oximeters and transcutaneous oxygen monitors are not always precise and accurate in their particular measures, but they are often useful for discerning important overall trends in a baby's respiratory maturity.

As the neonatologist observes your preemie's progress toward unassisted respiration, he or she will first make sure that your infant can breathe rhythmically—that is, can inhale and exhale steadily, with no incidents of apnea (see page 162). Once that has been accomplished, then gradually the number of breaths per minute that the respirator provides your baby will be reduced. When the support from the respirator is minimal and the baby has demonstrated the ability to begin to breathe on her own, then she can be removed from the respirator. But that doesn't necessarily mean that respiratory support is over for good. Once the infant is breathing on her own, she may be placed into a plastic bubble (hood) with oxygen piped in. The oxygen-rich air helps your baby breathe more easily during the first few days off the respirator. Alternatively, if the neonatologist determines that your infant may need a higher level of respiratory support, nasal prongs attached to the respirator may be inserted in your baby's nostrils. This implements a therapy called *nasal continuous positive airway pressure or NCPAP.* (Regular CPAP, which is more intrusive, is administered via an endotracheal tube, not nasal prongs.) In this treatment, the respirator's sole purpose is to deliver a steady flow of warmed oxygen under pressure while the infant breathes on her own. The pressurized oxygen serves an important function: to prevent the muscles in the infant's lower throat from collapsing and blocking the lower airway. These muscles, which have very little tone, can collapse and obstruct the airway, leading to incidents of apnea.

Usually before a preemie is taken off the respirator, she will be given either IV or oral caffeine or theophylline, drugs that sensitize the infant's respiratory control system to the presence of carbon dioxide (CO_2 levels increase if breathing isn't adequate). Supporting the baby's respiratory control in this way helps her breathe more rhythmically, thereby reducing the frequency of apnea.

After discharge, most infants will not need any further treatment with caffeine or require monitoring at home, since the most common causes of apnea are overall immaturity of the respiratory center and poor muscle tone in the lower throat. Both of these conditions tend to disappear with time as your baby matures. If the apnea persists beyond thirty-four to thirty-five weeks corrected gestational age (which is simply gestational age at birth plus the number of weeks since birth), then your baby will need a more focused examination to determine the cause of the breathing pauses.

Getting your baby off the respirator in the first seven to fourteen days is an important accomplishment. But it can be a more complicated process if she has simultaneous infections or if her patent ductus arteriosus (PDA) is still open (see page 215).

X-RAYS

X-rays are designed to take a picture of bones and air-filled structures such as the lungs or the intestine. When physical examinations and lab-oratory tests don't provide the answer, X-rays are a quick way to identify an underlying cause for your baby's symptoms or condition. If these tests don't identify a single cause of particular symptoms, they can help narrow down the possible range of causes.

Any radiology tests ordered by your infant's physician will be performed by a radiology technician. The specialized machinery needed for the X-ray is usually brought right to the infant's bedside, where the test will be performed. This is much easier and safer than taking the child to the X-ray department. An X-ray, which is painless to your child, will provide his caregivers a useful window on his health.

Since they are sensitive to the danger that radiation levels may pose to these tiniest of newborns, most neonatalogists will use X-rays sparingly, and only when important information can be gained from them. (The same philosophy holds true for echocardiograms, blood gases, and other tests typically performed on preemies.)

Parenting in the NICU

COMING TO TERMS WITH THE UNEXPECTED

Many of us have dreamed about becoming parents since our dating days. For others, it's something that's been anticipated since childhood. Though it's easy to believe, during the time immediately before and after delivery of a premature infant, that those dreams have been shattered, we hope to show you in this section how and why it is very possible that you can reclaim those dreams.

At first glance it seems that parents of full-term babies have an easy time realizing these dreams. The parent-child bond, which has grown and strengthened throughout the uncomplicated "perfect pregnancy," deepens when the baby is placed into his parents' arms immediately after delivery, and holding, cuddling, picture taking and breast-feeding take place within hours of birth. The closeness they share with their newborn is immediate, an unforgettable, transcendant experience.

As we have already pointed out, parents of preemies appear to be cheated out of most of these wonderful experiences. Susan, who delivered her 4-pound-4-ounce son at 31½ weeks after a difficult but successful bout with preterm labor, said: "I never got to experience the full-term pregnancy. My baby was in the hospital for three weeks after I was discharged. It was a very lonely, very empty feeling. In a way, I almost started thinking about having another child right away—I think I probably felt that I wanted to have the chance to do things right. I felt I was cheated out of a positive birthing experience the first time around."

Your pregnancy may have been beset with disturbing or debilitating complications. You may have spent weeks on bed rest, during which time you may even have come to resent your infant. After delivery, bonding with a preemie can be a much more gradual process, for often both mother and baby need to be hospitalized and medically stabilized before normalcy can resume for either of them. As a result of any or all of these factors, it may take days or even weeks or months before you are able to start feeling a real parental connection with your baby.

"It was drilled into me in nursing school that a mother simply had to spend time bonding with her newborn, so with Aaron I became afraid of being labeled as someone who was not able to bond with her son. I lived an hour away from the NICU and couldn't get there every day. And I was still sick. I cried and talked to a lot of the professionals at the hospital. They reassured me that this happens to many parents. By the time I had my second son, Ryan, I had learned that I needed to get well before I could worry about bonding, and I was able to rest easier about the whole bonding issue. I knew that the staff loved him. They also knew how sick I was. I did what I could to rest and get better. I took it as a chance to get rested and well before my babies came home. I learned to look at the silver lining on my black cloud."

—Kelly

"WHY DON'T I FEEL ANYTHING FOR THIS BABY?"

This feeling of loss—the loss of a long-dreamed-of birthing experience, and the bonding experience with the long-awaited newborn—is typical for new parents of preemies who have to spend their first weeks and months of life in an NICU. As you adjust your life to caring for the special needs of a preemie, the feeling of loss can affect the way you view your child long after she is born. There are a multitude of reasons for it. A person's true feelings about an experience—of joy, relief, happiness—can take time to evolve, especially in situations where the pregnancy has been high-risk throughout and your worst fears have been at the front of your mind for weeks or even months. Emotional withdrawal is a natural response to fear. If you have had a previous fetal loss or losses and are now trying again to have a child, you might reflexively dread the idea of re-visiting pregnancy—which you may associate with gut-wrenching emotions such as fear, anger, helplessness, loneliness, loss, and guilt. If you delivered prematurely in a previous pregnancy, you may not be looking forward to re-peating the experience. In such cases it is normal to build a protective barrier between your innermost emotions and the potentially harsh reality of premature delivery. When the fears go unrealized and a relatively healthy pre-mature newborn is in front of you, those barri-ers usually take a while to melt away.

There are other factors that can keep you from bonding with your preemie at the outset. A delay in bonding can be a precaution your psy-che takes to keep you from getting too attached to a baby whom you may think has a less than guaranteed chance of survival or who is at risk of having serious disabilities. Some parents we in-terviewed described a state of mind where they did not allow themselves to feel warm, parental emotions or anticipate their babies' arrival, all in the hope of avoiding pain and suffering should the worst happen. They got along the best they could, trying to keep a positive outlook, but all the while avoiding the attachments that might otherwise lead to bitter disappointment. For other people, to paraphrase a recent book, hope is a muscle. For them, an optimistic outlook, even a cautious one, is natural and even essen-tial. Such people may take comfort in family, in friends, or in faith as they hold out hope for a positive end to the story. Though such people may expose themselves to greater depths of grief if the worst happens, they may be more inclined to find joy in the moment after birth, no matter how hard the road that got them there.

Though some parents are able to pick them-selves up and parent their preemies like full-termers, experience has taught us that many parents need a lot of time and a lot of support to get to this place. We feel this is important to emphasize. We want you to understand that if you are having any of these feelings, you are not alone. And we hope that as you read this book, you will be able to take comfort knowing that you are in good company, and that in time you will be able to work past many if not all of these barriers to becoming emotionally engaged with your premature infant, no matter how big a challenge that may seem at this early stage in your parenthood.

The many parents we have interviewed have been very generous in sharing their stories with us so that you will better understand the rhythms of NICU parenting. It is important that you appreciate the essential importance of your role as a preemie parent and the special and unique bond that you will be working toward, a bond that will last a lifetime and be stronger for the difficulties you faced together with your child in his or her earliest days of life.

GETTING TO KNOW YOUR BABY

In the first few days and weeks of life in the NICU, you and your baby will gradually be getting to know each other.

Marie, a thirty-seven-year-old executive at a large consulting firm, remembers the first time she saw her daughter, Sonia, a thirty-four-weeker born at 5 pounds 8 ounces with Apgar scores of 7 and 8. "The reality of it all hit me when I finally saw Sonia. They had her wired up to everything, and I realized then that I wouldn't be able to hold her for at least several days. The whole time I was pretty unhappy about what was going on. But when I looked at the two-pounders in the nearby warmers, I realized it could be way worse.

"I stroked Sonia while she was lying in her bed. She didn't seem to like it. I seemed to be touching her too lightly, annoying her or tickling her or something. When I got to hold her

---

On Being an NICU Parent

Kelly, the mother of two preemies, offers these tips:

- Try to be involved in your baby's care as much as you can in the NICU. There are plenty of people to give you reassurance and guidance while you are there.
- Take special mementos and keep them by your baby's isolette. We had a special teddy bear and even hung a stocking on Aaron's bed because Santa had to visit him there.
- If your preemie has siblings, take them to visit [in line with your NICU's possibly strict rules about young visitors]. We weren't going to take Aaron to visit Ryan, but we were told that it might help him understand what was going on. He was only twenty-one months old, and it was the best thing that we could have ever done. He was so proud and so excited to see him. He washed his hands and touched Ryan through the isolette. He touched Ryan's little foot and said, "Look, Mama, he got little piggies." We were very busy with him and didn't get to take pictures, but it is just such a beautiful memory.

---

finally, I was nervous that she would fuss. But when the nurse placed her in my arms, she settled down immediately, as if to say, 'This is the way things should be.' Being rocked in my lap, she seemed to know where she belonged. It was a real rush."

Kimberly, the mother of twin girls delivered at twenty-four weeks, one of whom did not survive, said, "It was one thing to touch her on the warming table. It was another thing to hold her." Her daughter Mary McClain was on a respirator for about ten days, then on CPAP for forty more. She spent four months and four days in the NICU. Often infants on respirators can't be held by their parents. But because Kimberly, a teacher, had taught one of the children of one of the NICU nurses, she was allowed to do it. "It was all so overwhelming," she said.

As we have mentioned many times throughout this book, your baby's gestational age will play a large role in how much interaction he will be capable of in the earliest days of life. The more mature the infant, the longer he will be able to be held, the more interaction he will give you. But even for the most premature babies, some parent interaction is possible and indeed recommended. Even though in many cases you will feel as if you are doing nothing, sitting passively by the bedside, an important foundation is being built. You'll be getting to know your baby and learning what his behavioral cues are. Your baby, in turn, will learn to sense your presence and to learn your voice and speech patterns.

Your preemie's behavioral cues, or individual activity patterns, are the indicators we will focus on now as we continue to introduce you to the rhythms of life in the NICU.

CUES TO YOUR PREEMIE'S BEHAVIOR

To help you get more acquainted with your baby, in this section we will build on what you have already learned about your baby in relationship to his gestational age from chapter 5,

"Your Preemie's Growth and Maturation." We will discuss your baby's behavior in terms of his responses or cues to the stimulation he receives from the outside world. Additionally, we will discuss what behaviors can be specific to certain physical or emotional needs of your baby. We hope to arm you with indicators about your baby's needs, so that when he shows these behavioral signs, you will be able to assess the situation and step in as needed. Taking care of these simpler needs can be a great source of empowerment; anything you can do helps you grow into your role as an NICU parent. Of course, we also hope to help you distinguish even subtle differences about your baby's behavior that might indicate the need to seek professional medical intervention.

Learning to pick up on your baby's individual cues will take some time and patience. Your baby's individual character and behavior is already within him. All children are born with different ways of responding to the world, and two infants will respond to the same stimulus or express the same need in various ways. Understanding and distinguishing among different preemie behaviors is important because they are working so hard, expending so many valuable calories, when they try to communicate their needs. Therefore the more promptly their needs are met, the less effort they will exert conveying them and the more energy they can apply to more useful tasks such as growing and feeding and interacting with and getting to know their parents.

For the sake of simplicity, we have organized your baby's activities into three main behavioral categories:

• Awake/interactive behavior

- Sleep behavior
- Stress behavior

Awake/Interactive Behavior

Although it is natural for parents, first-time and experienced alike, to expect their infants to respond to voice, touch, and sight, preemies are seldom able to oblige. The twenty-four-weeker will probably not exhibit any of the signs we identify here that she is ready to interact with you. However, as your baby matures, she will grow in her ability to tell you when she is ready to play. A thirty-two-weeker will have short periods during the day when she is ready to "play." Of course, we don't mean "play" in the literal sense. But it is play nonetheless, in its own special way.

The following are interaction cues—the things preemies may do to express their desire to interact.

- Alert behavior
- Good eye contact
- Calmness when held
- Looking and listening, even if for brief periods
- Relaxed appearance

As your baby matures, her active/alert time periods will become longer and more frequent. These periods of interactive wakefulness can be some wonderfully special moments for parents who have waited patiently, week after week, for their preemie to "wake up." But the important thing to remember is, don't overdo it. Your preemie is still very easily overstimulated, so keep a watch out for her stress cues, even as she is exhibiting interaction cues.

"I remember how David would wake up from one of his long naps and just fix me with his flat, black little eyes," said Jim, the thirty-three-year-old father of a 3-pound-4-ounce preemie born at thirty-two weeks. "He seemed to be saying, 'I know you. I trust you. Please say something to me.' In moments like this, he would have this tremendous sense of calm about him. I remember his first sonogram. His bony little hand appeared to be giving us the thumbs-up sign. When he would look at me like that, lying there in his radiant warmer with an IV line stuck in his scalp, I knew he was keeping true to his word—that this was all going to work out all right."

TIP

Keep a journal or notepad handy so that you can write down important information about your baby's daily routine, including sleeping or feeding schedules, doctors' statements on your baby's status, or any questions you think of to ask the staff later. This way you won't forget your questions and you can easily give your spouse or family members a quick update on your baby's condition or progress whenever they ask (which will be all the time). You will also begin to develop a picture of your baby's sleep patterns.

Sleep Behavior

As we have previously discussed, your preemie will spend a very large portion of the day sleeping, at much as 75 to 80 percent of it in some cases. Since sleep is such a critical element of the growth and development of your baby, it is important to get to know your baby's schedule.

The NICU staff can help you develop a picture of your baby's sleep patterns. When you aren't in the NICU yourself (please take good care of yourself and don't succumb to the temptation to live there), they can make a running record of when your baby is asleep and awake. Talk to the staff about your wish to have this information, and write it down if you want to.

Once you have gotten a sense of the rhythms of your preemie's sleep life, work your schedule around your baby's. Visit when your baby is awake, and take care of errands (there will be a million of them) when your baby is asleep. Don't expect the NICU staff to let you hold or wake your baby in accordance with your own agenda or schedule. Remember, your baby is in the NICU for a good medical reason. It is therefore imperative to stay on the NICU's schedule. The around-the-clock administration of medications, feedings, assessments, and other NICU protocols and procedures must mesh with your baby's natural sleep schedule in order to minimize the toll it takes on his energy reserves. Since your baby will be sleeping most of the day, these procedures will need to be interspersed in between sleep periods whenever possible. When you consider that feedings alone will need to be given every two or three hours or so, you begin to appreciate the importance of giving your baby as much uninterrupted sleep as possible.

✤ Stress Behavior

Your preemie will give you a wide range of cues to indicate stress. These can take on many forms, and can convey a variety of particular messages: "I need a break from being held," "Something is not right," "I'm wet," "I'm hungry," "I need a new position," or "I'm overstimulated." As you get to know your baby better, and with the help of the neonatal nurses who care for her for hours at a time, you will become increasingly in tune with her different stress cues. Many things can stress your baby, and in time you will understand what you need to do to console her and make your baby more comfortable.

Remember: You're the Boss (but Be a Good Boss)

As you attune yourself to the busy rhythms of the NICU, remember this: You, as the parent, are welcome in the unit at all times (with the important exception of shift change). If you just want to sit by and quietly watch your baby while she is sleeping, if you want to be present for every feeding, even late into the night, the unit is open to you. A good NICU staff should encourage parent involvement.

Of course, it is important for you to communicate your plans to the NICU staff. If you intend to be present and administer the ten P.M. feeding, just let them know and they will make sure the necessary supplies are available. Likewise, if you make arrangements to visit your baby for a certain feeding and you can't make it, let them know if at all possible. For example, if they are counting on you to breast-feed for that ten P.M. feeding, they won't prepare anything at bedside. If you don't make it to the hospital for the feeding, your baby's delicate sleep and feeding schedule can be thrown off as the staff scrambles at the last minute to take care of the feeding themselves. Good communication with the staff (and this goes both ways) is the foundation of a good working relationship with them.

"The nurses would come over when I was doing skin-to-skin care (see page 196) with Sonia and tell me it was time to put her down so she could get some rest," Marie said. "I remember being annoyed once when they were sort of pushy about it. 'Go away,' I wanted to tell them, 'I'm rocking her, and she's getting plenty of rest right now.' "

Lisa, the mother of a thirty-four-week, 6-pound-6-ounce premature baby boy who had severe respiratory distress at birth, said, "Remember, this is *your* baby, not the hospital's baby. They were always telling me when I could pick him up, when I could feed him and couldn't feed him. Well, you don't have to slavishly obey every one of their whims. This is easier said than done. People often feel helpless and powerless. I was intimidated—by the system, by the atmosphere. Sometimes I felt like this was their child and I was a visitor."

On-the-Job Training

As we hope is clear by now, you won't be on your own while you are caring for your baby in the NICU. While we don't mean to gloss over the very real stresses and trials of neonatal ward parenting, it is true that the on-the-job training you get from the NICU staff is one of the unexpected benefits of being exposed to life in neonatal intensive care. If it's any consolation, picture the new parent who brought a full-term baby home two days after delivery, struggling to learn how to feed her baby. By the time you get home, you'll be a lot less likely to have such trouble, thanks to the instruction and demonstrations you'll receive in the NICU.

For the first-time parent, assistance from the pros is bound to be especially welcome. Try to make the most of your time as an NICU parent and learn all that you can about your baby's care from the staff. You'll have most of your contact with your baby's primary nurse. This is the person whom you will probably get to know the best. The primary nurse is a registered nurse who is responsible for tending to almost all of your baby's care and performing all of the procedures that don't require a neonatologist. The neonatal unit's nurses will be at your baby's bedside twenty-four hours a day.

It is important to develop a good relationship with your baby's nurse. Many parents have described to us how their relationship with the nurses while in the NICU helped them through the whole experience. When you leave to go home for the night, it's very comforting to know that your baby is in such good hands.

Jackie was thirty-seven when she delivered her older son, Ryan, via a cesarean delivery at thirty-three weeks. Of the several distinct miracles that the mother of two from Madison, Wisconsin, recalled during her preemie experience (not the least of which was the inexplicable "sealing over" of her membrane following a bout with PROM at twenty-four weeks, which probably saved her son's life), one of the most welcome was the entrance into her life of a veteran neonatal RN who went by the nickname "Grandma Donna."

JOE GARCIA-PRATS: "I once overheard one of my wise mentors giving some good advice to the parents of a newly born premature infant who had just been admitted to the intensive care unit. 'I would recommend that you get neither too excited on the good days of your infant's hospital course nor too disheartened when your baby has had a bad day,' he said. 'As long as things are better this week than last week, then that's progress and that is good indeed.' "

"She was this sort of Supernurse," Jackie said. "Everyone who's ever spent time in the NICU here knows her. She taught us everything, from how to get a preemie to latch on to a nipple, to how to dress and bathe him, to how to relax a little bit. She had this incredibly empowering attitude. She made *us* take charge. The other nurses were also very good, but many of them wanted to do everything for us. I really appreciated Grandma Donna's way of making us dig in like that.

"She was very good at letting you know what to expect around the next corner. After our son came home, he had the 'gruntsy groansies'—he'd make these grunting and groaning sounds almost constantly. It was the most god-awful thing you'd ever heard. This little guy did it all the time. I guess it was just part of his immature digestive system. Grandma Donna had warned us about that, which made it a lot easier to deal with. Too bad we never got around to taping it.

"If it wasn't for Grandma Donna, we wouldn't have gotten a lot of important information. She was very old school. It was very nice to have her as a resource."

Your baby will probably have several different nurses. Units that rotate nurses like that will strive to maintain continuity of care. And even if you have several nurses, you'll get to know them soon enough. If you visit frequently, you'll have the warm feeling of seeing familiar faces there.

WHAT YOU CAN DO IN THE NICU

Getting involved in your baby's NICU care can be a very rewarding job. This bond is en-

Doctors Are from Mars, Nurses Are from Venus

Doctors and nurses are often very different in their manner of dealing with you and communicating to you. Most physicians tend to focus on medical information and plans of care. They say things like "Your daughter had a great twenty-four hours. She came down on the oxygen, the anemia is under control, and her antibiotics are finished. Things are looking very good."

Nurses, on the other hand, often have a different perspective, as you would expect from people who take care of fundamental day-to-day needs as well as watching vital signs. (Nothing sexist is intended here: nurses are still closely involved in developing the goals and plans for the baby that day.) They are more inclined to say things like "You son seemed to be very alert today. He slept real well, though he was a little bit irritable in the morning. I think he misses you."

Because of their continuing daily involvement in the details of your child's NICU life, nurses can become among your closest friends. As one mother recalled, "When my son Timmy was in the hospital, there was one nurse who became extra special to us. She was very competent and professional, of course. But her warmth, caring, and empathy set her apart from everyone else involved in his care. There was a certain amount of tenderness and an understanding of our concerns as parents."

hanced as your baby matures and you are able to have more direct contact with her. As your baby's gestational age increases, her needs will progress from many of the life-sustaining measures of the early NICU days to more hands-on care such as feeding, diapering, bathing, holding, and even kangaroo care (skin-to-skin contact, see page 196). There are so many important firsts that will take place here: the first time you hold your baby, the first breast-feeding experience, the first diaper change. These activities are very important first steps to starting and continuing the bonding process with your child.

DIAPERING. Diapers need changing every few hours. Changing diapers at the start of each feeding is a good way to be sure it happens regularly enough. You'll be amazed by how many diapers you go through in the NICU, but it won't really hit you till you come home and you're the one picking them up at the grocery store.

CORD CARE. Infections can easily find a home in the little crevices around the remnants of your baby's umbilical cord. Until the last of your baby's cord dries up and falls off the abdomen, you will need to swab it with isopropyl alcohol every time you change a diaper.

CHECKING TEMPERATURE. If your infant is no longer hooked up to a monitor that records her temperature, along with other vital signs, you will need to check her temperature several times a day (at least once per shift). This is usually done in the armpit.

BATHING YOUR PREEMIE. In the clean environment of the NICU, your baby won't be bathed frequently. It won't be done at all, in fact, until your preemie is close to being ready to go home (see chapter 8, "The Intermediate Care Nursery"). At that stage, every three or four days your baby will be bathed in a small basin filled with warm water and a very mild soap solution. Extreme care must be used because wet little preemies tend to be slippery to hold. But this is good practice for you to have before your baby goes home.

🌿 TIP

Remember, the NICU is open to parents twenty-four hours a day. If you want to call in to check on your infant in the middle of the night, feel free. Keep the NICU's phone number handy for easy reference. A quick call to the unit for a nighttime report can provide just the reassurance you need to help you have a good night's sleep yourself.

HOLDING. It's one of the enduring mysteries of parenting: your baby will find comfort in your arms that no one else can provide. Even amid the distractions of life in the NICU, your preemie will know when you are near. Although removing your baby from the incubator won't be possible in the first few weeks of life owing to temperature concerns (this is particu-

larly true for very premature infants in the twenty-four- to thirty-week range), once your infant's temperature is stabilized, skin-to-skin care will be possible. Skin-to-skin care (sometimes referred to as "kangaroo care") is nothing more than placing your infant, wearing only a diaper, under your shirt so that skin-to-skin contact can take place. The benefits of this therapy are thought to be considerable. (See the more complete discussion of skin-to-skin care later in this chapter.)

Cori remembers her first cuddle with her twenty-four-weeker: "I wasn't able to hold him for almost two weeks, and when I did it was for only about five minutes. My mother and I had gone to visit, and the nurse (one of my favorites) told me not to have a heart attack, but that she was going to allow me to hold him. She reached in, picked him up, and handed him to me. It was shocking . . . exhilarating. It totally caught me by surprise. I don't think I took a breath through the whole thing. She ran around like crazy trying to find a Polaroid camera to preserve the moment. As she handed him to me that first time, my mom and I just stood there, crying and looking down at my beautiful son. Oh, what a joy."

POSITIONING. Your infant probably doesn't have enough muscular strength to roll over or move his head. Thus it is important to change your baby's position every few hours. This has a number of benefits:

- Turning his head from one side to the other may provide an enjoyable change of scenery from the bed—and also prevent the preemie's soft skull from molding flat on the side he prefers to lie on.

- Changing the positioning of the limbs, head, and torso will compel your baby to use different muscles and thus assist overall muscular development.

✹ TIP

If your preemie seems to have a preference for particular scenery, such as the light coming from a nearby window, reverse her position in the bed (flipping her around so her head is where her feet were). This forces her to turn her body the other way and use the muscles on the other side to continue enjoying the view.

DRESSING. Your infant should have her clothes changed at least once or twice a day. They get soiled frequently, and for sanitary reasons, it's smart to make sure your preemie is wearing clean clothes whenever possible. There is also a psychological benefit: It can be heartening for you and your family and friends to see your tiny little premature infant in a fresh set of clean clothes and in new colors. (You're never too young to have some style.)

SWADDLING. You will get used to seeing your baby all wrapped up in a square broadcloth. Keeping your baby so snug serves to keep him warm and also keeps the monitor contacts firmly in place. It won't take long for you to get good at getting your preemie wrapped up like a "baby burrito."

✹

While these "parenting" skills may seem elementary to you, when you add a preemie to the scenario, these procedures can take on a whole

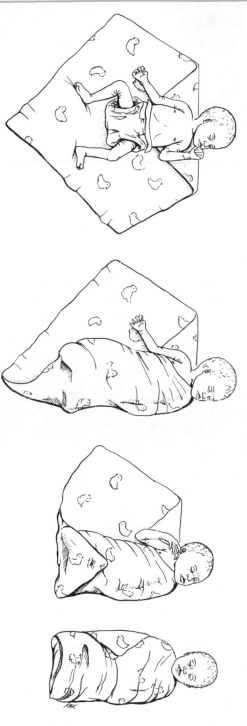

How to make a "baby burrito" (three frames)

more than you can imagine to make you feel like a parent and help you bond with your child while in intensive care.

✿ TIP

Remember, this is your baby. Get involved. Ask questions. Take the initiative to be an active participant in your preemie's NICU life. The more involved you get, the stronger the bond you will feel toward your child, and the more attached he or she will become to you.

"Until I got involved in the daily care of my preemie son," said Jim, "the NICU seemed like a mysterious, inscrutable place. But once I found out where the diapers were kept, where the breast milk was stored, and how to get that darn apnea monitor to quit squealing, I started to feel I belonged there, and I became a lot more confident that what was keeping my son alive wasn't the smoke and mirrors of modern medical technology, but his own little life force that would not be denied, no matter how many high-tech devices surrounded his crib."

new complexity. First, your preemie will most likely be attached to all sorts of wires and monitors. He may also have an IV line or central line, making some of these procedures difficult. Additionally, your preemie's muscles haven't fully matured so he'll be a little floppy and more difficult to hold and position. As frustrating as that might be, remember: Tasks like these are the job of the parent. It is better that you perform them than someone else. Mastering and performing these seemingly trivial tasks will do

FEEDING YOUR PREEMIE

Earlier in this chapter we described how nutrition is one of the most important aspects of your baby's treatment while in the hospital. We described how your preemie will make the transition from IV feedings to oral feedings. Once your baby has made the necessary progress—having gotten to the point where she can feed by nipple, be it breast or bottle—it will be time for you to make the transition, too. It will be time for you to become involved in your baby's feeding regimen. Feeding your infant becomes the next step toward becoming more involved as an NICU parent.

✒ The First Question: Breast or Bottle?

Once your preemie is able to take milk feedings, you should still be able to breast-feed if you are so inclined. However, due to your baby's immaturity and overall lack of strength, you may have to wait a little while longer to bring your baby directly to your breast for feeds. Most premature babies are unable to breast-feed directly because they lack the strength and coordination to do so. But don't worry, these skills will be learned in time. Until then your baby can still receive your expressed milk by gavage feeding (see page 158) or by bottle. If bottle feedings are used, special nipples are available that are rigid enough to help teach babies the sucking technique but flexible enough to allow for easier milk flow, preventing your preemie from having to work so hard to get these valuable nutrients.

Expressing (or pumping) your breast milk is a wonderful way to deliver valuable nutrients, as well as immune system stimulants, to your baby. Mother's milk is not only an excellent natural source of these nutrients, but also an invaluable link in the mother-baby bond.

If you have made the decision to breast-feed your preemie, you will need some guidance. For this you will need to see a lactation consultant. This is a nurse specially trained in assisting mothers with breast-feeding problems. Most hospitals will have one or more on staff to work with new mothers. You may have already had contact with a lactation specialist when you were on the postpartum floor. If not, don't hesitate to seek one out if you feel you need additional assistance. The NICU staff should be able to help you set up an appointment to see one in the unit.

Joan, the veteran obstetric nurse at a busy Canadian hospital, successfully held off preterm labor for seventeen weeks, delivering healthy twins at thirty-seven weeks. If that wasn't enough of a challenge, she had trouble breast-feeding, too. "Breast-feeding is a learned skill," she said, "not a natural one that happens automatically when we become mothers. When women grew up in families that lived close to each other, they watched their sisters and aunts breast-feeding, and they learned the skill. But it's not like brushing your teeth. Lactation consultants are routinely needed to help new mothers get up to speed." When you have a preemie who is probably not strong or mature enough to latch on right away, the need for help is only magnified.

As a new mom of a preemie, you will most likely need some education on breast-feeding and also on the use of the breast pump. There are two basic types of breast pumps: manual and electric. Both work equally well, though the electric is probably faster if this is an issue. The major difference in pumps is probably the price. Of course, the price is usually just rolled into your hospital bill. The manual pump is the least expensive. Electric pumps are much more expensive and can be either purchased outright or rented by the month. If you are planning on pumping for a long time or having more children, purchasing one might be more economical in the long run. If you are planning to continue to breast-feed after returning to work, or if you travel with your job, you might find

Tips for Success in Pumping/Expressing Breast Milk

- Borrow or rent an electric breast pump.
- Begin pumping milk within twenty-four to seventy-two hours of delivery in order to stimulate milk production.
- Pump every two to three hours: it will sustain milk production.
- Get plenty of rest—you'll be more patient and relaxed.
- Drink plenty of water (eight to ten glasses a day).
- Avoid alcohol, caffeinated beverages, and fizzy liquids, which can promote gas in the baby.
- Bear in mind that there is some evidence that cow's milk, cheese, chocolate, eggs, cabbage, caffeine, and heavily seasoned foods can cause gas and abdominal discomfort in the breast-fed baby.

Tips for Successful Breast-Feeding

- Breast-feed when your baby is most alert.
- Find a comfortable position.
- Place your feet on a stool.
- Position pillows for comfort.
- Try different positions until you find one that works best for you and baby. (The "football hold" is a popular one.)
- Squeeze a few drops of milk into your baby's mouth for encouragement.
- Take good care of yourself: get plenty of rest and fluids.

the electrical pump more convenient. But the choice is up to you.

As your baby matures and his condition stabilizes, he will eventually be able to breast-feed directly. This will most likely be a gradual process. This progression toward full breast feeds can be achieved by gradually introducing the breast to your infant between bottle feeds. This process of weaning the baby off the bottle and onto the breast has proven to be an effective way for babies to continue to get the needed nutrients while easing the transition to an unfamiliar delivery method.

For health-related or personal reasons, some mothers are unable or choose not to breast-feed. If this is the case, there are a variety of special infant formulas on the market that will provide your baby with needed nutrients. Even babies that are fed breast milk will often need to have their nutrition supplemented with formula, at least until the mother's milk supply catches up to meet all of the baby's needs. Ask your doctor for recommendations.

✍ TIP

Some larger companies have benefit packages that allow their employees to get assistance with the purchase of a breast pump. Also, check with your company to see whether any kind of private areas or rooms are available for breast milk pumping.

Whether you breast-feed or bottle-feed, the time spent feeding is an extension of the dependent physiological relationship that has existed between you and your baby since conception. If, as is common, you feel like an outsider in the NICU, you may find that the time you spend feeding your baby is especially rewarding. At the same time, the simple impossibility of being present for all of your baby's feedings during a twenty-four-hour period may become a source of frustration for you. If you wish to breast-feed but can't be there for all eight or ten feedings throughout the day, the NICU staff will arrange to store your breast milk in a specially designated refrigerator so that nurses can give your baby your milk round-the-clock. By replenishing the supply when you visit, you will ensure that your baby receives your milk at every feeding. Whether you feed your baby infant formula or breast milk, a staff nurse or nurse's assistant will administer feedings via bottle whenever you can't be there.

❧ TIP

When you're learning to breast-feed your preemie, pack a bagload of patience with the diapers. Remember, direct breast-feeding can be challenging at times even with a full-term baby. Your preemie may not be strong enough to latch on and suck steadily. Be patient with yourself and your baby. While you're in the hospital, don't hesitate to ask the nurses for help—or commiseration—and seek assistance from the hospital's lactation consultant as needed.

If you maintain a supply of your own milk in the NICU's refrigerator, be sure you clearly label each bottle with your name and the date the milk was pumped. The NICU staff has a procedure in place to double-check your milk for name and date, just as they would many medications, prior to administration. This will help to ensure that only your milk is given to your baby. Each institution will have a carefully detailed set of instructions for you on how to store your milk, how to label it, and where to bring it for storage and safekeeping. Be sure to inquire about your hospital's policy for the storing of breast milk.

Depending on their policy, a hospital will allow expressed breast milk to be stored for only a certain length of time. Forty-eight to seventy-two hours is typical if the milk is refrigerated directly after pumping. However, it can be frozen for much later use, in which case it can last for up to six months. Most hospitals have a policy about giving only fresh milk to preemies, not frozen, since they believe that milk loses its nutrients the longer it stays frozen. They believe that preemies, with their immature immune systems, need to have the most nutrient-packed meals possible. Once you get home, however, a ready supply of expressed breast milk in the freezer can be a tremendous convenience.

When defrosting frozen breast milk, let it thaw in a container of warm water for about thirty minutes. Microwaving it is thought to destroy nutrients. And never try to refreeze thawed breast milk.

❧ TIP

If you've provided expressed breast milk to the NICU to give to your baby when you are not available, always be sure to label each bottle clearly with your and your infant's names and the date you pumped the milk.

Whichever type of feeding you give to your baby, remember: Feeding time is important time, and some of the most special parent-baby moments are spent while feeding your baby.

The Advantages of Breast-Feeding

You may or may not be able to provide adequate quantities of breast milk for your baby. The use of mother's milk requires a great commitment by mom and a good deal of support from dad as well. If that commitment can be met, there are many health advantages that derive from feeding preterm infants breast milk (after they are stabilized), among them:

- Reducing the occurrence of necrotizing enterocolitis
- Improving feeding tolerance
- Strengthening your infant's immune system

If your baby is restricted as to how much milk she can take per day, breast milk fortifier may be added to your milk. The fortifier contains extra protein, calories, and minerals, which enhance the nutritional value of the breast milk when used at such low volumes.

TIP

Remember to keep your breast pump kit (and extra bottles along with ice packs and a small cooler, all labeled with your and your baby's names) handy at all times. This will allow you to pump and store the milk whenever you need to, thus relieving discomfort, keeping you on a pumping schedule if you are out and about, and ensuring you'll have milk handy when you visit the hospital. Most hospitals will usually have private, comfortable pumping rooms adjacent to the NICU that mom can use. Often these rooms are equipped with electric pumps. You simply attach your own tubing. If the busy NICU staff hasn't mentioned this to you, be sure to ask. These rooms can really be a nice convenience for NICU parents.

SKIN-TO-SKIN CARE (KANGAROO CARE)

Direct skin-to-skin contact with your baby is believed to be greatly beneficial to a premature infant's development. Your baby, clothed only in a diaper, is placed under your shirt on your bare chest. The time allowed for this care varies according to the status of the infant and the opinion of the doctor—anywhere from thirty minutes to an hour is typical. This is a wonderful form of bonding with your baby that more and more NICUs are adopting all of the time. Your baby will need to be medically stable before skin-to-skin care is possible. That means essentially that he should be able to maintain his heart and lung status and his body temperature while with you outside the incubator. But when he is mature enough, the staff will let you know. This can be an exciting time with the son or daughter with whom you have had so little contact. Ask the staff nurses from time to time to see when you can anticipate your baby's readiness.

Skin-to-skin care has been shown to achieve several purposes. Not only does it increase the parent-baby bond, but resting comfortably in the warmth of a parent's chest is believed to enhance the baby's overall well-being by stabilizing his heart rate, supporting him in maintaining body temperature while out of the incubator, and helping him maintain an even respiratory rate. It is a wonderful way for parents—mothers and fathers alike—to have some special time with their child. Through this contact the parents as well as the babies benefit, both with the emotional and the physical bond. This should really be no surprise. Human contact is an essential need, and babies are no different from adults. All living things thrive if nurtured.

One of the wonderful things about skin-to-skin care is its low-tech, holistic nature. Unlike the many other high-technology aspects of neonatology, skin-to-skin care treats the "whole person," both physically and emotionally. It supports and strengthens certain unmeasurable aspects of an infant's well-being. And it represents the love you have, and will increasingly feel, toward a little person who began life under less than optimal conditions.

Cori, mother of a twenty-four-weeker born after she'd developed placental abruption, remembers her first experience with skin-to-skin contact with her son. "One of my happiest days during his 104-day stay in the NICU was when they allowed me to 'kangaroo' him. Skin-to-skin contact encourages bonding through closeness. I was able to lay Bo on my bare chest with blan-

SHARON HORNFISCHER: "When our thirty-two-weeker, David, was a week or two old, the NICU staff said that we could perform skin-to-skin care with him. We didn't know what that was. But after they told us, the idea of holding our baby in such an intimate way sounded great, to say the least. Since I was either breast-feeding or present for most of the day feedings, it was actually my husband who usually performed the skin-to-skin care when he visited after work. We made a ritual out of it. Every evening after dinner, once the NICU's lights had finally dimmed after a busy day, it was time for my husband and his son to have their time together. Those moments make up some of our most special and tender memories of our six-week stint as NICU parents."

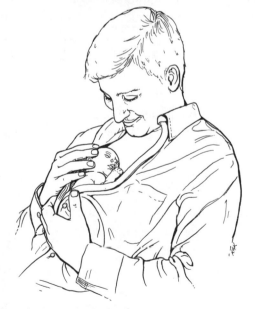

Skin-to-skin care (dad with baby tucked under his shirt)

kets draped over us. I was so thrilled when we did this, and my son handled it very well. His breathing became very regular and his body temperature raised several degrees, which was a good sign that he was tolerating it. There were other times that he didn't tolerate it very well, and it made me so sad. I felt that he was rejecting me and had to be taught that it didn't have anything to do with me. The problem might be that he was overstimulated, tired, or any number of things. I couldn't help feeling bad when this happened, though. We were able to increase our skin-to-skin contact to twice daily as his health stabilized, and I was so happy. He was tolerating it well and gaining weight much better."

Skin-to-Skin: Seeing Is Believing

JOE GARCIA-PRATS: "You look at the moms and the dads doing skin-to-skin care, and you can see that expression on their faces. 'This is so right,' they seem to be saying. It's good for both mom and dad and baby as well. Skin-to-skin care was first introduced in the early 1990s. Doctors didn't buy into it right away. There were concerns that taking the baby out of the warmer or incubator that she depended upon for heat might not be a good idea. Turning the baby over to another form of heat production seemed to have its risks. Some of us questioned whether mom and dad could maintain the baby in a proper thermal environment. Like anything else, however, it had to be tried and proven before it could be accepted. We all had to prove to ourselves that it was safe and positive. Only by seeing the successes did that happen. Then most of us became advocates."

❧ TIP

If your baby is mature enough to do kangaroo care with you, remember to wear a shirt that buttons up the front. (Women should wear bras with front snap closures.) This will make it easier to position the baby comfortably on your chest and easier to remove the baby without waking him or her.

Keeping the Home Fires Burning

Keeping the home fires burning while you have a child in the NICU can seem like an impossibility, even for the most conscientious of people. Your world is on hold, you may feel, so shouldn't the rest of the world also stop? Granted, life will slow down some for you after a baby is born. You'll have time off from work. Friends will forgive unreturned phone calls.

Housekeeping can slide for a week or two (maybe three or more). But expecting these accommodations is not generally a long-term reality. The world continues to come at you with all the speed it can muster. Bills will have to be paid, calls returned, clean clothes placed in the closets, and food stocked in the cabinets. Sooner or later you will need to get down to business. And if this isn't stressful enough, try adding other children at home to your list of responsibilities. Even though this great juggling act seems like an impossibility, if you break down your daily tasks, prioritize them, delegate, and take life one day at a time, it really can be manageable. Most important, don't forget to nurture your own spousal relationship. During the stress of a high-risk pregnancy or preterm delivery, it is often placed at the end of the priority list. Put it back where it belongs—at the top—and you may just find everything else falling into place.

TAKING CARE OF YOURSELF

Taking care of yourself both emotionally and physically is about the most important thing you can do as parents to prepare yourself for the challenges of preemie parenthood. Especially for mothers, the postpartum period can be very taxing physically. A cesarean delivery or any number of postpartum complications (such as high blood pressure or high or low blood sugar) can require a long time for recovery. There is a reason the American College of Obstetricians and Gynecologists recommends that mothers take six to eight weeks off work after delivery in order to recover from the demanding experience of pregnancy. And that six- to eight-week figure is barring further maternal health complications, the existence of which will only prolong this recovery period.

✣ TIP

Don't try to be Supermom too soon. Take time to regain your health first. Remember, if you are unhealthy, who will be there to take care of your baby? If you are at your best emotionally and physically, you will be able to give your child and family your best. And this is a job only you can do. Think of it as your first line of defense as you tackle the "great juggling act." If things are handled well in this area, you can move on to taking care of other important business.

HANDLING FINANCES

Handling finances remains an important part of your life while in the NICU, even more so as you incur the astronomical (and usually unex-

✣ TIP
If You Want to Just Shut off the World . . .

Family and friends will be eager to reach out to you when your child is in the NICU. They will offer assistance and support, but they will also want to have the very latest information. All well and good. Except that when you've told the same story about your preemie's medical condition for the tenth time in the same day, it can get exhausting (and, if the news isn't good right now, even depressing) awfully fast. If you have a large family with a high curiosity quotient, the volume of phone calls can be downright overwhelming. A good way to relieve some of this load (and reduce your phone bill) is to set up a phone or e-mail chain among your family and friends. You designate one person whom you will call with updates and information. This person is assigned someone else to call, who calls someone else, so on and so forth, until your whole network of loved ones has the latest. Of course, e-mail works well, too. It's not perfect. People who get the secondhand reports might feel left out. But you can make up for any hurt feelings later, when you're feeling less overwhelmed by life and are able to put some energy into talking to all your friends and family again.

A veteran NICU mom had another system that worked well for her. Kimberly said, "We got to the point that we'd change the greeting on our answering machine with updates: 'This is day such-and-such . . .' "

pected) expenses from a hospitalization, high-risk pregnancy, and NICU stay. Maybe your obstetrician pulled you off work early, forcing you to spend the last weeks or months of your pregnancy on bed rest, which put a sudden stop to your income stream. Or maybe you've chosen to leave a high-paying job for the full-time job of stay-at-home parenting. Though the emotional rewards are high, for many the pay is low. Credit card companies aren't like employers. They aren't in a hurry to add maternity time to your grace period. Getting along financially during this hectic time will require a businesslike approach to your family cash flow. Flying by the seat of the pants, which you might have gotten away with when two incomes were coming in, may no longer be an option. No matter what your circumstances are, cash-flow issues will probably come up during this transitional period in your life. You may need to cut expenses and find novel ways to earn additional income. Even if money is not an issue, the time it takes to manage it amid the demands of new parenthood needs to be considered and worked into your busy daily schedule as parent to a preemie.

One helpful thing to remember if you are feeling the crunch of managing your financial life during an NICU stay: Realize just how major this life transition is. Keeping matters in perspective is often the first step toward finding the sanity to tackle your situation head-on.

INSURANCE COVERAGE

Staying on top of your insurance coverage and bills is another very important ball to juggle. Most insurance companies require you to call them and add your newborn to your health plan within a few days of delivery. Many insurance carriers require preauthorization for certain medical procedures, while others may require letters from your baby's doctor confirming the need for special treatment or equipment.

It's important to file away in a safe place all records you receive in connection with your pregnancy and your baby's NICU care. This includes such things as medical records, financial statements, correspondence with the hospital or insurance company, and any bills relating to you and your infant's hospitalization and treatment.

An NICU can get very expensive. The estimated daily NICU charges ranged from $1,500 to $3,000 *a day*, and health care costs are only climbing. Keeping well-organized records can save money and time when dealing with an insurance company. You will be able to review the accuracy of charges and make the necessary inquiries. Having all the pertinent invoice numbers, statement dates, and itemized charges and diagnosis codes right when you need them will reduce the amount of time you spend on the phone with billing departments and insurance companies. During this trying period of your life, you won't want to spend a minute more than necessary talking to your insurance carrier.

✖ TIP

Remember to keep your insurance cards and numbers handy. A little sheet pinned by the telephone, or a small card in your wallet, will do the trick. To insure coverage for your newborn, remember to call your insurance company within a few days of the birth and add your infant to the policy for coverage.

Many companies are very strict about this policy, and failure to do so could cause important and valuable coverage to be denied.

Luckily there are resources that can help you with this. Your hospital billing department, social worker, or NICU parent liaison can help you sort out the often complicated questions regarding insurance coverage.

IF YOU DON'T HAVE INSURANCE COVERAGE

If you are uninsured, you should visit with your hospital social worker for assistance. They will be able to assess your individual situation and provide a list of possible resources for you to explore.

COMMUNICATE WITH YOUR EMPLOYER

If you are employed during your pregnancy and delivery, you should keep your employer informed of your plans for returning to work after your pregnancy leave. While employers don't have a right to know all of the details of your personal medical situation, it's good form to allow your employer to make arrangements in the event that you choose not to return at the end of your maternity leave. You may also find it helpful to review once again your benefits package and options for taking a leave of absence. If you delivered prematurely, you may not have had time to make all of the necessary arrangements prior to leaving the job. It's smart to wrap up those loose ends now.

The amount of paid leave you have will depend on your individual employer's plan and will likely be determined by your length of service with the company. Many women involved with high-risk pregnancies will have used up their paid leave during pregnancy and may have little or no paid time left after the delivery. This can seriously limit your options as you face a potentially long postpartum recovery period without the flexibility to take more time off.

Kimberly, the teacher, worked for a school district that had a policy that allowed other teachers to donate their unused sick days to a colleague for medical reasons. Creative approaches to time off are increasingly common today.

In 1993 the federal government enacted the Family Medical Leave Act (FMLA). This legislation allows men and women to take up to a maximum of sixty business days (twelve weeks) off in any twelve-month period for certain outlined family conditions without placing their job or insurance coverage in jeopardy. This additional time off is usually without pay if it is used to care for someone other than yourself—for example, a dependent minor child, as would be the case with a premature infant. The flexibility it offers you can be extremely valuable. After you are discharged from the hospital, you could choose to return to work while your infant is in the good hands of the NICU, then take FMLA and be at home for sixty days to take care of your baby on his or her homecoming.

Taking FMLA can be a real benefit to those who need extra time to parent their preemie. You can discuss FMLA and other benefit questions with your employer to see if you qualify and for any other questions you may have.

SHARON HORNFISCHER: "I knew there was no way that I could go back to work until my premature son was a little bigger and stronger and we had a chance to bond and establish a routine. In my situation, FMLA worked out great: even though I didn't get paid, it was good to know that I could be with my baby through those valuable first months and still have a job waiting for me when I returned."

Parent Support Groups and Other Useful Resources

During your NICU stay, ask a staff nurse or social worker whether your hospital sponsors a parent support group or any other kind of resource to ease your transition into premature parenthood. Such groups, which will meet regularly, usually once or twice a week, can be a great way to meet other parents who are sharing the preemie journey with you. Many parents we have spoken with have found these groups to be wonderful support systems. Their only complaint was that they didn't find out about them soon enough. If your nurse or social worker doesn't know of any such groups sponsored by your hospital, try calling another hospital in your area. If that doesn't work, introduce yourself to some of the other parents in the NICU and start a support group yourself. Because you all have the NICU experience in common, friendships can form quickly and deeply.

Some NICUs maintain reference libraries with impressive collections of materials on neonatal medicine. A resource like that is especially helpful for parents who aren't able to attend support group meetings because of schedule conflicts or aren't comfortable interacting in a group setting. Many such libraries will offer a collection of videos as well as books. Videos can be particularly useful when you want to see how breast-feeding is done or how infant CPR is performed and want to get the gist of it quickly.

Working the Web

Of course, in the age of the Internet your social network need no longer be limited to your geographic area. The on-line world is a great place to meet other parents of preemies who are eager to share their experiences with you. In fact, most of the parents we interviewed for this book were found on the Internet. Web sites such as Sidelines (an on-line organization that connects mothers with high-risk pregnancies with specially trained electronic pen pals who have been through the experience themselves) and the well-established Preemie-L discussion group (an electronic mailing list, or "listserv," that will put you in the middle of active, highly informative e-mail exchanges with other parents of preemies) are worlds unto themselves and helpful places to visit for anyone who's afraid of what lies ahead in their preemie experience.

Reference information also abounds on the Net. Seek and you shall find. There is information out there on just about any health condition. In Appendix C we list many of the Web sites that provide free information on almost every medical topic under the sun, including virtually any issue you might want to investigate in connection with prematurity and high-risk pregnancy. They vary from commercial, professionally oriented medical sites such as WebMD.com to parent-oriented resources such as the University of Wisconsin's "Parents of Preemies" page. Of course, it is important once again to point out that the operative slogan for Internet-based research is "Caveat emptor" ("Let the buyer beware"). While a great deal of authoritative, peer-reviewed research is available on-line, there is also a lot that is untested, experimental, anecdotal, or just plain wrong. Consider the source very carefully any time you are looking at information you obtain from the mixed bag of the Internet.

If you are looking for information on a particular topic, you can try entering the name of the topic into any of the excellent search engines available on the Web. These include, in alphabetical order:

- All the Web   www.alltheweb.com
- AltaVista   www.altavista.com
- Dogpile   www.dogpile.com
- Excite   www.excite.com
- Google   www.google.com
- Hotbot   www.hotbot.com
- Infoseek   www.infoseek.com
- Lycos   www.lycos.com
- Yahoo   www.yahoo.com

Since each collects or processes information differently, each of these search engines will return different results for a particular search query. You will probably settle on a favorite after you have had a chance to see which one provides the most useful hits.

See Appendix C for information on particularly useful medical and preemie-related Web sites.

7

SPECIAL CONCERNS IN THE NICU

WHAT YOU WILL FIND IN THIS CHAPTER

The eight most common conditions of prematurity

- Infection—early onset
- Intraventricular hemorrhage (IVH)
- Patent ductus arteriosus (PDA)
- Apnea of prematurity

- Necrotizing enterocolitis (NEC)
- Infection—late onset
- Bronchopulmonary dysplasia (BPD)
- Retinopathy of prematurity (ROP)

Other medical concerns in the first year

- Anemia
- Blood sugar instability
- Jaundice

- Respiratory distress syndrome (RDS)
- Temperature regulation

The Eight Most Common Conditions of Prematurity

Chapter 5 presented a very general view of preemies at three different stages of prematurity: twenty-four to twenty-eight weeks, twenty-eight to thirty-two weeks, and thirty-two to thirty-seven weeks. The assumption underlying the information provided there was that no intervening medical condition—problems reaching beyond the essential immaturity of the infant—would affect the baby's health. In this chapter we attempt to illustrate the range of risks for eight of the most frequently encountered conditions that preemies may encounter at each of the three gestational ranges of prematurity, any of which has the potential of complicating or extending your preemie's NICU stay.

As the risk threshold charts included in this chapter indicate, these eight conditions are as follows:

- Early-onset infection
- Intraventricular hemorrhage (IVH)
- Patent ductus arteriosus (PDA)
- Apnea of prematurity
- Necrotizing enterocolitis (NEC)
- Late-onset infection
- Bronchopulmonary dysplasia (BPD)
- Retinopathy of prematurity (ROP)

A quick comparison of the charts reveals the dramatic reduction in risk preemies gain as they spend longer periods in the womb. At the end of the day, these charts illustrate a simple idea and nothing more. They show that more mature preemies generally endure the rigors of prematurity better than less mature preemies. Beyond that, there is a considerable degree of variability among individual preemies. For instance, a twenty-nine-weeker whose lungs got a developmental boost with a series of maternal steroid injections may very well breathe better than a thirty-two-weeker who did not. Likewise, other factors such as gender and even ethnicity seem to influence how well preemies fare. Girls tend to do better than boys, and African American preemies tend to be more robust than Caucasian preemies. For reasons that are unclear but well established statistically, it takes longer, generally, for Caucasian male preemies to catch up.

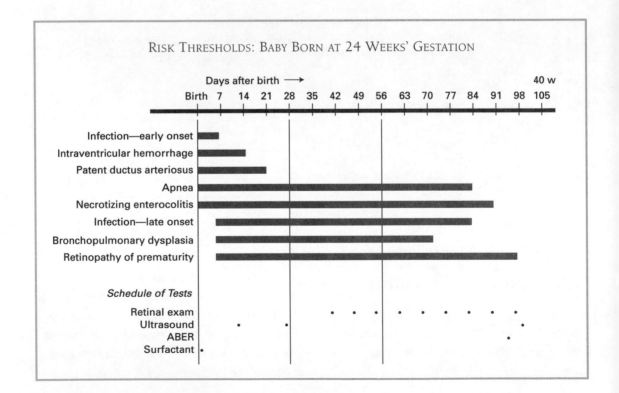

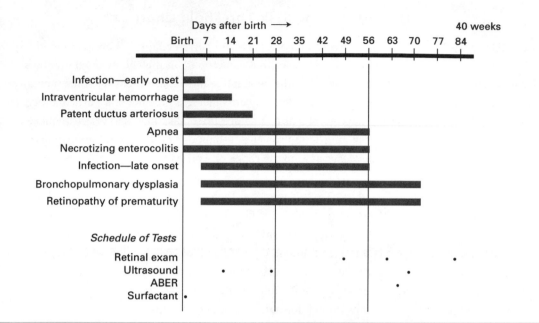

RISK THRESHOLDS: BABY BORN AT 28 WEEKS' GESTATION

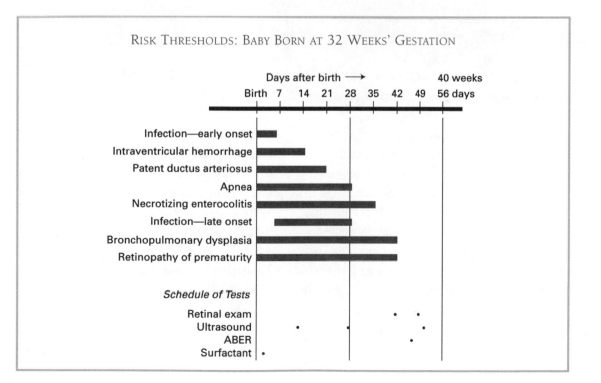

RISK THRESHOLDS: BABY BORN AT 32 WEEKS' GESTATION

How to Use the Risk Threshold Charts

JOE GARCIA-PRATS: "These charts (and the composite chart in chapter 4) are really nothing more than road maps of the kinds of obstacles that can crop up in the course of your baby's NICU stay. Your infant's neonatologist and the neonatal team will use them (or some mental facsimile thereof) to keep alert to the potential concerns facing a preemie of a particular age. Some of these concerns we'll have good treatments for. Others, like ROP and IVH, may have no treatments and may result in long-term problems. I think one of the helpful things these charts do is to place some *boundaries* around the range of worries that confront your premature infant.

"One father told me, 'I used to have this idea that there was an endless horizon of things that could go wrong for my son in the NICU. Seeing the chart, I was able to get my hands around his situation in a way that seemed to make it more manageable.' Others may feel differently, seeing that there is a range of potential problems that goes beyond what they were originally concerned about. At the end of the day, I think it's best for parents to have this information for the sense of empowerment it can provide. Nothing is easy when you have a preemie in the NICU. Not having good information at your fingertips doesn't really make it any easier."

So the charts, in and of themselves, should not be viewed as having significant predictive value. Nonetheless, we believe strongly enough in the simple proposition that they illustrate (see above) to include them in the book.

We are sensitive to the fact that any comprehensive discussion of the the full range of possible conditions and complications that can confront a premature infant can make for grim reading. Therefore we feel that the discussion that follows should be treated as a reference resource rather than a forecast. Few if any preemies endure all of these problems. But they are nevertheless common enough to be reviewed here.

Infection

When the body is invaded by a microorganism that it is unable to fight off, infection results. Infections can be common in premature infants—their immature immune systems make it much easier for microorganisms such as bacteria, virus, and fungus to enter and invade the bloodstream. Throughout the neonatologist's management of your baby, infection will always be suspected whenever something goes awry. The more immature the infant, the greater the risk of infection. This is because the transfer of protective proteins from the mother to the baby that usually takes place during the final weeks of gestation didn't have a chance to occur. Likewise, in preemies, white blood cells are restricted in their ability to migrate to a site of possible infection and to perform their germ-fighting task of ingesting and destroying bacteria. For this reason, preemies born at birth weights of 751 to 1,000 grams have a rate of late-onset infection of as high as 33 percent while in the hospital. Infants born at less than 751 grams have a late-onset infection rate of as high as 50 percent. Thus the staff will watch closely for any sign of infection, and your baby will be given antibiotics when unexpected or unusual symptoms that could indicate infection occur.

The emphasis on cleanliness and sanitary practices in the NICU underscores how immediate the risk of infection is. The vigilance calls attention to the threat and can cause parents to worry. Susan said that one of her biggests concerns while her son was in the NICU was infection. "I was lucky. All my son needed to learn was how to suck, swallow, and coordinate his breathing. But he had a neighbor who was on IV antibiotics, and all I could think about was finding a way to move him away from his neighbor. I didn't want him to catch some kind of infection. I was really pushing to get him out of there. I just wanted to bring him home."

Of course, the risk of infection is present everywhere. A friend or neighbor who visits you and your newborn at home is just as likely to carry infection as an infant in a nearby bassinet in the NICU. Infection is a fact of life in the NICU just as it is everywhere else. The particular concern in the NICU, however, arises from how fragile preemies are at this stage of their lives.

We discuss two general categories of infection here: *early-onset infections* and *late-onset infections*.

Early-onset infections manifest themselves, if at all, during the first three days after delivery. These infectious microorganisms reside in utero and also in the mother's vaginal canal. You will know within a few days of birth whether your preemie picked up an infection in utero or as he exited the womb through the vaginal canal.

Late-onset infections usually occur after three days of life, since they are caused by a wide range of pathogens that the baby may be exposed to after leaving the womb. The first indication of trouble could be very subtle, such as the baby not feeding or eating properly. He might have poor skin color or show signs of irregular breathing patterns such as apnea or labored breathing, reflecting the need for more oxygen. Irritability, lethargy, low blood pressure, and poor temperature control are more obvious signs of infection. (See the sidebar on page 210.)

Commonly found infections include *neonatal septicemia* (a bacterial infection of the bloodstream) and *pneumonia* (a viral or bacterial infection in the lungs resulting in inflammation or fluid buildup that makes respiration difficult and can compound other prematurity-related respiratory disorders). A less common but no less serious infection is *meningitis* (a viral or bacterial infection or inflammation of the lining of the layers around the brain). Another rather common infection is a *urinary tract infection (UTI)*. All infections should be taken seriously and treated promptly and aggressively. No matter how benign in nature, any infection could lead, if left untreated, to a serious problem for the immuno-suppressed premature infant.

An infection that your baby acquires in the hospital is called a *nosocomial infection*. Even though strict precautions are taken when deal-

> ### General Signs and Symptoms of Infection
>
> - Apnea or periodic breathing
> - Diarrhea
> - Feeding problems or loss of appetite
> - Fever
> - Irritability
> - Lethargy
> - Mottled skin
> - Pale skin color or cynanosis
> - Poor circulation (cold hands and feet)
> - Vomiting
> - Abdominal distention

ing with the premature infant—staff, parents, and visitors are typically required to perform a thorough hand/arm scrub upon each visit—no NICU is absolutely sterile. Infections such as pneumonia can be caused by bacterial growth in the respiratory tract. An outbreak of chicken pox may strike the NICU without warning. Germs spread, and they can get out of control in a hurry. When nosocomial infections occur, infants who are exposed may be placed in special isolation rooms where extra care is taken to prevent the spread of the infection in question. Additional precautions include requiring visitors to wear masks, gowns, and or gloves, or restricting visiting privileges to parents, grandparents, or young adults over sixteen years of age.

Bacteria cannot be controlled or eliminated, and indeed, it is virtually impossible to keep a baby sterile. The food the baby eats, the visitors the baby sees—everything external to the child is a potential source of infection. Infections can be managed only once the symptoms

manifest themselves. What we do know is that the fewer medical interventions the NICU medical staff performs—the fewer the IV sites, punctures, catheters, probes, surgical sites, and other invasive procedures—the stronger your baby's shield against infection will be. Any break in the baby's skin is a potential point of entry into the child and thus a potential site for infection.

When infections occur despite our best preventative efforts, they are generally treated with a course of antibiotics. Typically these will be given intravenously and administered for a specified treatment course—ten to fourteen days. There are a wide range of pathogens, and what your baby contracts will depend on where you live. For example, if you live in Detroit, your baby will get what's going around in Detroit at that time. So the choice of antibiotic must be made by your doctor with relation to the particular pathogen confronting him or her.

NEONATAL SEPTICEMIA

This is a potentially serious condition brought on by an infection, usually bacterial in nature, that has invaded the infant's bloodstream. The risk posed by infections of the bloodstream is that they can spread and infect many parts of the body all at once as the blood circulates through your baby's body. Septicemia needs to be quickly diagnosed and treated for the best outcome.

SIGNS AND SYMPTOMS. The symptoms of a septic infant can vary widely. As we said, the first indication of trouble could be very subtle, such as the baby not feeding properly. She might also have a poor skin color or show signs of irregular sleep patterns. More common, however, the infant will be very sick, showing signs of breathing difficulty, irritability, or lethargy, or temperature instability. If your child has been discharged home and shows any of these signs—especially an elevated temperature that is difficult to control—you should seek immediate medical attention. Diagnosis is usually made by blood culture and other pertinent laboratory data.

CAUSES. The immature immune system of the premature infant increases the risk for opportunistic infections to invade the body, which can in turn lead to septicemia. Infections such as pneumonia or meningitis may invade the body and enter the bloodstream, where it is difficult for the body to fight them off. It is not merely a single isolated organ or area of the body being affected, but rather every part of the body through which blood circulates.

TREATMENTS. Septicemia is treated with a course of antibiotics. Typically these will be given intravenously and administered for a specified treatment course. Other support measures may need to be taken, such as frequent analysis of vital signs. Particular attention needs to be given to the child's blood pressure. Special medication may need to be administered to your child to assist with the stabilization of the vital signs. Quick and aggressive treatment of neonatal septicemia is usually successful. But occasionally, even under the best of treatment regimens, the premature infant becomes just so sick, his immune system so weak, that he is unable to fight off the disease and the infection will prove to be fatal.

MENINGITIS

Meningitis is a serious but not terribly common infection of the covering of the brain (the *meninges*). There are two kinds of meningitis: bacterial and viral. If meningitis is suspected, your baby's neonatologist may perform a spinal tap to confirm the diagnosis. This is by far the best diagnostic tool for this disease. It involves taking a small sample of fluid from the infant's spinal canal, which is then analyzed in the lab for the presence of infection. Since the antibiotics and dosages used for treatment of meningitis are different from those used to treat other infections, your physician will probably want to perform a spinal tap to confirm (or rule out) meningitis as the cause of your baby's symptoms. Additionally, specialized tests such as ultrasounds, magnetic resonance imaging (MRI), or computerized tomography (CAT) scans of your child's head and brain may be performed to check for any lasting swelling or compromised blood supply to the brain or surrounding structures caused by the meningitis.

SIGNS AND SYMPTOMS. Irregular vital signs, poor weight gain, irritability, lethargy, unstable temperature, seizures, and even coma are possible symptoms of meningitis.

CAUSES. Meningitis is caused when a viral or bacterial infectious agent invades the blood and crosses over into the spinal fluid, where it travels to and infects the brain and its surrounding tissues.

TREATMENTS. Historically, the earlier the treatment for infection, the better the outcome. If the initial stages of the infection are serious in nature—involving, for example, seizures or loss of consciousness—the chances are greater of the child having some long-term neurological detriment, or even dying, from the infection. As with other types of infection, treating meningitis involves the administration of antibiotics. But since some antibiotics don't cross over into the spinal fluid, the antibiotic prescribed by your child's physician may be different from the antibiotics that your infant may have been given to fight other infections. When a baby shows signs and symptoms of an infection and meningitis is suspected, it is often difficult to document the infection until blood cultures and spinal fluid cultures, are back from the lab. This usually takes forty-eight to seventy-two hours. Thus, all suspected cases of meningitis, whether bacterial or viral in nature, are treated with antibiotics. These first few days are a critical time in the treatment of meningitis. If it turns out to be viral, the antibiotics the baby receives prior to that determination won't be harmful. The baby's vital signs will require close monitoring during the treatment and recovery from meningitis.

PNEUMONIA

A viral or bacterial infection of the lung, pneumonia causes inflammation or fluid buildup in the lung that can make respiration difficult and compound other prematurity-related respiratory disorders, such as respiratory distress syndrome (RDS). When diagnosis is made early, infants with pneumonia can have very successful treatments leading to a full recovery.

SIGNS AND SYMPTOMS. Pneumonia's symptoms usually include a change in the baby's vital signs—especially an increased pulse or respiratory rate—difficulty breathing, and temperature instability. Diagnosis is confirmed by X-ray or by abnormal breathing sounds audible to a physician with a stethoscope. Other signs of pneumonia may include an increased white blood cell count or positive microorganism growth in tracheal specimen cultures.

CAUSES. Your preemie's immature immune system puts him at increased risk for opportunistic infections, bacterial or viral, which can lead to pneumonia.

TREATMENTS. If the pneumonia is bacterial in origin, your preemie will be placed on antibiotics. Typically these will be given intravenously and administered for a specified treatment course. Other support measures may include frequent analysis of arterial blood gases and pulse oximetry. If oxygen levels are low, supplemental oxygen can be administered via face mask, oxygen hood, CPAP, or intubation. If the infection is viral, there is usually no therapy other than supportive care.

OTHER TYPES OF INFECTION

Your preemie's immunologic immaturity makes him susceptible to many other types of infection. Though these other kinds of infection are usually not as difficult to treat as pneumonia and meningitis and lead to fewer complications, they should nonetheless be taken seriously and treated promptly and aggressively. Any infection, no matter how benign in nature, could lead, if left untreated, to a serious problem for the immunosuppressed premature infant.

URINARY TRACT INFECTION (UTI). This infection of the kidney or bladder or other parts of the urinary tract can be caused by bacteria entering the urinary opening during urination or defecation or by the insertion of a catheter into the urinary tract.

MATERNAL CHORIOAMNIONITIS. This is an infection of the placental membrane. It can be caused by premature rupture of membrane (PROM), which leaves the *chorion* and *amnion* (the sacs and fluid surrounding the fetus) vulnerable to opportunistic infection. Likewise, the reverse is true: infection can cause PROM. This type of infection can be transferred to the child before or during birth. Because of the circulatory role performed by the placenta, chorioamnionitis can lead to neonatal septicemia (see page 210).

Intraventricular Hemorrhage (IVH)

Also commonly called an *intracranial bleed,* this is a potentially serious condition that occurs when there is bleeding in the brain tissues near the ventricles of the brain. The vessels of the premature infant's brain, initially both fragile and immature, are prone to damage or rupture. Rapid changes in blood pressure, for example, can alter the pressure and blood flow within these fragile, immature cerebral blood vessels, possibly exerting enough stress on them to cause a bleed into the surrounding brain tissue. Until about thirty-four weeks' gestation, your preemie will have a large number of blood-rich capillaries in the brain, which help the brain develop. The more premature your baby, the more fragile cerebral vessels she will have, and the longer the exposure to risk of IVH until she reaches the thirty-four-week threshold at which the brain has developed sufficiently to have significantly fewer of these immature vessels.

FREQUENCY OF IVH

Gestational Age	Frequency
32 weeks	<10 percent
28 to 31 weeks	10 to 20 percent
26 to 27 weeks	30 to 40 percent
24 to 25 weeks	50 to 60 percent

Several medications help prevent hemorrhage. One of them is steroids—the same medication you may have been given to help your baby's lung development. The prenatal administration of steroids by obstetricians and perinatologists has increased significantly since the issuance of the official consensus report at the 1994 National Institute of Child Health and Human Development Conference.

Two other medications can help avoid hemorrhage after your baby is born: phenobarbital and indomethacin. Phenobarbital, which sedates the infant, is thought to offer protection from the wide swings in blood pressure that would otherwise damage the delicate cerebral blood vessels. Some premature infants have trouble maintaining a steady flow of blood to the brain. This fluctuation of blood flow with variation in blood pressure is thought to cause bleeding in the brain. Sedation can alleviate the impact of these fluctuations on the baby.

Indomethacin is believed to protect the brain from the effects of prostaglandins, hormones that are released during stress, like that caused by labor and delivery. Prostaglandins can cause the immature and poorly supported blood vessels in central areas of the brain to dilate. These expanded blood vessels are at risk of rupturing when blood flow to the brain is reestablished after the stress of birth.

THE FOUR CLASSIFICATIONS OF BRAIN BLEEDS

Brain bleeds are classifiable into several types. The mildest ones, which usually reabsorb, are called grade I. The most severe are called grade IV. Depending on the severity, symptoms may include irregular vital signs, poor skin color, vomiting, unusually rapid increase in head circumference, bulging fontanels, lethargy, irritability, and in some cases even seizures. It is also possible that the infant may have no symptoms at all. Frequent neurological examinations will be performed on any child who is suspected of having intracranial bleeding. Additionally, a brain ultrasound or sonogram will be performed to confirm the diagnosis.

The smaller brain hemorrhages (grades I and II) are usually not associated with long-term neurological problems. On the other hand, more severe hemorrhages (grades III and IV) may increase the likelihood of long-term problems (mental retardation and/or cerebral palsy).

A grade I or II bleed most likely will not have any complications, so there is no need for additional treatment. These bleeds usually reabsorb within two to three weeks, and the condition completely resolves on its own.

Grade III and IV bleeds have a greater degree of variance in their associated complications and outcomes. Some of these bleeds reabsorb on their own, some cause some temporary ventricular enlargement that eventually resolves, and some lead to persistent ventricular enlargement. The enlargement results from an imbalance between the production and reabsorption of spinal fluid that occurs in the ventricular system. This complication, called *hydrocephalus,* causes increasing pressure on the brain itself. Premature infants who develop hydrocephalus do not have an "abnormal" appearance since it is known that the ventricles in the brain dilate long before the size of the infant's head begins to grow. So although your infant's head size may be measured weekly, an enlarging head size in excess to what is expected is a very late sign. Ultrasound of the head is used to assess the size of the ventricles and is performed weekly or every other week. Should your infant's head size begin to grow, another sign that the head size is growing too fast is that the space between the bones of the skull (*sutures*) become separated. This can be felt by carefully running the tips of your fingers along the edges where the bones of the head meet. This condition may resolve on its own over the course of weeks, and the neonatologist may consult a neurologist and/or neurosurgeon in the assessment and possible treatment of this increase in the ventricular size. If serial ultrasounds, which will be done weekly or every other week, indicate that the fluid is still accumulating and the brain tissue is being compressed, then the neurosurgeon will perform a ventricular tap, a procedure that drains off the extra fluid inside the ventricles. This procedure, which can be done at the patient's bedside or in a treatment room, entails placing a needle into the ventricular system and removing the spinal fluid. This procedure will have to be repeated until the spinal fluid protein content is low enough for a more permanent drain to be placed into the ventricle. This more permanent drain uses a tube that is placed into the ventricles and drains the extra fluid into the abdomen. This is called a *VP shunt* or *ventriculo-peritoneal shunt*. It is difficult to predict how long an infant will require a VP shunt to treat the hydrocephalus—increased accumulation of cerebrospinal fluid. One can assume that it may be years before the condition reestablishes a balanced production and absorption of the cerebrospinal fluid. Some grade IV bleeds lead to serious damage in the brain tissue itself. As the blood is eventually reabsorbed after being put under pressure from the ventricular swelling, pockets caused by the blood remain, leaving holes in the brain tissue. These holes are called *porencephalic cysts*. The location and size of the cysts will determine whether any treatment will be needed and whether they will cause any complications in brain function.

The developmental prognosis for children with IVH varies greatly. Some experience no developmental delays at all. At the other end of the spectrum is mental retardation and cerebral palsy. There are no guarantees with IVH. One child can experience any grade of hemorrhage with little or no known developmental delays. Another might have never experienced a bleed of any type and still show signs of developmental delay. Though this uncertainty offers a parent little comfort, children born today have much better chances of a positive outcome due to continuing advances in prenatal and postnatal care.

Patent Ductus Arteriosus (PDA)

This is a cardiac condition common in premature infants where the blood vessel that connects the aorta and the pulmonary artery (the

A condition related to IVH is *periventricular leukomalacia (PVL)*. PVL reveals itself when small densities or cysts in the brain are found when a head ultrasound is performed. These cysts or densities are a sign that the baby's brain suffered from a restricted blood flow or an infection that occurred while the baby was still in utero or shortly after delivery. The cysts vary by their location on one side or both sides of the brain and by their size. In cases where the cysts or densities are small and disappear quickly, the prognosis will be very good. However, cysts that appear on both sides of the brain and take a long time to go away have been linked to cerebral palsy. When these cysts appear in the bundle of nerves that connects the brain's cortex to muscles, damage can result that leads to the breakdown in muscle control that characterizes cerebral palsy.

main blood vessel carrying blood from the heart to the lungs) does not close as it should after delivery. It is important for the ductus to remain open while the baby is in the womb in order to allow oxygenated blood from the placenta to bypass the lungs (which are collapsed and water filled) and be pumped to the rest of the body. The mother's placenta provides oxygen and nutrients to the fetus. At birth, the PDA in all babies is still open. Usually it will close spontaneously during the first one to two days of life. The ductus needs to close in order for proper oxygenation of the blood to take place.

SIGNS AND SYMPTOMS. Upon initial assessment, the neonatologist will listen to the infant's heart sounds. If he detects an abnormal blood flow (a heart murmur), he may suspect a PDA. Occasionally a "silent" PDA occurs, where you can't hear the abnormal flow. In this case the doctor has to use other clinical observations and diagnostic tools. The signs and symptoms could include difficulty breathing, irregular vital signs such as a bounding pulse, and an increasing need for oxygen or a deterioration of lung function whereby the respirator has to do more for the baby. PDA may also be diagnosed by chest X-rays, which may show an enlarged heart and/or increased blood flow to the lungs. The confirmatory test is an *echocardiogram*, a sonogram that creates a visual image of the structures and function of the heart. The neonatologist may ask a pediatric cardiologist to become involved to assist in the diagnosis as well as to recommend treatment choices and to ensure that there are no other structural defects in the heart. The heart ultrasound is usually done by the cardiologist or an echocardiogram technician who works under the supervision of the cardiologist.

TREATMENT. The primary treatment goal is to improve the oxygenation of the baby by keeping her lung function normal. This means reducing the flow of blood through the PDA so that fluid doesn't accumulate in the lung and affect its function. For some babies, time and patience are all that is needed for the PDA to close. This is especially true with larger, more mature preemies. However, it may be necessary to administer supplemental oxygen to the infant by means of an oxygen hood, CPAP, or respirator. Babies on oxygen will also be monitored by

pulse oximeter. Chest X-rays and frequent arterial blood gases will also be analyzed. These tests, along with the findings of the echocardiogram, as well as the baby's overall status, will help the physician assess the effectiveness of this treatment.

Medication may be used as the treatment of choice in some cases. The drug of choice for PDA is indomethacin (Indocin). In 50 to 70 percent of cases, Indocin (a nonsteroidal anti-inflammatory, like aspirin) has been known to produce dramatic results within twelve to twenty-four hours of administration. Your baby may also be given diuretics—drugs that decrease the fluid in her lungs and increase her urine output. Your baby's fluid intake and urine output will need to be observed closely. For some infants who are very sick because of the effect of the PDA on lung function, or who have abnormal kidney function or problems with bleeding (which would place them at some risk by using indomethacin), surgical closure may be the best option. This consists of placing the baby under general anesthesia while a pediatric surgeon or cardiovascular surgeon closes the ductus with a metal clip. This procedure has few side effects, and the baby usually recuperates fully within two to four days. However, this relatively short procedure is never taken lightly.

Apnea of Prematurity

Apnea is a common problem in premature infants. Generally defined as an interruption in breathing that lasts for fifteen to thirty seconds, coupled with a drop in pulse rate below one hundred beats per minute and the infant turning cyanotic (a blue pallor to the skin), it is the consequence of the preemie's immature respiratory control system.

SIGNS AND SYMPTOMS. While in the NICU, your baby will be on twenty-four-hour respiratory and cardiac monitors with alarms set by your neonatologist according to your baby's individual health profile. Long pauses in breathing associated with drops in heart rate will cause an alarm to go off. These "apneic episodes" may cause a change in your baby's skin color from rosy pink or brown to dusky gray or blue (this of course is more easily detectable in Caucasian infants). These will also be detected by pulse oximeters and cardiac monitors. It is important to distinguish apnea from mere "periodic breathing," which is characterized by shorter pauses in breathing of five to ten seconds that do not lead to heart rate drops or changes in color. Periodic breathing does not require therapeutic intervention. However, the more periodic breathing a preemie experiences, the greater the chance that apnea will occur.

CAUSES. The immature central nervous system of the premature infant seems to be a principal cause of apnea. Obstruction of the upper respiratory tracts is also associated with it. Other contributing factors can include poor temperature regulation, patent ductus arteriosus, and infection.

TREATMENT. Treating a spell of apnea can be as simple as lightly tapping your baby on the foot. This gentle stimulation may "remind" him to breathe and effectively remedies many apenic episodes. If your baby doesn't respond to manual stimulation, it may be necessary to give him oxygen via a hood or a nasal canula. NCPAP is a common way of administering continuous pressure and oxygen to a preemie. Frequent occurrences of apnea can be remedied with drugs such as caffeine or theophylline, which promote regular breathing patterns. Alternatively, he may be placed on a respirator as the physician checks for other possible causes of the apnea, such as hypoglycemia (low blood sugar), infections, or a central nervous system disorder.

Necrotizing Enterocolitis (NEC)

Once a premature infant begins feedings, the NICU team will be constantly on the lookout for symptoms of *necrotizing enterocolitis* (*NEC*). This is an inflammation of the intestinal tract whose symptoms include abdominal distention, feeding intolerance, emesis (vomiting), bloody stools, and some of the symptoms of infection—including lethargy, low blood pressure, fast heart rate, and apnea. Severe instances of NEC can lead to necrosis (death) of tissues in the bowel, thereby reducing the infant's ability to absorb nutrients from feedings.

CAUSES. The causes of NEC are not known, but associated factors appear to be overall immaturity and reduced blood flow to the intestinal tract. All newborns are susceptible to it, but premature infants make up about 95 percent of the cases reported annually.

TREATMENT. The initial treatment of NEC entails stopping oral feedings and supplementing the baby with IV fluids, or possibly TPN (total parenteral nutrition). A naso-gastric (NG) tube may be used to decompress the infant's gastrointestinal tract and remove any old milk or formula that remains in the intestinal tract. This tube also continues to remove any gas or mucus that the infant's intestine can't pass owing to the NEC. Frequent X-rays and blood analysis will be used to assess the extent of damage to the bowel. Since infection occurs frequently in association with NEC (because the protective lining of the intestine has been lost, bacteria may pass from the intestine into the bloodstream), intravenous antibiotics will be given. If these treatments don't reverse the problem and your baby's doctor is concerned about the extent of the intestinal damage caused by the NEC—the most severe of which involves perforation of the small bowel or colon and the possible spread of infection elsewhere in the body—surgery may become necessary. Perhaps the most severe long-term problem associated with NEC is *short bowel syndrome*. Occurring in infants who have had to have significant portions of their intestine removed because of the necrosis, short bowel syndrome impairs their ability to absorb nutrients from food.

A growing number of studies are pointing to the benefits of breast milk in NEC prevention. There is an increasing amount of information in the literature that demonstrates the advantages of utilizing expressed breast milk (EBM) to reduce the occurrence of NEC. The use of EBM as the milk for feeding premature infants appears to reduce the occurrence of NEC but does not prevent it totally. So the use of EBM may be protective but not preventative.

Another strategy that has been noted to reduce the occurrence of NEC is the antenatal administration of steroids to mothers in premature labor. The initiation of steroids in the mother to reduce the occurrence of HMD and IVH in her premature infant may also play a role in reducing the occurrence of NEC. Again, the exact mechanism of how this protection works is not known.

Bronchopulmonary Dysplasia (BPD)

If your baby cannot be taken off the respirator in the first seven to fourteen days of life owing to RDS (see page 225), then the neonatologist may become concerned about the risk of his developing *bronchopulmonary dysplasia*, a type of chronic lung disease. Preemies who need prolonged respiratory assistance on a ventilator, or who are very immature when they are born, often undergo detrimental changes in their lung anatomy. These changes involve the air sacs, the airways, and the accompanying blood vessels and result in fluid buildup in the lungs as well as degeneration in the lung tissue that can lead to chronic lung disease. Any baby who requires prolonged respirator use is at risk for developing BPD, although ultimately it is unclear why some babies develop BPD while others don't.

SIGNS AND SYMPTOMS. The presence of BPD is detected when mechanical ventilation or oxygen becomes required for an extended period of time because the baby is unable to be weaned off the respirator. Chest X-rays are used to assess the severity of the BPD. They may reveal a bubbly appearance to the lungs, which indicates areas of *atelectasis*, and/or overexpansion.

CAUSES. This condition most likely is the result of the infant's immaturity and possibly the inability to protect himself from different naturally occurring forms of oxygen called oxygen-free radicals. These exist normally in our tissues, and the body is typically able to dispose of them. However, infants who develop BPD may lack this ability. The likelihood of BPD developing has been linked to the degree of an infant's prematurity and to the severity of his lung disease. There is increasing evidence of a possible link to a family history of asthma. This disease is confirmed by X-ray, the infant's age, and the need for continued oxygen or respirator use beyond the expected therapeutic period.

TREATMENT. If your infant develops BPD, his stay in the hospital could be as long as several weeks to several months. BPD can take months and in extreme cases years to fully heal. Your infant will be kept stable on the respirator. While he is on the respirator, adequate amounts of oxygen will be administered to reduce the chance that areas of the lung will be exposed to low oxygen levels. Likewise respirator pressures will be chosen to produce adequate-size breaths so that the lung receives the oxygen concentration that was ordered. These are important treatment goals since adequate oxygenation and ventilation of the lung reduce strain on the right side of the heart. The right side of the heart pumps blood into the lung, where it picks up oxygen and releases carbon dioxide. If adequate ventilation and oxygenation are not achieved, then the blood vessels in the lung constrict. This causes increased resistance to the function of the right side of the heart, thus causing it to work harder (strain). Should this continue for prolonged periods, the right side of the heart will fail, causing the infant to die.

Reduction of the oxygen delivered and reduction of the respirator pressures needed to provide an adequate breath will be imple-mented only when the neonatologist notes consistently high oxygen levels as recorded by transcutaneous oxygen monitoring or pulse oximetry measurements. In addition to good respiratory support, good nutrition will be the focus of care as well as support of your baby's development by using assessment and intervention by nurses, occupational therapists, physical therapists, and play therapists. Treatment for BPD may also include scheduled chest physiotherapy (CPT), which entails using either vibration (using battery-powered toothbrushes) or percussion (small rubber doughnuts that are used to gently strike the chest) to all areas of the chest or to specific areas of the chest where lung collapse has occurred. This will be determined by your baby's neonatologist. In addition to the chest physiotherapy, there will be adequate suctioning of any mucus that is dislodged from the lung during the treatment. Premature infants are very sensitive to overstimulation by light, sounds, and touch, so procedures can often lead to increased heart rate and labored respiration. Because these fluctuations in vital signs can hurt the preemie with BPD, he will often be placed on stimulation precautions designed to keep him calm and relaxed. Don't be alarmed if this is recommended for your child. The precautions will stay in place only until your infant's respiratory status stabilizes.

Certain medications may also be administered to counter the effects of BPD. These can include bronchodilators and inhaled steroids, which aid in opening the bronchial tubes, thus making breathing less strenuous. Most infants with BPD experience episodes of wheezing and chest retractions due to the narrowing of the small airways of the lung. They generally require the same medications that asthmatic children would use—inhaled bronchodilators and steroids. Diuretics may also be given to help decrease the amount of fluid buildup in the lungs. Recent studies have also shown the benefit of the use of steroids given intravenously. It is thought that this therapy reduces inflammation caused by BPD and may reduce the amount of oxygen the infant needs to receive, thus reducing the amount of respirator support he needs or even allowing its discontinuance.

Retinopathy of Prematurity (ROP)

A disorder of the eye associated with immaturity, ROP involves the disruption of the normal growth pattern of blood vessels in the retina (the light-sensitive "photoplate" at the back of the eye). This can lead to scarring or detachment of the retina, thereby causing vision impairment or even blindness. In most premature infants, some changes in the retinal blood vessels occur normally as the infant matures. Stress caused by the baby's prematurity can disrupt the natural growth of these tiny capillaries from the center of the eye out to the edge of the retina. Many times this disruption proves to be harmless as the blood vessels of the retina resume their normal development. However, when the capillaries stop growing, or resume growing too densely in one area of the retina, damage can result. Most of the severe instances of ROP are found in infants who weigh less than 1,000 grams (2.2 pounds) at birth or are born at gestational ages of less than twenty-eight weeks. A study of more than 2,500 infants of less than thirty-seven weeks' gestation, pub-

lished in 1999, showed the overall incidence of ROP to be 21.3 percent among all premature infants. However, in this study no instances of ROP were noted in infants born after thirty-two weeks, and no infant born after twenty-eight weeks needed retinal surgery.

Although 66 percent of patients who weigh less than 1,251 grams at birth develop ROP (any stage of the disease), only 11 percent of the infants in this weight group develop severe stages of ROP that warrant intervention. The rate of severity of the ROP is inversely proportional to the baby's birth weight (and gestational age). One study demonstrated that infants with birth weights between 1,001 and 1,250 grams had a less than 5 percent chance of developing severe ROP, whereas infants with birth weights between 751 and 1,000 grams and birth weights less than 750 grams had an incidence of severe ROP of 12 percent and 24 percent, respectively. If these infants develop severe ROP and require laser treatment, favorable outcomes are noted in 85 percent to 95 percent of the infants treated. Most long-term visual problems are associated with infants who had the more severe stages of ROP, although all preterm infants with ROP may be at some risk for long-term associated eye problems, including myopia, astigmatism, anisometropia, and strabismus.

Most of these problems are more often seen in the infants with the most severe stages of ROP; however, follow-up with your baby's ophthalmologist is critical. Myopia, astigmatism, and anisometropia are all related to vision problems owing to the shape of the globe of the eye or differences in the shape of the globes. All can be treated with glasses. Strabismus (lazy-eye, cross-eye) can be treated with patching of the eye: simple treatments when started early.

CAUSE. It was once mistakenly thought that the administration of excessive amounts of oxygen was the only factor causing eye problems such as ROP in the premature infant. It was thought that the vessels in the eye couldn't handle the additional oxygen in the blood. Today, however, additional causes of ROP have been suggested—notably immaturity itself. During normal gestation the fetus receives her nutrients as well as her needed level of oxygen from the placenta (these oxygen levels are relatively low compared with the oxygen levels that the baby will achieve when her lungs expand and begin to function after birth). After birth the increased level of oxygen that the baby either breathes herself or is given supplementally may alter the development of the immature blood vessels of the eye. Today doctors are acquiring new insights into the delicate balance that exists between oxygen administration and retinal development.

There is a current controversy over whether ROP can be caused by fluorescent lighting in the NICU. A major study published in the May 1998 *New England Journal of Medicine* found that reducing light levels in the NICU did not reduce the incidence of ROP among infants at high risk for the disorder. However, critics have disputed the validity of the study. Both sides agree, however, that it cannot be a dangerous thing to make nurseries more friendly to babies by reducing light and sound—whatever the actual connection between light levels and ROP.

TREATMENT. Six or seven weeks after birth, your baby's retina will be examined weekly or every other week by an ophthalmologist. These exams will continue until it can be confirmed that the retinal vessels are growing normally and will soon complete their normal development from the center of the eye out to the edges of the retina. Several outpatient visits may be needed to insure that normal growth has occurred. However, if any abnormal growth of the retinal vessels is detected, or if any bleeding is noted, then spontaneous resolution will most likely not occur. Abnormal findings can include the cessation of development of the retinal blood vessels, formation of abnormal blood vessels, and bleeding of the abnormal vessels. If the condition is allowed to continue, damage to the retina could lead to severe visual impairment or even loss. The treatment for this "threshold" stage of ROP is surgery to destroy the abnormal blood vessels in the retina. In the past the preferred technique was *cryotherapy,* which involved freezing these blood vessels. However the preferred method now is *laser surgery,* during which lasers burn the abnormal blood vessels. The advantage of the laser is twofold: it is a very precise way to alter blood vessel growth in the eye, and it causes much less inflammation than other kinds of treatment. Approximately 30 percent of babies diagnosed with ROP need to undergo laser therapy. Of this group, only about 10 percent will develop severe vision impairment.

Let us emphasize that surgery is seldom necessary. In approximately 90 percent of cases of ROP, the eye changes will correct themselves. Nonetheless, early assessment, diagnosis, and treatment are essential to minimize the risks. It is important to follow your physician's directions and keep all scheduled appointments with your infant's ophthalmologist. Treatment of ROP decreases the chance of blindness but does not always prevent it. In the long term, premature babies will more frequently need corrective lenses than full-term infants, whether they have experienced ROP or not.

Other Medical Concerns in the First Year

The first part of this chapter discusses the seven most common conditions of prematurity, as illustrated in the risk thresholds chart (see page 206). In the remainder of this chapter we will discuss some other medical conditions that you may encounter while your infant is NICU bound:

- Anemia
- Blood sugar instability
    Hypoglycemia
    Hyperglycemia
- Jaundice (or hyperbilirubinemia)
- Respiratory distress syndrome (RDS)
- Temperature regulation

Anemia

Anemia is defined as an abnormally low percentage of red blood cells in the blood. Red blood cells perform the crucial function of carrying oxygen to tissues throughout the body. The anemic baby may experience more difficulty transporting oxygen to the body's tissues due to his very low red blood cell concentrations. The blood's reduced oxygen-carrying capacity forces the heart to work harder. The heart's extra work reveals itself through in-creased heart and respiratory rates and the presence of a soft heart murmur. Some physicians believe that an infant's weight gain can be affected by the hemoglobin levels, but this has not been widely accepted. Many physicians also believe that prevention of anemia reduces the rate of apnea of prematurity. This has likewise not been conclusively proven. The consequences of anemia range from trivial to very serious, and as a result your baby's medical caregivers will watch his hemoglobin levels very closely. If the anemia becomes significant, a blood transfusion may be necessary.

All full-term babies normally experience a *physiological anemia* at about six to ten weeks after birth. This is the time in the infant's development when most of the red blood cells are beginning to be recycled and the red-blood-cell-generating activity of the bone marrow has not quite started yet. This type of anemia actually stimulates the baby's bone marrow to make more red blood cells. In the premature infant, this process is exaggerated owing to the loss of blood from blood tests, the rapid breakdown of immature red blood cells, and the low baseline level of red blood cells that the infant started out with. On occasion, the baby may need blood transfusions as well as oral iron supplements (which are already present in special premature infant formulas). Caution: Too much iron can be deadly, so follow your doctor's orders precisely if you're told to give your baby iron supplements.

SIGNS AND SYMPTOMS. Anemia is often visible from the pallor of the baby's skin. Actual diagnosis is done by laboratory testing, which will determine the level of hemoglobin in the blood. This is a routine test performed on all newborns, full-term and premature alike. A premature newborn's hemoglobin level is approximately 15 grams at birth. The blood sample can be drawn from the infant's heel, a central line, or an umbilical line.

CAUSES. The main causes of anemia in the premature infant are intrauterine complications or anemia of prematurity.

INTRAUTERINE COMPLICATIONS

If a child is born anemic, it is often due to blood loss that occurs while he is still in the uterus, not due to delivery. This can be caused by maternal complications such as placenta previa, which causes intrauterine bleeding. Anemia is also caused by blood incompatibility. If a mother is Rh-negative and the baby Rh-positive, the mother will make antibodies, which cross the placenta to destroy the baby's red blood cells. Incompatibility of blood type, so-called ABO incompatibility, is another cause of anemia.

ANEMIA OF PREMATURITY

Anemia is sometimes the result of the baby being robbed of the full third trimester in the womb, the gestational time when his iron stores are being maximized. These iron stores are essential for red blood cell production. The condition can be exacerbated by the frequent blood draws preemies often require, which can reduce the number of red blood cells in the blood faster than they can be replaced. It can also cause a loss of critical iron, which is contained in the red blood cells.

Other causes of anemia can include infections that trigger the breakdown of red blood cells and bleeding that reduces the number of red blood cells in circulation.

TREATMENTS. The treatment goal is to raise the level of hemoglobin in the blood so that the body's tissues can remain properly oxygenated with a low expenditure of energy. The infant may only need to be treated with iron-fortified formulas or oral iron replacement. He may be placed on cardiac and respiratory monitoring. In some severe cases of anemia, blood transfusions are needed. On the other hand, in most occurrences anemia is self-correcting: when it occurs during the first three months of life and there is no bleeding or infection to cause blood loss, it is often merely a matter of time before your baby develops his own ability to generate new red blood cells.

Blood Sugar Instability

Glucose is a sugar that serves as the fuel that our bodies, notably our brains, burn for energy. The term *blood sugar* refers to the amount of glucose in the bloodstream. Glucose is a critical source of energy for your baby, but only so much of it can be used before an excess becomes a problem. Premature infants are often unable to regulate their blood sugar levels properly. If left untreated, this may cause sudden and severe problems for your baby.

HYPOGLYCEMIA

This is an abnormally low level of glucose in the bloodstream.

Signs and Symptoms. The symptoms of hypoglycemia are nonspecific and thus difficult to diagnose. Some infants show no symptoms at all. Others have symptoms similar to those indicating an infection, such as lethargy, listlessness, tremors, or temperature instability. Apnea, convulsions, and coma are possible if the hypoglycemia is severe. Prolonged hypoglycemia may cause seizures and possibly congestive heart failure or persistent pulmonary hypertension.

Causes. Your infant's immaturity can cause her to have very low stores of complex sugars (glycogen), which can be broken down to supply glucose to the body. The baby's system may not be sufficiently developed to regulate its glucose level. The premature infant's general lack of body fat means her system does not have a major source of blood sugar. The breakdown of fat that occurs naturally during metabolism creates blood sugar. Mothers with diabetes require special perinatal care to minimize the risk of blood-sugar problems for their fetus.

Treatments. Your baby's physician will initiate some form of glucose solution as soon as possible. This could be in the form of IV fluids or oral feedings, depending on the child's overall health and maturity level. Also, keeping the baby warm, well oxygenated, and as stress-free as possible will aid in keeping her glucose needs to a minimum. Your baby's blood sugar level will be sampled after birth. It will then be checked periodically until it stabilizes.

HYPERGLYCEMIA

This is a term that describes an abnormally high blood sugar level.

Signs and Symptoms. There are no symptoms that are specific to this disorder except for a possible increase in urine output—a high sugar concentration spills into the urinary tract, carrying water with it. If it is not diagnosed quickly, dehydration may occur. A persistent, extremely high glucose level may affect brain metabolism if it is not brought down very carefully.

Causes. The overall immaturity of the child can lead to hyperglycemia. Additionally stress, steroid treatments, and infection can be causes of hyperglycemia.

Treatments. The hospital staff will do close monitoring of your baby's blood glucose levels. Careful monitoring of IV infusions and administration of insulin (a medication that assists the body in controlling high levels of blood glucose) may be needed.

Jaundice

Also known as *hyperbilirubinemia*, this disorder occurs when there is an overabundance of bilirubin in the body. Jaundice is fairly common among newborns and is not usually a serious condition, but with some babies, especially premature ones, there can be special concerns. Normally bilirubin is released into the bloodstream when red blood cells break down. Then the bilirubin binds to protein molecules that transport it to the liver, where it is metabolized and then excreted. But as the level of bilirubin in the blood increases, it moves into the tissues, thus causing a yellowish skin color and sometimes causing the whites of the eyes to turn yellow. If the bilirubin level is allowed to continue rising beyond certain levels, it can pass through the blood-brain barrier and can result in irreversible brain damage, also called *kernicterus*.

SIGNS AND SYMPTOMS. There is no exact value above which an infant's bilirubin level is said to be too high. It seems that the more premature the child, the lower the danger threshold of bilirubin. Thus each child must be evaluated individually, with factors such as gestational age, birth weight, and overall health determining his "normal" bilirubin level. Since bilirubin levels are most likely to peak within seven to ten days after birth, doctors and nurses will be closely observing your child at this time.

CAUSES. All newborns have large numbers of red blood cells at birth. As these cells break down, the level of bilirubin increases. Premature infants' livers may not be developed enough to process this amount of bilirubin, leading to an excess. Additionally, premature infants tend to have less protein in the blood for the bilirubin to bind with en route to the liver. As a result, an excess amount will stay in the bloodstream. In some instances breast milk can actually increase bilirubin levels in infants. Known as *breast milk jaundice,* this rare condition (affecting only one in one hundred breast-fed newborns) usually occurs a week or less after birth, peaks at three days after birth, and can persist for as long as sixty to ninety days. Although it is seldom necessary to stop breast-feeding altogether, some neonatologists will elect to treat this condition with a twelve- to thirty-six-hour halt in breast-feeding. The consequences of breast milk jaundice are not known to be serious. Of course, it is prudent to watch bilirubin levels closely if any type of jaundice manifests itself.

TREATMENT. If needed, the baby may be treated with phototherapy or an exchange transfusion. *Phototherapy* involves exposing a baby's skin to special blue or green fluorescent lights ("bili-lights"), which have been found to reduce the bilirubin level. Special care needs to be taken to shield the infant's eyes during phototherapy, as it is suspected to cause visual problems in some children.

Exchange transfusion involves slowly exchanging a healthy donor's blood for the premature infant's bilirubin-laden blood. The procedure is usually performed in the NICU at the infant's bedside and takes approximately two hours to complete. Occasionally more than one transfusion may be needed before the liver is mature enough to remove bilirubin on its own.

Respiratory Distress Syndrome (RDS)

This is a respiratory condition very common to the premature infant. It causes the child to have difficulty breathing and is related to the premature infant's overall immaturity, in particular the immaturity of the infant's lungs.

SIGNS AND SYMPTOMS. Respiratory difficulty is the most obvious sign of RDS. Laboratory studies to analyze arterial blood gases will often show impaired carbon dioxide and oxygen exchange.

CAUSES. RDS is caused by overall immaturity factors and the fact that the infant has an insufficient amount of surfactant in her lungs (surfactant is a chemical that helps the small air sacs in the lungs called alveoli to remain expanded).

TREATMENTS. Prenatally, one of the greatest advances for RDS came in the 1960s with the discovery of steroid medications that could be administered to the mother once delivery of the preemie was imminent. The steroids enhance fetal lung development. After delivery, support measures include careful monitoring of the child's respiratory status, including vital signs and analysis of laboratory data, and administration of surfactant via an endotracheal tube. Medical management through ventilation therapy and oxygen monitoring are also continually performed.

Temperature Regulation

Since premature infants often have trouble regulating their core body temperatures, intervention is usually necessary by the use of radiant warmers or incubators.

SIGNS AND SYMPTOMS. The infant is unable to maintain his body temperature. A normal range of temperature for an infant is 96.6 degrees Fahrenheit to 99.6 degrees Fahrenheit.

CAUSES. These infants usually have an immature hypothalamus, the area of the brain that assists with body temperature regulation. Additionally, preemies have very little fat to act as an insulator and very thin skin, making thermoregulation difficult. Energy sources needed for burning, such as fat and complex sugars, are also limited in preemies.

TREATMENTS. Initially, radiant warmers or incubators aid the baby in maintaining his body temperature. As he grows, he will build the necessary energy reserves that will help aid in maintaining body temperature. Temperatures are usually taken by a probe attached to the infant's body, or with a thermometer placed under the armpit. These methods are less invasive than rectal methods but will be adjusted accordingly to provide an accurate core reading. Your baby will be weighed daily to determine whether he's gaining weight properly. It is also important that the preemie's environment is very controlled. By decreasing light and noise from the outside environment, the conditions inside the womb can be partially simulated, thus promoting growth and development.

❧

This chapter has discussed the basics of various conditions that might affect your newly born preemie. Given the rapid pace of developments, you should rely upon your infant's own physician as the primary source of current information. Your child may experience none, one, or more than one of these conditions during his NICU stay into his first years. This list is not intended to be all-inclusive, but simply to give you an overview of what you might expect during your baby's NICU visit.

8

THE INTERMEDIATE CARE NURSERY: YOUR BABY'S FIRST STEP HOME

WHAT YOU WILL FIND IN THIS CHAPTER

- Life in the step-down unit
- Guidelines for discharge: Your baby's ticket home
- Medical concerns to deal with before your baby comes home
- Medical treatments that may continue in the intermediate care nursery
- Developmental care in the intermediate care nursery
- Discharge planning
- Rooming in before discharge: Dress rehearsal for life on your own
- Your discharge debriefing

Your premature baby may have spent anywhere from half a day to several months in the neonatal special care nursery. If your baby's time there was on the longer end of the spectrum, you may have become accustomed to—and even comforted by—the rhythms of life there. In Chapter 6 parents spoke of the reassurance that comes from specially trained nurses always being near and neonatologists and other specialists hustling in and out of the unit. As you get to know the individuals charged with your baby's care, that feeling has only grown. But there will come a time when

the close monitoring and twenty-four-hour supervision will no longer be necessary. Preemiedom isn't a place; it's a journey. And your baby is slowly making her way toward doing by herself all of the things the "artificial womb" of the NICU once did for her. Before being discharged home, your baby will spend some time in a way station to discharge: the intermediate care, or "step-down," nursery (also sometimes called a *level II nursery*). The name of this area may vary from hospital to hospital. Sometimes it is not even physically separated from the main NICU itself. But no matter what it is called or where it is situated, step-down units all serve the same basic purpose: getting your baby ready for her long-awaited journey home.

Life in the Step-Down Unit

Some babies are brought here directly from the labor and delivery area, and if that is the case with you, you are fortunate indeed. Your baby simply needs a higher degree of care than what is provided in a full-term newborn nursery.

But if you are a veteran of the NICU yourself, you may not be sure that this move was

> JOE GARCIA-PRATS: "You might expect parents to breathe a sigh of relief once their child is far enough away from danger to be transferred to a step-down unit. Instead I find that most families spend a very unsettling several days there. The pace and intensity are very different. The number of staff present in the unit is very different. The impression often is that the level of care is inadequate. It's not. You've simply moved on. Your baby doesn't need to have vitals checked every hour. Urine doesn't have to be measured regularly. Your baby doesn't need to be handled as often. Parents are frequently unnerved by that. They've become used to all the activity, to seeing doctors and therapists wandering in and out. Now all of a sudden it's quiet. The hustle and bustle goes away. And parents have an opportunity to spend more time with baby. Which is what being a parent is all about."

such a good idea. You may have to wean yourself off the dependency that can emerge from having relied for a potentially long time on the unit's specialists and high technology to keep your baby well. By comparison with the NICU, the step-down unit may strike you as too quiet. There isn't as much going on. The nurses appear to be so much more laid-back compared with those in the NICU. There aren't as many doctors around, either. The slower pace of life may make you wonder whether you and your baby have been abandoned by the nurses, technicians, and doctors who did so much for you and your baby in his moment of greatest need.

Intermediate care nurseries are designed to provide basic care to slightly immature or moderately sick newborns. Babies who require hourly monitoring or respirator care are not placed in this unit. In many hospitals these units are physically part of the NICU, enabling the babies to move from one area to the other. In such facilities there may be walls separating different bays, and the babies in the step-down area are kept in open cribs instead of warmers or incubators. In other hospitals the step-down or intermediate care unit is a separate nursery altogether. Since the infants staying here are usually much more stable, the nurse-to-patient ratio is higher. In the NICU it was one to one or one to two. In the intermediate care nursery it is often one to four.

Accordingly, it is not uncommon for parents to have some anxiety about the care their baby will receive here. But try to take that as a source of comfort rather than fear: your infant is not the same critically ill newborn who first came to the NICU. If the absence of doting medical staff, relative to the NICU, causes you to worry about a lack of attentiveness on the part of staff to your baby's progress, please know that it is a sign of his budding independence and strength. Recognizing that will allow you to appreciate the change of pace. The less hectic environment, with fewer voices and mechanical noises to distract or overstimulate your child, may very well enable you to get to know your baby better. The bonds you forge with your infant during the trying times of the NICU will be strong. But when the pressures of the NICU are a thing of the past, you may find that you can get to know your baby in a whole new way. If you find that this is the case, your preparation for going home will be all the more complete.

Guidelines for Discharge: Your Baby's Ticket Home

Once you've made the adjustment from the NICU to the intermediate care unit, it is only natural to begin thinking about the next steps: discharge and homecoming. Your baby will be moved only when he is stable enough to be safe in the level II environment. Your baby's neonatologist will make sure that the plan of care initiated in the NICU is continued, so that your infant can come home as quickly and safely as possible. The neonatologist will explain your baby's particular situation and needs and outline the benchmarks that must be met before discharge is possible.

There are some general discharge guidelines around which you can orient your thinking. Most institutions previously used the so-called 5-pound rule as a guide to when a preemie was ready to be discharged. It was thought that an infant was ready to go home only when her weight exceeded 5 pounds. Of course, as we

have said throughout the book, measuring an infant's health generally defies reduction to a single number, be it weight, gestational age, or what have you. Today neonatologists use a much more comprehensive and individually tailorable set of standards for determining when a baby may be discharged.

The broader view includes the following functional goals that a baby must reach before he can go home.

First, your baby's medical problems should be resolved or made manageable on an outpatient basis. Obviously, any condition or problem requiring hospital care precludes discharge.

Second, the baby should be able to tolerate being in an open crib and to maintain his own body temperature. This is partially a function of weight, insofar as body fat serves as a good insulator. However, many babies are able to maintain temperature before they reach 5 pounds.

Third, your infant should be gaining weight steadily while taking a standard diet of infant formula or breast milk. Ask your doctor to show you your baby's weight progression to date. It is charted daily.

Fourth, as a parent, you should be proficient in the technical aspects, if any, of your baby's home care. This can include parent training on any monitors that may need to come home with the baby. Prior to discharge, the hospital will assign a nurse or other specialist to train you in the operation of any such equipment. It is important that you take an infant CPR course geared for parents of preemies, if it is available at your facility. If not, call the American Red Cross or American Heart Association to find out where you can take a course.

Fifth, your home must be ready for the new infant. This can include preparing a nursery with proper medical supplies, ensuring the air quality in your home by changing air filters, removing carpets that contain pet dander, and so forth.

Sixth, follow-up medical care should have been arranged before discharge. This usually means you've selected a pediatrician who will assume care of your infant after he goes home with you.

Clearly, some infants weighing less than 5 pounds will be robust enough to meet these criteria. Others won't meet them until they are much heavier. Remember that each child is an individual, and this individuality becomes apparent even in prematurity. Support your child's individuality and don't be frustrated if his progress is not "by the book."

Medical Concerns to Deal with Before Your Baby Comes Home

By now your baby has come a long way on the journey toward discharge. The intensive care nursery is a thing of the past. Mechanical respiration, if she ever needed it, is history, too. It is no longer necessary to apply day-to-day vigilance over every vital sign. Nonetheless, a number of medical concerns will remain until the day your baby is finally discharged.

APNEA

Control of breathing is one medical concern. If your child had apnea in the special care nursery, caffeine or aminophylline was probably prescribed. Both are thought to make the baby's respiratory control center more sensitive to carbon dioxide. This means that the respiratory control center will trigger more regularly, resulting in regular, steady breathing, and not allow carbon dioxide to accumulate in the baby's system. That is what happens in our mature respiratory control center. The respiratory control center matures with time, and usually the infant has no apnea after the thirty-fifth week. Should apnea continue beyond thirty-five or thirty-six weeks postconceptional age, then usually further investigation is warranted. The next step is to do a "multichannel" study that integrates heart rate, respiratory rate, pulse oximetry, and the baby's respiratory effort. The objective of the test is to determine whether a problem exists with your baby's respiratory control center or whether there is a problem with a blockage in your infant's airway (so-called obstructive apnea). Obstructive apnea is usually caused by muscles in the infant's lower throat that aren't strong enough to keep the throat open. It is important to discover the cause of apnea because the way each cause is treated is different.

Your baby will continue receiving the caffeine (or aminophylline) until he is apnea-free for a certain period of time determined by the neonatologist in the context of the baby's overall health. This usually happens after thirty-three to thirty-four weeks postconceptional age. Once the apnea is resolved on medication, the medicine will be stopped and the baby will

Gastroesophageal Reflux (GER)

GER is a condition where the infant regurgitates very often. This may be due to overfeeding (rarely) or to some problem with the sphincter valve where the stomach joins the esophagus. This valve stays closed after feeding and keeps milk in the stomach until it is pushed into the lower intestine. Since a preemie's sphincter may not be as tight as the older infant's, small amounts of reflux are often quite normal. Reflux becomes a problem when the volume of vomiting is such that the baby's nutritional intake and the rate of growth are impinged. Also, the acid that is refluxed into the lower esophagus from the stomach can cause the infant pain and discomfort, and the vomiting can block the infant's airway, causing apnea.

Usually as the baby matures, the problem goes away since the muscle in the sphincter becomes tighter with age. In the meantime, several steps can be taken to reduce or prevent the reflux:

- The infant can be placed on the stomach and the head of the incubator raised, thus using gravity to slow the reflux.
- The volume of milk can be reduced or its caloric density increased.
- The time over which the milk enters the stomach during feedings can be lengthened (60 to 120 minutes).
- If the baby is receiving feedings by gavage, staff can reduce or discontinue the caffeine or aminophylline that is being used to treat the apnea, since this may reduce sphincter tone and increase stomach acid secretion. The milk can be supplemented with an antacid or H_2 blocker.
- Medications can be administered that increase gastric emptying or sphincter tone.

be watched for one to two weeks. Most neonatologists are comfortable with an infant being apnea-free for just one week after the caffeine dosage has fallen to a level that does not affect the baby.

If apnea continues and the multichannel study shows an abnormality, then the neonatologist and/or pediatric pulmonologist (a specialist who often consults in connection with apnea) will recommend a *home apnea monitor*.

This monitor, which you'll set up at home, will record your baby's heart rate and respiratory rate, and sometimes his oxygen saturation, sounding an alarm if they become too low. If your baby has such a monitor, you will be trained, prior to discharge, in how to either stimulate the infant to breathe or begin CPR.

When your baby is attached to an apnea monitor, it will take you a while to return to a "normal" home life. You can't just ask the teenager from down the block to come and watch your child while you run to the store. Indeed, anyone caring for your infant, even for the shortest time, must be trained in CPR. As a result, stories like Kimberly's will be the exception rather than the rule. Apnea monitors are generally recommended only when your physician believes that this would be helpful in managing a medical problem. How long your baby needs it will depend on the cause of the apnea and how quickly your infant's respiratory center matures. On average, most infants will require the monitor for three to six months after hospital discharge.

NUTRITION AND WEIGHT GAIN

Your baby's nutrition and growth are a fundamental concern throughout his journey through the NICU, and equally so after he reaches the home stretch toward discharge. Your doctor's goal is for your baby to achieve the same rate of growth that he would have had in utero: a gain of 15 to 30 grams per day. This is no small task. If your infant is making satisfactory progress in his feedings and nutrition, he will be more likely to thrive after discharge. Here we review the progression that a baby must make through the course of his NICU stay.

The first variable in the type of nutrition your baby received was what type of nourishment he could tolerate in his intestinal tract. If you decided to provide breast milk, then the milk was probably fortified to increase the calorie and mineral content in order to accelerate your child's rate of growth. If you decided not to breast-feed or couldn't provide the volume of milk the baby requires, then formulas specially made for premature infants were probably used. How your baby gets the milk or formula depends on how mature your baby is. Maturity determines whether there is a suck and swallow reflex and how well the two are coordinated. Coordination is usually achieved at about thirty-four weeks postconceptional age, but this varies. Most likely your infant receives milk or formula by gavage, a small tube placed into the stomach through the mouth or nose. The initial amount of milk or formula is very small. It is increased over the course of care. Some infants proceed very quickly and others very slowly. From gavage feeding, your baby progresses to the point where he can take one feeding per day by nipple.

Some researchers believe that using a rubber nipple causes the infant to use a different tongue movement than is used when feeding at the breast. It is thought that these infants have a harder time making a transition from the bottle to the breast. Lactation consultants are often available for those mothers who would like to breast-feed but have difficulty either producing enough volume or helping their infant make the transition from bottle to breast.

As your baby successfully takes the single feeding by nipple in fifteen to twenty minutes, then another feeding can be added until he is taking all the feedings in the required time. Again, how long it will take your infant will vary. Don't get discouraged if your child is a slow feeder. It will probably work out just fine with time. Some physicians will recommend tube feedings at home until your baby can feed well by nipple. If you need to learn how to place the tube into your baby's stomach, the nurses will show you how. It is not hard, and both parents will be taught. It will allow your baby to come home while he is learning to nipple-feed.

What Is a Breast Milk Bank?

As this is being written, six hospitals across the country have set up breast milk banks, facilities where breast milk is donated and stored and given to mothers who wish to give their babies breast milk but aren't able to produce it themselves. The American Academy of Pediatrics issued a policy statement in 1997 that read, "Human milk is the preferred feeding for all infants, including premature and sick newborns, with rare exceptions."

Donor mothers tend to be mothers who are currently breast-feeding their own infants but have a surplus. The donors are screened meticulously for drugs, infections, and lifestyle. The milk is pasteurized and stored for use by mothers who need it. Since breast milk's composition changes to suit a growing baby's evolving needs, the milk banks try to give infants milk that comes from donors who have babies of the same age.

Though breast milk banks have yet to be accepted into the medical mainstream in this country, our advice is to stay tuned to this development and ask your doctor's advice.

The paramount criterion of your baby's maturity is weight gain. It will do no good in the long run if your infant is nippling all feedings but not gaining weight. Remember that growth is like a checkbook register: if your baby expends resources (calories) working hard to nipple-feed, fewer calories will be left for growth. So advancing the number of nipple feedings depends not only on how well your baby feeds, but also on how rapidly he grows while expending those calories. Moving your baby to an open crib has the same kind of dynamic. Lying there in the open air, he may appear as if he's one step closer to going home. But if he has to burn more calories to maintain body temperature in the crib, then the move works against him in the final analysis. When your baby is gaining weight *and* is nippling well, it is time to consider placing him into an open crib.

Medical Treatments That May Continue in the Intermediate Care Nursery

Several treatments that started in the NICU will need to be continued in level II. Some of these treatments may even become necessary after discharge. Arrangements for outpatient treatment will be completed before you go home, however.

One lung problem that will be managed in the level II nursery is BPD. If BPD is present, your infant may be off the respirator or CPAP but still require oxygen by nasal prongs until the physicians know that her lungs are in good enough shape to keep the oxygen level in her blood at normal levels. Removal of the oxygen is done very slowly, since doing so too soon could place strain on your baby's heart. Part and parcel of any oxygen treatment regimen is the maintenance of good nutrition and growth. Without good nutrition, the infant's lungs will not grow and repair themselves. As the baby with BPD continues to grow, the chronic lung disease should fade away owing to the amount of normal new tissue that is rapidly forming in the lungs. After discharge, your baby's medications or oxygen needs will be monitored closely.

Two other disease processes that will still be watched for in the level II nursery are *infection* and *necrotizing enterocolitis* (*NEC*). We wish that leaving the neonatal ICU meant we wouldn't have to worry about those two major problems. It is true that increasing maturity does reduce the chances of your baby's having any more bouts of infection, but it doesn't eliminate them. The same symptoms the staff watched for in the NICU can still appear: difficulty tolerating feedings, lethargy, poor temperature regulation, low blood pressure, apnea, and so on. Likewise, NEC is still a potential problem until your baby is mature enough to go home. For this reason, each feeding is charted carefully. Your baby's chart will record the number and character of stools and any incidence of blood in the stool, vomiting, or distension of the abdomen. All could be hallmarks of NEC. Currently there is no way to prevent infection or NEC, other than supporting your baby and waiting for her to mature out of the risk period.

Another medical issue that will be monitored weekly while your infant is in the level II nursery is the proportion of red blood cells in the blood; too little means *anemia*. In a preemie, the trigger that starts the infant making red blood cells is blunted, and the baby will therefore have very low proportions of red blood cells. As long as the infant is gaining weight and the heart rate and respiratory rate are normal,

there is no need to transfuse the infant. As the infant matures, the trigger to begin making red blood cells will engage and the anemia will gradually abate.

Developmental Care in the Intermediate Care Nursery

In the context of discussing all of these issues that you may confront in the level II nursery, you probably noticed that several other practices and procedures of the NICU have followed you into the level II area. The lights are dimmed as much as possible. The noise level is kept low. Incubators are covered with decorated covers or blankets to reduce light and noise even further. Each infant has a small rolled blanket or other object supporting his positioning to simulate the close surrounding of the uterus, and many of the premature infants are swaddled as well. The nurses, though they aren't as immediately present as they were in the NICU, intervene quickly when they notice that your infant is uncomfortable, beginning to cry, or growing hungry. To make sure your baby isn't stressed, the nurses are careful to avoid doing anything that could disturb him. All of this is part of a "developmental" approach to the premature infant. It goes beyond the pathology of illness to recognize that general comfort and well-being are critical elements in a preemie's overall care. The medical literature appears to support the long-term benefit of this approach.

There will also be some "normal baby" issues to deal with in the level II nursery, depending on how long your infant is in the hospital. One is *immunizations*. The first will come when your child is about two months of age. If your baby is home by that time, then your pediatrician will arrange for that to be done in the office. While in the hospital, in some states, parents will have to sign a consent for immunizations to be administered. Subsequent immunizations will be organized and directed through your pediatrician's office.

Another normal baby "must" is the newborn screen—which in most states is mandated to be done when a full-term infant leaves the hospital and then again about seven to ten days later. This blood test looks for diseases that occur early in the infant's life and that require rapid intervention, such as hypothyroidism or sickle cell anemia. Your preemie will have at least two of these newborn screening tests while in the hospital, the first at one week of age and then again at about one month. Results of these tests are usually available within two weeks after they are sent to the state lab for testing.

Your infant will get one other screening test before he leaves, a newborn *hearing screening test*. This is usually done in the nursery, where is it quiet. If your baby fails the test, then a more sophisticated test will be ordered to confirm the findings. If the test is still not normal, then your infant will be referred to an ear, nose, and throat specialist and the audiologist who works with him or her for further recommendations.

Discharge Planning

As many of the issues just mentioned begin to be dealt with successfully, the discharge planning process will begin. In addition to ascertaining that the baby's health is appropriate for discharge, this planning involves assuring that the parents are informed about or trained on all

> ### Will My Insurance Company Pay for Home Nursing Service?
>
> Remember that in some instances, if your infant's problems are complex, insurance plans will provide some home nursing support. As the planning process gets under way, the discharge nurse or coordinator can help you find out what your insurance company will help pay for. As is typical where a question of insurance coverability arises, you or your baby's neonatologist will likely need to communicate to your insurer that the home nursing service is medically necessary.

discharge needs of their baby. This can include parent education in CPR, training on the use of home monitors that your baby may need, and general care of the premature newborn. These are all an important part of the care that you'll give your child at home. That being the case, both mom and dad need to be prepared to learn what is needed; most nurses are wonderfully helpful in teaching you what you need to know. Learning things like the times and methods for administering medications, though intimidating at first, is easily mastered.

Usually a team of several individuals is involved in your baby's discharge plans. This team can include the neonatologist, nurse practitioner, registered nurse, dietitian, social worker, ophthalmologist, and possibly other specialists. First they'll discuss what type of medical follow-up your infant will need after she goes home.

Some preemies need only to be followed by their pediatrician. However, sometimes a specialist of one type or another will need to see your baby on an outpatient basis. Ophthalmologists, otolaryngologists, pulmonologists, dietitians, and lactation specialists are frequently called in in the first year of a preemie's life.

If any equipment needs to go home with baby, you'll need to master its use before your infant leaves the step-down unit.

Choosing a Pediatrician

Choosing a pediatrician is one of the most important decisions you will make regarding your baby's health care needs after discharge. The relationship that you are able to foster with your pediatrician is very important, because she will be your baby's primary caregiver for years to come. You need to feel comfortable knowing that she or her staff will be available twenty-four hours a day, seven days a week. The choice of a pediatrician is a very personal one. We have compiled the following list of questions and considerations to assist you in making this important decision.

Questions to Ask When Choosing a Pediatrician

- Do you care for many preterm infants in your practice?
- What are your opinions/recommendations on bottle-feeding vs. breast-feeding?
- What is your recommended immunization schedule?
- Do you always see your own patients?
- How are after-hours calls handled?
- With whom do you share calls?
- Where do I go for emergencies?

- What hospital do you use for emergencies should this be necessary?
- Do you accept my insurance?
- Do you file insurance claim forms?
- If specialists are needed, what is the referral process?

Other Things to Consider When Choosing a Pediatrician

- Is the office close to your home?
- What hospital is used for admission? Is the hospital close to your home?
- Do you have a good rapport with the doctor?
- Does he explain things clearly and simply?
- Are the other office staff and nurses helpful and courteous?
- Is the office convenient to your work location or child care facilities?

❧ TIP

Once you have chosen a pediatrician, be sure to give the pediatrician's name, address, and fax number to the neonatologist. This will assist in the transfer of records to the pediatrician's office prior to your baby's first visit, which will take place within the first few weeks of discharge. It will make for a smoother transition if the pediatrician can review the records well ahead of time.

Predischarge Procedures and Testing

LAB TESTS. Prior to discharge, your baby will have additional labwork performed as necessary. This could include a complete blood count and white blood cell count to test for conditions such as anemia and will probably include, per your state's law, a newborn screening. This screening commonly tests for the following conditions:

- Sickle cell disease
- Hypothyroidism
- Phenylketonuria
- Congenital adrenal hyperplasia (CAH)
- Galactosemia

CIRCUMCISION. A circumcision is the removal of the foreskin from the tip of the penis. The opinion of the medical community about its value has vacillated over the years. Additionally, most parents have strong personal opinions about this. Individuals with certain religious or personal beliefs may choose not to have their baby circumcised, or they may prefer to make special arrangements for this to be performed on an outpatient basis. If you are undecided, review the literature, seek medical guidance, and be sure all of your questions are answered prior to consenting to this procedure. Remember, this is an elective procedure and will need your parental consent to be performed.

If you choose to have your baby boy circumcised, this will usually be performed in the hospital. Circumcision is generally performed by the OB/GYN who delivered your baby. As discharge approaches, the nursery staff will help coordinate and schedule this procedure with your OB/GYN or pediatrician. Your physician will discuss the procedure beforehand. You will need to sign a consent form to authorize the procedure. There may be some reluctance on the part of your baby's physician about performing a circumcision on your premature infant. This comes from a concern of having a procedure performed associated with some risk

(very small) in a baby who has survived many more procedures associated with greater risk. There is no data demonstrating any increased risk of circumcision in the healthy premature infant. Likewise there is no reason why this could not be performed by a mohel at a bris.

The circumcision site will heal within a few days, and the nursery staff will train you in the proper techniques for keeping the site clean and protected until it heals completely.

VISION EXAMINATION. This may have been performed earlier in your baby's NICU stay, but your baby's vision will continue to be assessed throughout the admission. This is primarily because premature infants are statistically much more prone to visual disturbances than full-term babies. (See the discussion of retinopathy of prematurity [ROP] in chapter 7, "Special Concerns in the NICU," page 205.)

Additionally, at discharge your doctor will recommend you follow up with an ophthalmologist usually around three, six, and nine months and again at one year. These frequent eye examinations will help the physician determine whether the muscles and vessels of your baby's eyes are maturing satisfactorily.

THE CAR SEAT TEST. Most car seats on the market today are designed for full-term babies and may need to be modified for use by a preemie. Thus a car seat test will be performed on your preemie prior to discharge. The test will help determine if your chosen car seat is appropriate for your baby. The factors to consider are support, angle when carried, angle when stationary, and enough support to properly position the baby while riding in the car. The main concern with positioning is making sure the baby's airway doesn't become blocked if his head moves during transit. A preemie very often doesn't have head or neck muscle control until he is many months old. Therefore he can't move his head by himself if it gets placed in an awkward or dangerous position. It is common for preemies to assume a slumped position in a car seat, where the chin comes to the chest. Breathing can be difficult in this position.

For this test, you will be asked to bring in your baby's actual car seat, the one he will be using at discharge and after. During the test, which will take place right in the step-down unit, your baby will be positioned in the car seat, surrounded and cushioned by the padding. He will then be attached to a cardiopulmonary monitor to evaluate his heart and respiratory status. The test will take approximately an hour to perform. The goal of this testing is to simulate riding in the car seat.

A Note about Car Seats

It is very important that any infant younger than one year of age sit in a rear-facing car seat. It is also recommended that the seat be certified for infants of up to 30 pounds.

If your vehicle is equipped with a passenger-side air bag, do *not* use the car seat in the front seat. The explosive force of the air bag can injure and even kill an infant.

Preemie sitting in a car seat

If your baby passes the test, and your car seat is appropriate for him, you are one step closer to discharge. If your baby flunks the test (by having any apneic episodes or breathing pauses during the test), most likely the car seat will need additional padding. Various types of padding or head supports can be purchased in stores that sell the car seats themselves. After the adjustments have been made, your baby will be retested until he passes.

Rooming In Before Discharge: Dress Rehearsal for Life on Your Own

Many parents find it useful to have a "rooming-in" period before embarking on life as their preemies' sole caretakers. "I had her all to myself for two days," Melissa said. "They would make sure I was feeding her often enough and keeping her temperature warm. I thought it was great. I would have been terrified if I had to take her home cold turkey from the nursery to my house after waiting all that time. I was very comfortable taking care of her by the time we went home." How this practice is handled varies from hospital to hospital. Most likely its feasibility

will depend on how complex your baby's needs will be at home and how well trained you need to be to meet them. Rooming in entails living with your baby in a hospital room, usually very close to the nursery. You and your spouse take care of the infant with no help from the nurses, the purpose being to simulate what it will be like taking care of your child by yourself. The nurses are always available for help, but the idea is for you to learn to fly without a net.

Many parents discover that being on their own like this makes for a heady, unforgettable experience. Cori, the mother of a 1-pound-3-ounce twenty-four-weeker who spent 104 days in the NICU, recounted for us some of the details of her rooming-in experience. "Finally the day came that we were able to bring him home. We 'roomed in' at the hospital in a room that was directly across from the NICU and were given training on the apnea monitor that we'd take home with Bo. It was like, 'They finally let us have our baby.' For so long he had been theirs. They made the rules. They told us when we could hold him. Now we could shut the doors and do whatever we wanted.

"My husband and I were so nervous. We were afraid that something would go wrong, that we would damage him for life, and that they wouldn't let us take him home. We knew how well taken care of he was in the NICU. But now we were responsible! I felt fear as I've never known fear before.

"Bo was brought to the room, and the nurse left. What happened then was sort of funny. My husband and I found ourselves 'fighting' over which one of us could hold him. I would lay Bo down and my husband would go pick him up. I'd tell him rather sternly that Bo needed to lie in his crib. But as soon as my husband would lay him down, I'd find a reason to pick him up again. I think it was the freedom from the nurses' eyes that made us this way. We hardly slept a wink that night with each of us getting up constantly to check on him. His alarm never did go off that night, which was really a blessing in disguise. If it had, we probably would have told the doctors to keep him a little longer—not!

"The next morning, Bo was discharged. He weighed a whopping 4 pounds 8 ounces. He got his picture taken by the newborn baby photographer. The nurse then put me in a wheelchair with Bo in my lap. She wheeled us to the NICU and we said our good-byes, with lots of hugs and kisses and well-wishes. One of the nurses took a picture of our 'going-home day' to be put up on the 'graduates' picture board. She then wheeled us down to the car, with my husband taking pictures.

"We were so happy that day. All we'd ever wanted, dreamed of, and wished for had finally come true. We were going home."

Your Discharge Debriefing

On the day of your baby's discharge, you will meet with the neonatologist and primary care nurse for the last time. You may also meet with a discharge-planning nurse. They will debrief you on your baby's condition and recommended treatment plan. This is your last chance to ask questions face-to-face with your baby's health care team, so come ready to listen and armed with any questions that have yet to be answered.

TIP

Remember that the NICU staff wants to help make your transition home with your baby as smooth as possible and will encourage you to call the unit with any questions that you may have. Don't hesitate to take them up on that offer. You will have a tremendously valuable resource at your fingertips while you make the transition of turning over your baby's medical care to the pediatrician. Your first visit with the pediatrician will most likely be scheduled within a week or two of discharge from the NICU.

How formally the discharge process unfolds will vary from hospital to hospital. Some NICUs conduct a comprehensive review of your baby's condition and treatment, as well as a thorough discussion of caring for a preemie at home. At other facilities the only real review is of the medical issues still in your baby's picture during the final week.

In any event, you will want to have answers to the following questions:

- Who is your baby's pediatrician?
- How are you going to feed your baby?
- Are you clear on the medical procedures you need to implement: putting in a tube for feedings, administrating oxygen, handling apnea and heart monitors?
- Have you made the other necessary appointments for your baby—hearing screenings, vision tests, times for the home health nurse to visit, and the like?
- Have you completed your infant CPR training?

9

BRINGING YOUR PREEMIE HOME

WHAT YOU WILL FIND IN THIS CHAPTER

- Good-bye to the NICU
- The home environment
- Breast-feeding vs. bottle-feeding
- Life at home with multiples

- Meeting the pediatrician: The first-year checkups
- Dressing your preemie
- Preemie support groups
- Keeping dad involved

It's official discharge day, the day when it's time to take your child home from the special care nursery. You've been debriefed for discharge, and you're ready to go. This is a day you may have dreamed about ever since you first imagined yourself becoming pregnant. Most likely you never guessed it would have taken so long. But the wait has probably done little to diminish the excitement of finally being able to be a full-time parent. From the time this unexpected whirlwind began, the NICU staff has been helping you plan for this day. And you probably found a certain level of

comfort in the knowledge that your child was safely sequestered in the NICU. While it was initially hard on the nerves, the close twenty-four-hour monitoring by highly trained professionals gave you confidence that your premature baby's every need would be quickly met. Then your baby graduated to the step-down unit. Though infants don't come with owner's manuals, it was easy to believe otherwise in the structured, measured world of the special care nursery. Now you're on your own. For many parents, the prospect of taking their fragile preemie home sometimes gives life to the phrase "Watch out what you wish for, you just might get it."

Throughout your baby's stay in the special care nursery you have watched her pass through stages of development that most parents never see. If at times you have felt distant from your baby, not fully bonded, as many parents report, you may have later found that going through the experience of prematurity with your baby has helped you forge a bond that will deepen as time passes. Some parents have spoken of the NICU stay as "bonus time" with their babies. The process of surviving and coping with this experience can strengthen the connection you feel with your child.

Advice for Parents on Discharge Day

JOE GARCIA-PRATS: "Though it can be stressful, discharge day is a fun day that you will likely remember for the rest of your life. It's full of lots of little odds and ends to take care of—stocking up on vitamins, medicines, and other supplies. It has a feel that's similar to graduating from high school or going off to college. It's a major life transition for your child, and it brings out the same emotions. Of course, worry is foremost among them. But then, parents are going to worry about their children. Indeed, parents of preemies get quite a jump start on worrying. I try to make parents realize, as subtly as I can, that even if their child wasn't a preemie, they'd probably still be worrying."

For your baby's entire stay in intensive care, the discharge date has been a goal for you to focus on, a light at the end of the tunnel. Typically the neonatologist will peg that date to your baby's original due date. For example, if your infant was delivered at thirty-two weeks' gestation, then she would stay in the NICU for about eight weeks, or until she reaches the full-term gestational age of forty weeks. Some children have special needs that require longer hospitalizations. And others who gain weight rapidly and stabilize their temperature and respiration may be discharged prior to their due date. To allow for the unexpected, and to avoid getting your hopes up, your neonatologist and other staff may have been rather guarded about specifying a particular discharge date.

Whatever the particular criteria your baby must meet in order to be cleared for discharge, and no matter how much advance notice you have of your baby's progress toward those criteria, discharge from the NICU or step-down unit may give you mixed feelings. While you'll be eager to begin your family life at home, you'll be saying good-bye to a comfortable and secure world. You'll be leaving behind the friendships you may have forged with those who have cared for your child at this critical time in her life. And you'll be moving on without benefit of the professional support and expertise of the NICU staff that you have come to depend on. In a way, your baby is being born again, entering a new world for the first time: your world, your home, with surroundings quite different from those of the only world that she has ever known, the hospital NICU.

How David Came Home

SHARON HORNFISCHER: "Our son had been having what the NICU nurses and doctors called 'A's and B's.' That stands for apneic breathing, or pauses in respiration that come with drops in pulse rate. The rule was that every time a preemie experiences A's and B's, his NICU stay is automatically extended by a week. A baby has to be apnea-free for a full week before he can be discharged.

"On the afternoon before we were due to bring David home, my husband and I worked to get everything ready for David's homecoming the next day. All the while I was quite anxious about the what-ifs of bringing a 4½-pound baby home. Can we really do this? What if he has A's and B's at home? I was basically second-guessing myself at every turn. I remember praying that if he was going to have any more apneic episodes, I wished for them to happen today, while he was under the constant watchful eye of the NICU staff, and not when he was home. Well, we went back to the hospital for his last evening meal as an inpatient. Immediately after we scrubbed in, David's nurse came up to us and said that he had actually had an apneic episode while we were out. At first I thought she was kidding. Then I realized the implications: he, and we, would be staying another week. I had a rush of guilt—did I somehow *will* this to happen? What a bad mother I must be. I was upset with myself and at the same time glad that he would be staying where he needed to be for just a little while longer. But exactly one week later we brought our son home. And this time we were ready, and so was he."

Good-bye to the NICU

As exciting, elating, and liberating as your baby's discharge day is, it may also be filled with other emotions: fear, self-doubt, insecurity. These feelings are all very normal. Just know that coming home with your baby from the NICU is like a commencement, an ending and a beginning. And you, like many people before, will be able to do it—to take your preemie home to a loving, safe, and nurturing environment in which your child will grow and flourish. And you will be able to get down to the long-awaited job of becoming a full-time parent to your child.

The Home Environment

VISITORS AND GOING OUT

Once you finally get your child home, you probably won't want to go out too much. Even after their discharge, preemies are still playing a game of catch-up. Their immune systems are still developing, and they are therefore more susceptible to infections than full-term babies. As a rule of thumb, it's a good idea to avoid public places where the environment is uncontrolled. Many preemies are still delicate at this stage, and even exposure to a common cold or another relatively innocuous illness could set them back considerably and cause additional doctor visits or even rehospitalizations.

Just staying put at home with your newborn can be refreshing and relaxing. But at times duty calls—or sheer claustrophobia—and you need to go out. When this happens, it is best, if possible, to make arrangements to leave your baby at home with a qualified caregiver rather than expose him to possible infection in a public place.

Of course, finding help may not be easy, es-

pecially if your baby came home on a monitor or regularly requires any special procedures. Kristi's thirty-two-week son, Jacob, came home on an apnea monitor and three medications—Propulsid, Zantac, and caffeine—to treat his apnea. "The big thing for us was, even when we wanted to leave him with a baby-sitter, we had a lot of trouble finding someone who was able to take care of him and deal with his medical needs. Because of this, we almost never went out. We got used to his apnea monitor going off all the time. But it scared other people really badly."

The same thinking applies to all those well-meaning aunts, uncles, co-workers, friends, and their children. Though they may be motivated by nothing other than love or concern, and

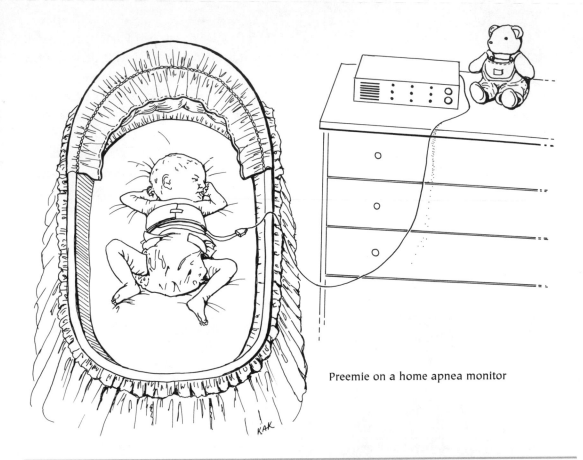

Preemie on a home apnea monitor

SHARON HORNFISCHER: "After David was home for about six weeks, I finally felt comfortable enough to take him out with me. Because preemies, like all babies under twelve months of age, have to sit in rearward-facing car seats, I couldn't see him in the rearview mirror. So I was always checking him to make sure he was breathing. I'd reach back, one hand on the steering wheel, to feel for his breath on his lips and to see if he would grasp my finger reassuringly. Occasionally, if he was slumped in the seat or needed repositioning, I'd stop the car to adjust his posture. I eventually wised up and bought a mirror that attached to the backseat, which allowed me to keep an eye on him while I watched the road.

"Once I got home after a few hours at the grocery store, the mall, or the doctor's office, my first impulse was to whisk him into the bathtub as quickly as possible. Who knew what kinds of germs he'd come into contact with? I felt that this ten minutes of bath time was a good insurance policy against sickness."

FAQ:

"Given her immature immune system, how should I manage my preemie's exposure to other children?"

The risk your baby faces from public exposure depends largely on her health status. A preemie who is discharged after a bout with a serious infection such as necrotizing enterocolitis may be rather fragile and should probably have less exposure to the public than a baby who had no complications.

After a long NICU stay, you might want to rush out and introduce your new family member to every corner of your world. But try to control that impulse. Remember that your baby might just need a little extra time before the real world can come to visit. This is not to say that you should completely isolate yourself and your new bundle from her adoring fans. It's just to say, use common sense and good judgment, and be aware of potential exposure to infections or other contagious ailments that can easily be transmitted in public places. Before you know it, your child will be ready to accept any and all visitors and will be able, at last, to go out and meet the world in person.

Consult with your pediatrician. Your baby's doctor will have the best knowledge of the strength and resilience of your preemie's immune system.

though they have your best interests at heart, it is important to limit these visits, especially if any of your well-wishers have any illnesses.

Naturally, in small doses, visits from family can make for special times. This is a time of life that you will never forget; including your family and friends, on your and your baby's terms, can strengthen your family bonds and create wonderful memories. Kelly said, "Make it a special time for the immediate family. We had one grandma home with Aaron when we brought Ryan home, and we did not want a big homecoming. It made it more special, and it gives you a chance to spend quality family time."

Finding a baby-sitter can be tough work, especially when you've just come home and are feeling protective toward your newly liberated preemie. Lining up a sitter is generally a private matter for you to handle through your own network of contacts. Grandparents, aunts, and uncles are prime candidates—especially those with experience handling small children.

However, if your baby has special medical needs, such as apnea monitors, oxygen, or feeding tubes, the hospital social worker may be able to help you find specially qualified help in the home, such as nurses or specially trained nannies depending on the needed level of care. This help will be at your expense, unless home nursing care was required by your physician and your insurance covers home health visits. Your baby's physician will direct any such care.

"A FULL NIGHT'S SLEEP? WHAT'S THAT?"

"Will we ever sleep through the night again?" This is a question frequently asked by new parents of preemies. In fact, it's been said that the sleep difficulties a woman experiences during her third trimester of pregnancy is Mother Nature's way of preparing her (and her husband) for the many sleepless nights that come after the baby arrives. While this has probably never been clinically proven, it is an interesting theory that has a certain Darwinian logic.

Sleep for the parents of newborns is almost always catch as catch can. Veteran parents recommend that if at all possible you should attempt to sleep when your child sleeps. Of course, this may be more than a little idealistic if you live a fast-paced, twenty-first-century life that requires you to use the peace and quiet of your infant's naps not to sleep, but to focus on work that can't get done when baby's awake. If you're running a home-based business of any kind, your baby's nap time may be your only opportunity to make phone calls to people who may think it less than the hallmark of professionalism to hear an infant crying in the background.

Some full-term infants are able to sleep through the night right away, or as early as six weeks after birth. Many more can sleep for long stretches: five, six, seven hours at a time. A preemie, on the other hand, will most likely be get-

ting you up several times at night for the first few months he's home. He doesn't have the fat reserves that would otherwise serve as an energy source to carry him through the night's long stretch between meals.

Preemies need to eat on a regular schedule—day and night—so that they can maintain a steady rate of growth. Due to the small size of their stomachs, preemies will consume a

Surviving Those Late-Night Feedings

SHARON HORNFISCHER: "We were told to feed our eight-week-premature son every two hours around the clock, even if we had to set an alarm to wake us up. Since the discharge nurse in the NICU stressed the importance of this, we wanted to follow her instructions to a tee. It could be a little hard to wake a sleeping baby, especially at three in the morning, but we did. And it served our son well. Today he sleeps through the night—as he has since he was four months old. Now that he's left his preemie days behind, the only alarms that go off at our house are the ones that have a newspaper and cup of coffee at the other end."

When You Have Multiples and Other Children at Home

Pam's advice is, "Just try to enjoy it. Our philosophy is that babies are the most important thing. We should do everything possible to make them happy. If there are things you can postpone or get away with doing a halfway job on, like cleaning the house, go ahead."

smaller amount of milk at each feeding. And since they have faster metabolisms than full-term babies, their meals are digested faster and they will need to replenish their food energy stores with greater frequency. It is often recommended that preemies continue their every-two-hour hospital feeding schedule even after discharge. Proper growth is essential to the child's overall health profile. That will come at the expense of a good night's sleep for you.

If you are expressing your breast milk to be stored and fed to your preemie later, you have availed yourself of one of the best time savers (and sleep savers) a mother of a preemie can have. You can alternate late-night feeding duty with your husband. You'll be able to catch up on your sleep, and your husband can take advantage of a great way to bond with his newborn.

IF YOU HAVE OTHER CHILDREN

If you have other children in the house to care for while you're looking after your preemie, try to share the responsibility with your spouse or other family members. Older children may have a tough time adjusting to the presence of a new baby in the family. All the extra attention your preemie receives may make that transition hard for the older child. This puts added pressure on you not only to take good care of your premature newborn, but to spend extra time making your older children understand their new brother's or sister's situation and acknowledging their feelings in a way that is appropriate for their age.

If you have it available and feel that it's necessary, hire outside help. Baby-sitters aren't just for your nights on the town anymore. A good sitter can be invaluable in taking your older children off your hands for an hour or two while you breast-feed your preemie or just take a nap. Because preemies often lack the strength to breast-feed efficiently, nursing them can be an almost round-the-clock exercise. The intensity of that commitment can make it difficult to look after other children. Bringing in a helper, whether it's a family member, friend, neighbor, or other paid help, can spell the difference between rest-harmony and exhaustion-chaos.

Before you leave the hospital, the staff may assess your home situation to determine whether you have sufficient resources at your disposal to care effectively for your preemie. If needed, the hospital may be able to assist you in locating someone to help with special needs. For example, if you or your child has ongoing medical problems, the hospital may arrange for a home health nurse to visit and carry out the doctor's orders—including administration of medication, dressing changes, health assessments, and evaluations of your baby's progress. A hospital social worker may be able to provide you with a list of child care resources to assist in caring for your older children, if necessary.

During the first few months at home with your premature infant, it is crucial to remember: This stage will pass. Preemies eventually outgrow their need to be fed every two to three hours. Their sleep periods will start to lengthen at about four or five months of age, until one morning you will awaken, look at the clock, and realize with a shock that you have slept through the night uninterrupted. After you get past the initial alarm and run to check on your little one, you will breathe a sigh of relief and realize that you (and your baby) have graduated from one of the toughest stretches of parenthood.

PROVIDING A HEALTHY HOME ENVIRONMENT

It isn't enough to provide a loving home for your baby. You also need to provide her with a *healthy* home. To promote the growth and development of your baby, here are some simple things you can do to maximize her chances of overcoming the setback of prematurity and get her on her way to a healthy, robust childhood.

- *Establish a smoke-free environment.* As a general rule, you should keep your child's living area as smoke-free as possible. The detriment of secondhand smoke is sufficiently well established to recommend caution in this area. Children who are exposed to tobacco smoke have a higher than normal incidence of respiratory infections. Smoke residue builds up in carpets, sheets, drapes, and blankets and can be irritating to the baby's respiratory system long after the air has cleared. Ideally your whole house should be smoke-free. If you or your spouse do smoke, however, try to keep your baby's nursery away from the smoking areas of your home. If visitors smoke and you are trying to keep your house smoke-free, don't hesitate to ask them to step outside. They should understand. After all, it's a baby's health you're standing up for, not the mere preferences of an adult.

- *Keep your baby's room as dust-free as possible and avoid the use of powders,* which can also irritate the child's lungs. If your house has a central air conditioning or heating system, use pleated filters, which catch more dust particles and allergens than regular fiber mesh filters. Replace them monthly.

- *Always wash your hands with antibacterial soap before handling your child.* The importance of good hygiene does not disappear when the NICU's doors close behind you. Additionally, try to keep clean any items that your baby touches or plays with. Unless your doctor tells you it isn't necessary, sterilize your bottles and nipples. At the very least, be sure they are cleaned with hot soapy water and rinsed and dried well between uses.

- *If other children are in the house, make sure they understand the importance of good hygiene,* particularly hand washing and the importance of not spreading germs. Siblings with colds need to be taught how to prevent the spread of infection.

Breast-Feeding vs. Bottle-Feeding

You may hear the phrase "Breast is best," and indeed there is ample evidence that breast milk is very beneficial for the full-term infant. The

American Academy of Pediatrics (AAP) has collected abundant data that supports the idea that breast-feeding is optimal for a baby's and mother's health. "The AAP now recommends that women breast-feed for at least the first year of life, since the longer you breast-feed, the more benefits your baby will derive," wrote Joel J. Alpert, M.D., president of the AAP, in 1999. Most practicing pediatricians agree about the benefits of breast milk, among them:

- Protein, sugar, fat, and other vitamins needed to be healthy
- Antibodies that help protect against disease and infection, including NEC, pneumonia, bronchitis, meningitis, ear infections, and allergies

- Possible reduced risk of sudden infant death syndrome (SIDS)
- Physical closeness and warmth, which can help create a bond

According to a survey of 1,137 pediatricians published in the March 1999 issue of the AAP's journal, *Pediatrics:*

- 65 percent of pediatricians recommended breast-feeding exclusively for healthy, full-term babies in their first month of life.
- 20 percent made no recommendation.
- 13 percent recommended breast-feeding with formula supplementation.
- 2 percent recommended exclusive formula-feeding.

Premature Infants and Breast Milk—Weighing the Benefits

- Your breast milk is custom-made for your baby. Your body manufactures the antibodies that are best suited to combating the proteins found in the foods you eat and fighting the bacteria found in your body.
- Researchers have found that breast milk produced by mothers who are nursing premature infants is higher in fat content than the milk produced by mothers of full-term infants.
- Breast milk produced for premature infants also has higher levels of nitrogen, sodium, lactose, chloride, protein, and enzymes (lipase) than full-term mother's milk. These additional nutrients aid the development of your preemie's nervous system and brain.
- Breast milk is easier for your baby to digest. Premature infants, whose digestive systems are often delicate, have an easier time digesting breast milk due to the softer curds it forms in the stomach.
- Breast-fed babies tend not to get diarrhea or constipation and have varying degrees of protection from pneumonia, bronchitis, influenza, polio, middle ear infections, and hyperthyroidism.
- Breast milk does not cause allergic reactions (though substances transmitted through the breast milk via your diet may).

Most pediatricians believe that breast-feeding should be used whenever possible. The survey showed the following responses from 657 pediatricians whose children were breast-fed and 435 others who had no personal experience with breast-feeding.

PEDIATRICIANS' VIEWS ON BREAST-FEEDING

	Pediatricians with personal experience	Pediatricians with no personal experience
Breast-feeding and formula-feeding are equally acceptable methods for feeding infants.		
Agree	40	53
Disagree	44	28
The benefits of breast-feeding outweigh any difficulties or inconveniences mothers may encounter.		
Agree	74	62
Disagree	12	19
In the long run, formula-fed babies are just as healthy as breast-fed babies.		
Agree	31	39
Disagree	43	32

Please note that the above opinions are with reference to *full-term* infants. Though there is a consensus among pediatricians in favor of breast-feeding full-term infants, it has been a matter of some controversy among neonatologists whether breast milk or a high-potency formula is ideal for very premature infants in the first days and weeks after delivery. The controversy arose out of the uncertainty about how rapidly such an infant should be growing at that early stage of life. Now agreement is emerging, however, that breast milk has certain bene-

Why Preemies Have Trouble Breast-Feeding

- Immature suck and swallow reflex
- Overall muscular weakness and poor coordination

fits that make it an attractive alternative once the preemie is able to nurse on his own. Breast milk contains approximately one hundred ingredients not found in cow's milk. Research has revealed breast milk's surprising potency in killing intestinal parasites. Though modern manufactured formulas are a very good overall nutritional source for your child, they will probably never perfectly duplicate the full range of benefits found in breast milk, several of which go beyond simple nutrition.

As the parent of a preemie, therefore, the method of feeding you choose is a personal decision that is highly dependent on individual circumstances. Although it is important to get input from your physician, your baby's pediatrician, nurses, and even family members, ultimately it's your choice. Don't let anyone make you feel like less of a mother if your choice is not their choice.

Breast-feeding a full-term infant can be frustrating enough without having to confront the particular difficulties that a preemie presents. In addition to their essential underlying prematurity, which limits their strength, preemies have difficulty coordinating their suck and swallow reflexes. Logistics are another issue. Because your preemie is too immature to breast-feed by himself, you may decide to pump your breast milk and administer it via bottle or tube.

Don't give in to this frustration. These difficulties aren't a personal failing on your part. They go with the territory. Focus on the fact that prematurity is a *temporary* condition, whereas breast-feeding is something that you can do for your baby long after his condition stabilizes in intensive care. If your baby is unable to breast-feed at the outset because he simply lacks the strength for it, focus on the fact that he probably will be able to breast-feed in time.

Your own overall health may be a factor in deciding on a feeding method, too. Your health may be too delicate for you to be able to breast-feed, even after the baby has been discharged.

BREAST-FEEDING AND THE WORKING WOMAN

If you're a professional woman who works outside the home, the need to go back to work at some point is a significant one. Though the demands of balancing motherhood with a profes-

sional life are high, increasingly today, employers are learning that family-friendly policies encourage employee loyalty and the retention of experienced personnel—and make for good public relations as well. Many companies that have on-site child care—which is increasingly prevalent in corporate America—now have designated private areas where mothers can pump or direct breast-feed in comfortable settings. Other ways companies are allowing new mothers to spend time with their babies include increased use of part-time positions, four-day work weeks, and telecommuting. Check with your supervisor or human resources specialist to see whether these and any other special arrangements are available for new mothers. And be prepared to make the case for why these arrangements will benefit not only you, but your employer as well. Remember, you will never know unless you ask.

Life at Home with Multiples

As exciting as it was to discover that you were carrying twins or more, now is when reality hits home. Can you handle them on your own, without three nurses to call on for help? For all its special rewards, life with multiples can be very challenging. Multiples are not only twice or thrice the expense, but they create more dirty diapers, bottles, laundry, and overall workload for the parents. Two newborns are said to be more than twice the work of one. (Most mothers of multiples acknowledge, though, that with the extra doses of love, hugs, and smiles, basically everything evens out.)

Before you leave the hospital, a social services professional will try to assess your home situation to determine whether you have sufficient resources at your disposal or whether you might need a bit of assistance in managing the first few weeks home. You will be asked how much assistance you will receive from family or other community support. The staff will try to establish whether your household income and insurance coverage are sufficient for you to meet the responsibility of caring for your babies. If you or one of your newborns has ongoing medical needs, the hospital may

Grandparents to the Rescue

"Our twin boys were born at twenty-four weeks' gestation, at 1 pound 3 ounces, and 1 pound 9 ounces," said Tara. "They spent a total of about four months in the NICU. When they were finally discharged home, they were still in need of various pieces of equipment such as apnea monitors and oxygen tubes. They also needed extra help with their feedings. My husband was already back into his work routine, and I needed twenty-four-hour help with the boys. Luckily for me, my parents lived close by. And even luckier, they agreed to help us out by letting me and the boys camp out at their house for a while. One child who requires special needs is a lot for new parents, but two was simply more than I could manage on my own.

"Today the boys are into their second year. No matter how many times I thank my parents for their help during that time, words never seem to adequately convey my appreciation for all that they did for us. Needless to say, they get my vote for grandparents of the year."

arrange for a home health nurse to stop by and perform procedures or simply evaluate your child's progress. This could involve a hospital-based home health nurse, or nurse's assistant, or a third-party child care provider to help watch the older children a few times a week while you and your new bundles catch up on your sleep.

If you are fortunate, you will have family, religious ties, neighbors, friends, or other resources to help you make the transition from hospital to home.

MORE TIPS FOR PARENTS OF MULTIPLES

"Get help if you need it," said Tara. "No one is an island. Take care of yourself so you will have the energy and resources to be able to take care of you children.

"Do everything together: feed them at the same time, bathe together, nap together. Keep them on a tight, coordinated schedule, if possible."

MULTIPLES AND BREAST-FEEDING

If you have had a multiple birth, you might very well be asking, "Can I really provide enough milk for two, three, or more children all at the same time?" Although there are certainly limits to what a body can do, it is clearly established that the more milk that is demanded from you, the more you will produce. There is also the issue of time. Breast-feeding just one baby can keep you on duty round-the-clock, especially in the beginning, when the baby is learning to feed, a process that takes longer when the baby is an immature preemie. Breast-feeding twins or triplets may prove to be even more challenging.

For your own convenience, you will likely find it best to feed two of your babies at a time. This time can be relaxing for all of you. Once you have become accustomed to the process, your babies' feeding time can be an opportunity for you to lie back and take it easy. Feeding time can be a good time to read, listen to the radio, indulge yourself with a sitcom, or simply clear your mind of all of the clutter of the day. Most important, however, it is a time to bond with your babies. Many times one of them will be asleep while the other feeds, allowing you to focus on one baby at a time. One baby may be hungrier than the other, and one may develop a preference for one breast over the other. This is normal. However, you may notice one of your breasts becoming larger than the other if this pattern is allowed to persist. Try alternating breasts.

The bottom line on breast-feeding is that you need to recognize the trade-offs between the benefits for your children and its demands on your time and your energy.

As mentioned earlier, your baby's health status may rule out direct breast-feeding. She may have special health or feeding concerns that make her too weak or otherwise physically incapable of breast-feeding. She may simply have trouble with her sucking reflex and need to mature to the point where she can breast-feed properly. The hospital can provide you with a lactation consultant to help guide you through these issues.

NAP TIME OR MEALTIME . . . GETTING TOO COMFORTABLE

A mother said, "Though my premature baby daughter was strong enough to direct breast-feed, she just kept falling asleep on me. The doctors and nurses in the NICU were always stressing the importance of frequent feeding, saying how important it was to her overall health, growth, and development. But every time we were all snuggled up, she would latch on and feed for about five to ten minutes—then invariably get too cozy for her own good and fall fast asleep. It was so frustrating. I had no idea how much milk she was receiving. As a result, I just kept pumping breast milk and bottle-feeding it to her. This way I knew that she was getting well nourished and knew exactly how much she was receiving."

Though the frustration is understandable, it is usually best to allow your baby to determine just when enough is enough. Just to make sure the amount of milk your baby is getting is adequate, check the following indicators that your baby is getting enough to eat:

- Six or more wet diapers per day. The urine should be a pale yellow color.
- Regular bowel movements. Frequency and quantity will vary.
- Stretches of two or three hours between feedings. Your baby knows when she is hungry and will let you know it.
- The weight gain will vary considerably. However, a typical rate is 4 to 6 ounces a week during the first month and up to 8 ounces per week in months two, three, and four. Review your baby's weight progress with your pediatrician.

Meeting the Pediatrician: The First-Year Checkups

By now you are quite familiar with the role your infant's neonatologist will play in the early weeks of life. But upon discharge, the medical care of your child will be handled by your child's pediatrician, with occasional visits to specialists as well. The first visit to the pediatrician's office will fall approximately one to two weeks after discharge from the NICU. This initial appointment is typically longer than most follow-up appointments. It's a time for the pediatrician to review your child's hospital records while building a relationship with you that will hopefully last for many years to come.

✤ TIP

Soon after you first take your preemie home, your baby may have so many appointments with the pediatrician and various specialists that your calendar could well begin to resemble that of a corporate CEO. (One mom told us: "It's killing my self-esteem—my infant has a busier calendar than I do!") Try to coordinate your appointments so that you can take care of more than one in a single outing. This will economize not only your time, but your baby-sitting expenses (and goodwill with any friends and family who may be helping you out).

Depending on your child's age at the time of this visit, the procedures will vary. All children will have a full head-to-toe assessment, including measurements of height, weight, and head circumference. The physician and her staff will review with you various developmental milestones for the present and upcoming months (see Appendix A, "Developmental Milestones"). Bring your list of twenty questions for your physician and her staff—invariably you won't remember everything that you had planned to talk about. Without a list, you may get frustrated once you arrive home without all the answers.

Depending on your baby's age at this visit,

it may be time for him to start his immunizations. If his health permitted, he may have started receiving immunizations while still in the NICU. In either case it will be the pediatrician who takes over these all-important immunizations at this time. Following is a list of the immunizations that your child, like all newborns, will be receiving. Your baby's own immunization schedule may vary somewhat. Any number of health concerns—including a fever at the time of a scheduled immunization—may lead the pediatrician to delay their administration. But each child should eventually get back on schedule and receive all of the necessary immunizations.

SUGGESTED IMMUNIZATION SCHEDULE

Age	Vaccines
2 months	HgB, DTaP, IPV, and HibCV
4 months	HgB, DTaP, IPV, and HibCV
6 months	HgB, DTaP, IPV, and HibCV
12 months	Varicella (chicken pox) and TB
15 months	DTaP, IPV, HibCV, and MMR
4–6 years	DTaP, IPV, HibCV, and MMR
14–16 years	Tetanus
Thereafter	Tetanus every 10 years

DTaP (Diphtheria, tetanus, and pertussis)
IPV (inactivated polio vaccine)
HibCV (haemophilus influenza type b conju gate vaccine)
MMR (measles, mumps, rubella)

The AMA's suggested immunization schedule may be modified by your physician as necessary to meet your baby's needs.

Source: American Medical Association.

In the event of an emergency, have your baby seen immediately by the pediatrician or your closest emergency department. Most pediatricians in medium- to large-size practices have a partner on call twenty-four hours a day. In the remote event that emergency situations come up in the middle of the night, it is comforting to have medical advice a phone call away. Remember, you will know your child better than anyone else, and if something isn't right with his health, seek medical advice right away. It is often best to err on the conservative side.

Dressing Your Preemie

New parents are often anxious to dress up their new bundles in the newest pink or blue outfits they just got from friends or family. With preemies, the trouble often is that nothing fits. You may be frustrated that all of the adorable newborn shower gifts you received are still months away from being the right size for your preemie.

The good news today is that many manufacturers are making clothes especially for preemies. The brands and selections are somewhat limited, and these clothes are a little expensive given how little material they use, but they are increasingly available through retail and mail-order outlets. Major department stores and stores such as Babies "R" Us and J. C. Penney are increasingly offering lines of such clothes. Check with your local children's retailers for advice about where you can find clothes for your preemie, or run a search using an Internet search engine using keywords such as "baby clothes." Sites such as Parent Soup and Prematurely Yours sell preemie-size clothing and other items.

❦ TIP

Don't invest too heavily in preemie clothing or clothing of any particular size. Your baby will grow faster than you expect and will be wearing those regular newborn clothes before you know it. After that happens, keep one or two of your child's preemie outfits for posterity. When you pull them out a year from now, it'll be hard for you to believe that your child was ever this small.

Preemie Support Groups

The pressures and worries of caring for your preemie at home, especially in the first few months, can be greatly alleviated if you can find other parents to share your experiences with. Today there are many parental support groups for parents of preemies and special needs children. Traditionally, new parents find good sources of support from family and close friends. If that is the case, you may be content with that. Sometimes, though, the well-intentioned efforts of people who have experience with only full-term infants will fall short of what you need. Many hospitals sponsor weekly or monthly parent support groups where parents of preemies or multiples meet to discuss their experiences and share their insights. These groups usually start while your child is still an inpatient in the NICU. A special bond of friendship can form among parents who have gone through the preemie experience together. You may find that the support meetings continue their usefulness well past your child's hospital discharge date. Baby-sitting cooperatives or play groups can be a great way to build a support network in your community with other parents in your situation.

Additionally, as the home computer continues to make the world a smaller place, it is increasingly possible to find the support you need on the Internet. It's not difficult to venture on-line and find people in your situation looking for advice and support. Every day more and more preemie Web pages and support group chat rooms pop up on the Internet. On-line resources such as Preemie-L, ParentsPlace.com, and ParentSoup.com—see Appendix C for further information—can be virtual lifelines for parents of preemies who feel isolated, misunderstood, or alone. Additionally there are many excellent Web-based medical journals, newsletters, and on-line informational clearinghouses that offer the recent information on just about any medical subject you could desire. These include the American Academy of Pediatrics's Web site (www.pediatrics.org) and WebMD (www.webmd.com). (See Appendix C page 335 for more details.)

When driving across town to that weeknight support group is just out of the question, your home computer can be a wonderfully convenient alternative. It's an especially useful resource for parents living in rural areas where populations aren't large enough to sustain regular support groups or provide libraries with complete collections of medical literature. And some people find that the anonymity of the Internet makes it easier for them to open up and expose themselves emotionally.

"I found a lot of comfort in just having other parents in my shoes to talk to," said a mother of triplets. "They understand what you're going through. Even an electronic shoulder is helpful to cry on, if that's all you've got."

Keeping Dad Involved

Please forgive the gender bias in our presumption that it is the mother who is the primary user of this book. Whether or not that is the case, an active, engaged father is a good father. The more closely dad is involved in the daily care of his premature infant, the better the experience for everybody. Your baby will grow up with a feeling of security that can only come from the participation of two adults in his upbringing. You will have a backup on those days when the world just seems to close in on you with responsibility. And dad will find new dimensions of manhood as he embraces the challenge of taking care of a premature baby whose needs are all the greater because of his prematurity. We have come a long way from the days when fathers were shut out of delivery rooms while their wives were giving birth. The more the father is able to contribute despite the challenge of balancing work and family—a challenge that many women are confronting at the same time—the stronger the bond that will develop to hold the family together through this sometimes difficult transition period.

10

TAKING CARE OF YOURSELF

WHAT YOU WILL FIND IN THIS CHAPTER

- Rest
- Exercise
- Eating well

- Lifestyle issues
- If you are thinking about becoming pregnant again

The special demands you face while caring for your premature infant can change the day-to-day flow of your life in ways you could have scarcely imagined just a short while ago. Even if your baby spent only a brief time in the NICU, and even if you have suffered no ill health yourself, you have probably experienced a disorienting sense of altered expectations—all the more so if your baby spent several months in intensive care or if you had to bring breathing monitors or other special equipment home with you. Whatever the exact circumstances, you have very likely recalibrated your entire life around the fact of your infant's prematurity.

During the first months of your preemie's life, you will focus almost all of your energy on tending to her needs. Extra trips to the doctor, special dietary considerations, frequent nighttime feedings—it can take a lot out of you. While our willingness to change our lives for our children is a wonderful testament to the priorities of our species, it is also true that during the first few months of a preemie's life at home, many parents are prone to neglecting *their* own needs. That works not only to their own detriment, but to the detriment of their babies, too. It requires a substantial expenditure of emotional, physical, and financial resources to parent a preemie. And that expenditure can't be made when your tanks are dry.

If you had health problems that led to your baby's prematurity—including, for example, pregnancy-induced hypertension, diabetes, or delivery complications—you may pay an even heavier toll. Bouncing back from a bout with pregnancy-induced illness while caring for a premature infant can be draining in ways that may not be immediately evident to you. If your obstetrician or perinatologist put you on bed rest prior to delivery, you may find that your overall level of energy and fitness have suffered. You may find it will take months to recover your former vigor. But during those months, your parenting responsibilities won't go away.

This chapter is rooted in the principle that what's good for mom and dad is good for baby: rest, good nutrition, physical fitness, and emotional well-being. Throughout the trying period of your infant's prematurity, it is important not to lose sight of the importance of taking care of your infant's main source of wellness and security—yourself. Find a workable balance between selflessness and self in those frightening first months home from the hospital. Kelly said, "Moms and dads: Rest! This has been traumatic, and you need to take care of *you* as well. Especially if you have other children. I know that a lot of parents make a daily trip to the NICU, and this is hard both emotionally and physically. What better hands could this baby be in? Take time for yourself. I didn't get to see Ryan much while he was in the NICU because we lived far away. But he is very close to me today. He's Mommy's little boy, and I love every minute of it."

Rest

Studies have shown that babies take many of their behavioral cues from their parents. If you

are exhausted, stressed, or flustered, your baby may reflect it by becoming irritable or withdrawn. We can't emphasize strongly enough how much good rest can influence the perspective you bring to the task of parenting and the quality of your emotional relationship with your preemie.

Finding time to nap, or even just relax with some good reading material, can be difficult. As we've said, preemies may need to be fed as frequently as every three hours. And since feedings can take as long as twenty minutes, due to some preemies' weakness and slow rate of consumption, you may find yourself with only two hours to spare until the next feeding is due. Then there is the small matter of diaper changes. And feeding yourself. And maintaining some semblance of control over the housekeeping. Even if you have a partner who pitches in with all of this, you may still find yourself without time to yourself to rest.

Following are some of the best secrets that parents who survived the first months of preemie parenthood have shared with us:

- *Nap when your baby naps.* "As soon as I heard her sucking air from the bottle and she started looking ready for another nap, that was my cue to put her in her bassinet and go lie down myself," one mother said of her eight-week-premature daughter. It may not be possible to nap simultaneously more than once a day. But even then, that one small stretch of rest can mean the difference between feeling stressed and feeling on top of the world.

- *Put a sign on the door to greet well-wishers who might stop by—and ask them to come by an-*

other time. "My friends and family seemed to have a knack for visiting whenever I was too tired to see straight. I would soldier through the chitchat, then collapse. It was actually an easy problem to deal with. I have a message board with Velcro on the back, and when I'm too tired for company I'll just hang the sign on the door and go take a nap. The fun part is that when I woke up sometimes there were gifts at the door." The message might read: "We are deeply grateful for the support we are receiving from our loved ones throughout the difficult period. However, right now we are catching up on some much needed rest and would appreciate it if you would stop by another time."

- *Turn off the ringer on your telephone.* "It seemed like the phone was ringing all the time when David first came home. When I napped, I would simply switch off the ringer. I decided that that hour or two of sleep was mine, and no one was going to take it from me. I always called them back as soon as I could."

- *Hire a baby-sitter—then stay home and nap.* A friend or a family member may be willing to help out for a few hours while you catch up on your rest. If you're lucky enough to have a baby-sitter you have a lot of confidence in, hire her for an afternoon to cover for you and take care of two or three feedings and diaper changes. Your sitter might take less money, given that you'll be home (albeit blissfully comatose).

- *Let your baby cry for at least five minutes before going to her assistance.* Sometimes sleeping babies cry out suddenly, only to fall back into dreamland right away. Make sure your baby is up for the duration before going into her room.

Exercise

If you had a surgical delivery or complications of any kind, or if you have continuing medical problems, you should consult your physician for advice about when you may resume exercising and what kind of exercise would be useful to you. To regain your prepregnancy physical condition and to offset the stretching that occurs in your abdominal muscles during pregnancy, you will want to exercise regularly. You will want to start exercising as soon as it's medically safe. It's not just about losing weight. Most women lose their added pregnancy weight with little effort within six weeks of delivery. Exercise will help you to restore your physical toning and improve your ability to relax, handle stress, and fight any signs you may be experiencing of postpartum depression.

The physiological benefits of exercise are well documented. Abdominal exercises will improve your circulation (reducing the risk of dangerous clots) and strengthen your lower back. You will also experience fewer cramps, varicose veins, and less swelling of the feet and ankles. Perineal exercises—Kegels—will help you reduce the risk of stress incontinence—the postpartum leaking of urine that some women experience. A good general workout regimen will help restore your bones and joints (preventing osteoporosis and even arthritis), as well as your pelvic and uterine muscles, to their prepregnancy strength and resilience.

Embarking on a comprehensive exercise program may not be an idea you relish in the days and weeks following your infant's NICU discharge. If your baby is still somewhat ill, you may feel selfish worrying about your own health. That feeling should be alleviated by the fact that your good health contributes to your baby's. Moreover, improving your fitness does not require an all-consuming exercise program that takes you away from your baby. It's possible to get back into some semblance of fitness by doing just one or two exercises a day while you lie in bed, after you've eaten, or while you watch your baby sleep. Focusing on one or two areas of your body (say, your abdomen, buttocks, or thighs) and going for a twenty-minute walk every day can be enough to bring you the benefits of exercise without unduly cramping your schedule.

EXERCISE GUIDELINES FOR MOMS OF PREEMIES

- If you had medical problems that led to your premature delivery (including hypertension or diabetes), or if you are recovering from a cesarean section or a difficult labor and delivery, be sure to consult with your doctor about when and how to begin exercising. Ask your physician what your maximum heart rate is and how not to exceed it while exercising.

- Once you are cleared medically, commit yourself to a regular schedule for exercise. Anything other than sticking to a routine will be a waste of your time—the results just won't be there. Every week fit in at least three 20-minute aerobic exercise sessions— walking, biking, or swimming are three popular aerobic activities. For muscle toning (sit-ups, weight lifting, and so on), shorter, more frequent workouts are more effective than fewer, longer ones.

- Since your joints and ligaments are still loose from carrying your baby, stay away from exercises that involve sudden, jolting motions or stressful extensions of the joints during the first two months postpartum. Before beginning to exercise in earnest, always warm up by stretching gently or doing some nonstressful exercise such as stationary biking with low resistance.

- Build your number of repetitions slowly over time, and don't push your limits. Starting slowly will acclimate your body to the routine. Don't deviate from your scheduled number of repetitions, and quit when you start feeling exhausted.

- Avoid overheating. If you must work out in the sun, exercise in the morning or evening and wear white, lightweight clothing and a cap to protect your head. Drink plenty of water before, during, and after your exercise session.

- If while exercising you experience dizziness, nausea, blurred vision, pain in your back or pubic area, shortness of breath, heart palpitations, or difficulty standing, stop exercising immediately and contact your physician.

- Use exercise as a way of bonding with your baby. Strap your infant up against you in a baby carrier while you are on the stationary bike or treadmill. Let him watch you do stretching, sit-ups, crunches, or leg lifts.

- If you're breast-feeding, feed your baby before you exercise. Research has shown that many babies refuse their mother's nipples after their mothers have been exercising. This may be due to increased levels of lactic acid, which is caused by exercise, which makes the milk taste sour. Wait at least ninety minutes after finishing before feeding your baby. Until that time it might be best to pump milk before you exercise and feed your baby from a bottle.

<table>
<tr><td colspan="2">CALORIES NEEDED TO MAINTAIN YOUR PREPREGNANCY WEIGHT (NON-BREAST-FEEDING MOTHER)</td></tr>
<tr><td>Lifestyle</td><td>Multiply Your Prepregnancy Weight By</td></tr>
<tr><td>Sedentary</td><td>12</td></tr>
<tr><td>Active</td><td>15</td></tr>
<tr><td>Very Active</td><td>22</td></tr>
</table>

For example, a sedentary 130-pound woman would need 1,560 calories daily to maintain her weight.

Eating Well

You need all the nutritional fortification you can get in order to recover from the rigors of pregnancy. Finding the energy to be a good mother in the days following the trying experience of adjusting to premature parenthood makes it doubly important to eat well. And if you're nursing, it's crucial for your baby's nutritional needs that you not neglect your diet. Your nutritional intake will have a bearing on the quality and quantity of your milk output. In that event your own nutrition and your baby's remain interconnected, if not as tightly as they were when your baby was in utero.

Following are some general guidelines for eating well. Though they are guidelines to follow at any stage of your life, they take on additional urgency in the months following delivery. The first list of dos and don'ts is for mothers who are breast-feeding. If you are breast-feeding, you are still eating for two, to a degree. What you eat affects your baby. If you aren't breast-feeding, there isn't that direct connection between your nutrition and your baby's. Mothers of bottle feeders have different nutritional guidelines (see box).

IF YOU'RE BREAST-FEEDING

While you're breast-feeding your baby, you don't need to monitor your diet quite as carefully as when she was still in utero. Nonetheless you should be prudent in your eating habits, since it's still possible to affect the quantity and quality of your lactation through your diet. Your diet cannot change the essential formulation of your breast milk. If your body doesn't get the protein and calories it needs to lactate from your diet, it will tap your own body's supply as necessary. The quality of your diet and other habits can, however, affect your milk's vitamin content and even its flavor.

Most things you eat contain substances that will find their way into your breast milk to one degree or another. Some of these substances

Your Breast Milk Is What You Eat:
How Your Diet Can Affect Your Breast-Fed Baby

- *Garlic, cabbage, beans, onions, cheese, chocolate:* Foods such as these may cause your baby some gastric discomfort. They may also change the taste of your milk and affect your baby's willingness to breast-feed.

- *Alcohol:* Studies have shown that even a small amount of alcohol can hinder a baby's motor development. Of more immediate concern is alcohol's dehydrating effect—it saps body fluids that are necessary to milk production.

- *Caffeine:* A diuretic—it extracts fluid from your system that is otherwise needed for milk production. Coffee and caffeinated soft drinks are okay in moderation, but in excess they slow your lactation and can cause irritability and sleeplessness in you and your baby. Read labels; caffeine hides in teas, chocolate, even cold preparations.

- *Chemical food additives:* While none of the FDA-approved food additives most commonly used today has been shown to be harmful to your baby when delivered via breast-feeding, you would be wise to minimize your baby's exposure to additives, including artificial colors, flavors, sweeteners, and preservatives.

- *Herbal drinks:* These would seem to be a healthy, natural part of your diet. However, some of the herbs generally used in beverages are powerful drugs that can have harmful effects on a breast-fed baby. Chai teas, herbal soft drinks, or similar beverages should be cleared by your doctor before you consume them with any regularity.

- *Seafood:* Fish are only as healthy to eat as the waters they live in. Thus be wary of any type of seafood that may come from a water system with significant pollution levels. Shellfish are prone to absorbing contaminants from the waters in which they live. These are unnecessary risks to take during the relatively short time you will be breast-feeding.

- *Pain relievers:* Acetaminophen and aspirin should be taken only at the advice of your doctor and only in the dosages prescribed. Ibuprofen (Advil and the like) is somewhat safer, since it is less likely to pass from your bloodstream into your breast milk.

- *Laxatives:* These can have a laxative effect on your nursing infant and are best avoided. If you're constipated, eat more fruits, vegetables, and whole-grain foods.

- *Prescription medication:* Any medication you take while nursing should be taken only at the direction of your physician. Little is known about the actual effects of most medications on the nursing mother's milk. Where the known benefits of a drug outweigh the unknown but potential risks, your doctor will likely permit you to take it. Always make sure your doctor knows you are breast-feeding when you are discussing a possible medication.

- *Cigarette smoke:* Although not part of your "diet" per se, cigarette smoke contains toxic substances that can enter your bloodstream and therefore also your milk.

will have no effect on nursing, some will have a minor effect, and some will have a significantly harmful effect.

✒ Don't

- *Don't eat an excess of sugar.* Sugar is nothing but empty calories—energy for you without sustenance for your baby. You'll find sugar in surprising places in your diet. Obvious foods such as cookies, ice cream, and candy are only the tip of the iceberg. Processed foods such as soups, salad dressings, cold cuts, and frozen dinners are often full of sugars such as fructose, corn syrup, and dextrose. Be aware of their sugar content, and keep it to a minimum. Chocolate has been thought to cause gastric discomfort in nursing babies.

- *Don't get caught in the fat trap.* During your pregnancy you needed a steady intake of fat to maintain your and your baby's health. Now you'll want to keep your fat–calorie ratio to 30 percent or less. This means that less than a third of the calories you consume should come from fat. You'll find the fat–calorie percentages on the side panel of packaged foods, as required by federal law. This means that for a normal, 2,000-calorie daily diet (this "normal" number will vary with your weight—see the formula on page 263), no more than 600 calories should come from fat. That equates to about 66 grams of fat per day (there are 9 calories in a gram of fat).

- *Don't overuse the salt shaker.* Like fat, salt is a nutrient that was important during pregnancy, but one you should cut down on now. Making a couple of nonnegotiable dietary decisions can cut down on your salt intake dramatically. For starters, don't allow potato chips or salted crackers in your house. Replace them with rice cakes and unsalted table crackers. Your baby will quickly acquire a taste for salt if he's exposed to it early.

- *Don't give in to temptation.* During pregnancy you may have been accustomed to indulging your impulses. It comes with the territory, to a degree. (French vanilla with pickle juice may not be the special at Baskin-Robbins, but sometimes it's just what a pregnancy orders.) Now that your responsibility to your child includes keeping up your own health, it's time to cut back. And remember: Good eating is a habit learned by example; your child's own eating habits can be formed around yours—for better or worse.

- *Don't give in to vices.* Even though you are no longer carrying your infant, as long as you are breast-feeding you should avoid any use of alcohol, tobacco, or caffeine. All of these substances pass to the baby through your breast milk.

✿ Do

- *Eat three meals a day.* Missing a meal after delivery may not rob your baby of as much nutrition as when she was in utero, but it is still important to have a regular, nutritious meal plan in effect to maximize the quantity and potency of your breast milk.

- *Eat a sufficient quantity of complex carbohydrates.* Whole-grain cereals, breads, legumes (beans, peas, and so forth), pasta, and rice provide important unrefined fiber in your diet as well as vitamins and minerals that tend to be missing from "refined" grain products. Have six or more servings a day—a couple of pieces of whole-wheat toast at each meal is an easy way to accomplish that.

- *Drink plenty of fluids.* If you're nursing, drink at least eight 8-ounce cups of water daily to provide your body with a plentiful reservoir from which to produce milk. (If you're nursing multiples, increase that to 12 cups a day.) Other drinks such as fruit juice, milk, and soft drinks are okay, but generally their higher sugar content makes them harder for the body to absorb.

- *Get your iron.* Beef, spinach, dried fruit, sardines, soybean products, liver, chickpeas, and iron-fortified cereals are sources of this important nutrient. Have at least one serving a day.

- *Eat at least three servings of fruits and vegetables daily.* Five or more is even better.

- *Calcium.* Though your own calcium intake while breast-feeding won't affect your milk's calcium content, it is important to replenish the calcium drawn from your body to produce that milk. If you do not do so, you may increase your odds for osteoporosis later in life. Have five servings daily if you're nursing (add one serving for every additional infant you may be nursing simultaneously). Milk (skim or 1 percent), nonfat or low-fat cheese, cottage cheese, broccoli, collards, or sardines are good sources. For mothers on a dairy-free diet, calcium supplements are a good idea.

- *Protein.* Three servings a day are recommended for breast-feeding mothers, two for mothers who aren't breast-feeding. Milk, yogurt, cheese, fish, meat, and poultry are excellent sources of protein, as are peanut butter, tofu, legumes, and cottage cheese.

Lifestyle Issues

Rest, nutrition, and exercise are three of the basic building blocks of your well-being, which in turn is essential to your ability to be a good parent to your premature infant. But those three elements alone aren't sufficient to create a balanced life. Following are some reminders that may be helpful to you as you make the adjustment to the sort of intensive parenthood that your premature baby needs.

RECREATION

It may strike you as somewhat self-indulgent to do anything recreational while you are caring for your premature infant. The feeling is surely understandable. If you had any regular commitments prior to your baby's arrival—a dinner club, a sports league, a book group—it is likely that you have temporarily retrenched around the higher priority of caring for your premature newborn. Hobbies and pastimes tend to fall by the wayside once baby comes home. You may find that the frequent late-night feedings a preemie requires concentrate the mind on matters more important than personal recreation.

But by your baby's third or fourth month home, you may find yourself once again with the privilege of sleeping through the night. With that privilege comes your own responsibility to rest in order to be a more attentive parent. If recreational activities were an important part of your life before your baby came, you may find that once you're getting the sleep you need, finding time for those activities after delivery can make you a more patient, tolerant, engaged parent.

YOUR MARRIAGE

Joseph Garcia-Prats: "We don't mean to diminish the importance of marriage to a healthy family environment by including it as a subtopic under the heading 'Lifestyle Issues.' Indeed, in our previous book, *Good Families Don't Just Happen,* my wife, Cathy, and I described our view of marriage: as the center of the family and the foundation on which its strength and vitality rest. Marriage takes work

How Dad Can Help

- *Get involved in the day-to-day.* By helping out with diaper duty, you will not only relieve your wife, you'll build a closer bond with your baby too.

- *Give your wife an evening off.* Whether it's a quick shopping trip or coffee with some girlfriends, nothing recharges the parenting batteries like some time off. It shouldn't be a regular thing, and she probably won't care to leave the baby in the first days and weeks home. Nonetheless, in time a break from the routine every now and then will prove beneficial.

- *Encourage your wife to take a nap.* It can be hard for a committed mother of a preemie to slow down and realize that her own level of relaxation affects her ability to be a good parent. Help her adopt this perspective by insisting that she just lie down and forget about the world for a couple of hours every week.

- *Give her a full night's sleep.* If you work during the week, compensate her on the weekend with a night off from late-night duty. Tell her that you'll take all of the feedings on a given night. You might even move a cot into the baby's room so as not to wake her when the baby starts crying.

and commitment, and the relationship evolves and grows as we do."

Parenting a preemie will test your marriage's strength and resiliency. It will change your family dynamic and require compromise and some sacrifice from both husband and wife. By rising to its challenge, you will be helping both your spouse and yourself to grow—and to strengthen your marriage along the way. As you watch your spouse embrace the new challenge, rising to the task of caring for a delicate and fragile premature infant, you may find your love renewed. Try not to lose sight of the fact that whatever pressures come to bear on your family as a result of the late-night feedings, the frequent doctors visits, and the other duties that go with preemie parenthood, your spouse and you are the foundation of everything to come.

HELPING YOUR OTHER CHILDREN COPE

The introduction of a new baby into a household will invariably dilute the all-encompassing attention to which your older child or children may have been accustomed. The extra attention and concern that premature infants typically receive from their parents may strike your other children as unfair. If your other child or children are very young, they may not be able to articulate their jealousy in a way that allows you to address it. They may simply act out. Try to defuse any potential jealousy by explaining to the older children how much their new preemie brother or sister needs them. Pay special attention to the older children whenever you have a break from your preemie. It can also be helpful to involve them in the new baby's care, whether it involves

holding him and stroking him while you change a diaper or playing with him gently after mealtime and before going to bed.

Note: older siblings up to age two or three should be carefully monitored in their interactions with your preemie. Their innocent play can sometimes involve unintended roughness, which a delicate premature infant is not equipped to handle. Try not to let this protectiveness seem obvious. You don't want it to appear to your other children as unfair doting.

FRIENDSHIPS

When you come home with your preemie, your life will very naturally turn inward as you focus your energies on tending to her needs. If this is your first child, you'll likely find your priorities changing dramatically. The days when you could go out on a whim will be a thing of the past now that you have to consider the risks of exposing your preemie in public places. As your social calendar melts away and the imperatives of premature parenthood take hold, you may fear that a certain distance will develop between you and your friends. It's natural to worry about that. But just remember: Your true friends aren't going to go anywhere. They will understand the changes taking place in your life. In fact, they may very well help you celebrate them.

"During my first few months home, I found out who my friends really were," one mother said. "When I stopped going to them, they not only didn't mind—they started coming to me. The kind of 'party' we had changed completely. Whenever we had a get-together at my house, the baby was the main attraction. Our gatherings were completely refreshed by the baby. In some ways we all felt we were advancing into a new stage of maturity together."

If You Are Thinking about Becoming Pregnant Again

This chapter has an important purpose: to emphasize the connection between your own health and well-being and your baby's health and well-being. It also has an implied, more far-reaching connection: the issue of any future pregnancies you might want to have. If you are planning to have more children, you need to consider your health very seriously and weigh the likelihood, based on what your obstetrician tells you, that the same complications that caused this baby to be delivered prematurely will recur. If the prematurity was the result of pregnancy-induced hypertension or another of the unexpected syndromes that continue to cause prematurity despite our most strenuous

efforts to understand and correct them, it is not at all a foregone conclusion that your next pregnancy will result in premature birth. The incidence of PIH is quite low in subsequent pregnancies, although medicine does not yet have a good answer as to why.

However, if your baby's prematurity was the result of a chronic or congenital health condition you suffer from, whether it's chronic hypertension or an abnormally shaped uterus, you need to assume that this condition will likely affect your next pregnancy as well. Mothers whose first children were full-term have a 4.4 percent chance that their second pregnancy will be premature. If your first baby was premature, however, those chances increase to between 20 and 30 percent. If you do have a chronic condition and have decided to get pregnant again, it is very important to take scrupulous care of yourself in order to protect yourself and your future baby. If it turns out there is little you can do to manage the condition, you may decide that it's wisest not to run the same risk again.

11

LATER-LIFE DEVELOPMENT OF THE PREMATURE INFANT

WHAT YOU'LL FIND IN THIS CHAPTER

- Health
- Growth
- Neurological disorders
- Cognitive and psychological development

- Behavior and social competence
- School performance
- A caveat for the concerned parent
- What a parent can do

When your premature baby is finally out of danger in the hospital, or perhaps after he has come home to become, at last, a full-time member of your family, you might find your concerns shifting to the longer term. New types of questions may begin to preoccupy you: Are children born prematurely subject to later-life developmental difficulties? Are they at risk of not realizing their full physical, intellectual, and emotional potential? If premature birth represents a shattering of our expectations of pregnancy, might it also represent a threat to our hopes that our child will grow into the vigorous young adult we envision, years down the road? Questions like these are on the minds of most parents whose babies are born prematurely.

We wish we could provide airtight responses to these questions. Unfortunately answers are very hard to come by. While comforting anecdotal information may be available to you in the form of a neighbor who confides that her successful, athletic son or daughter was born prematurely, and while a cautionary note might be sounded by the parent of a preemie with cerebral palsy, dyslexia, or attention deficit disorder, clinical research into long-term development requires many years to take meaningful shape. And even then there is a paradox. Neonatal medicine does not stand still. During the necessary wait for study results to emerge, new breakthroughs continue to occur in the science of caring for premature babies. This progress, while heartening, can mitigate the results of studies conducted on children born during a time when the new lifesaving or life-enhancing therapies were not available. In that sense, researchers studying later-life development of preemies are continually trying to capture lightning in a bottle.

We are tempted to concede that finding solid answers to such questions would be tantamount, on some level, to unraveling part of the mystery of life itself. For indeed, the prognoses for most premature babies are so individualized—so particular to the baby's biological and environmental circumstances—that sweeping answers to basic questions about later-life development are elusive. Stories of very-low-birth-weight premature newborns who miraculously survive and go on to grow into childhood without complications are common enough that it would be unjustly disheartening for some parents to be told that it's highly probable their child will suffer from one or another serious neurological disorder. Respecting the mystery of life requires that we allow it to surprise us every now and then.

But that is not what the practice of medicine is all about. It is the duty of medical professionals to unravel as many of these mysteries as possible. Ever since it was developed in the early fifties, the Apgar score has stood as the most commonly used composite indicator of a newborn's need for immediate support. But researchers today are attempting to develop better techniques to predict a baby's later development. In a study jointly run by Stanford University and the University of North Carolina at Chapel Hill, researchers devised a simple correlation known as the Neonatal Health Index. It uses just two numbers—length of stay in the hospital/NICU and birth weight—to compare a premature newborn's status relative to other preemies.

Some disorders, such as severe forms of cerebral palsy, can be discernible shortly after birth. Others, including behavioral disturbances such

Kristi was twenty-nine when she delivered her son Jacob at thirty-two weeks, weighing 4 pounds 11 ounces. Jacob was almost two years old when we interviewed her. "Developmentally he's fine. He's speaking in sentences now. He walked at fourteen months," she said. But Jacob's colds tend to be severe. "Every other month, he doesn't just get a cold; he gets a cold and it turns into bronchitis or pneumonia. He gets asthmalike symptoms. He constantly has a runny nose." Kristi's own diminutive stature (she's five feet one) may partially account for Jacob's small size—fifteenth percentile for weight and height—but he's showing a steady increase. "We're not worried about it," she said. "He eats like a horse. When he had his NEC scare, he was getting his feeds intravenously. He started eating again two weeks after that. He can eat, but he's still pretty skinny."

as attention deficit hyperactivity disorder or mild cerebral palsy, can take years to manifest themselves. Your baby's neonatologist or pediatrician will watch for signs of irritability, anxiety, apathy, or unresponsiveness to stimulus, which in the absence of an illness could signal some sort of possible developmental problem. Your premature baby cannot be expected to function like a full-term newborn from birth. Accordingly the physician will typically wait a few months, until your baby has passed his due date, in order to have a basis to compare what your baby is capable of with what a full-term baby of that gestational age would be capable of. If signs of developmental delay are evident, the physician may choose to reevaluate your baby at regular intervals to track his progress. A physical therapist may be assigned to work with your baby to promote his developmental growth.

In this chapter we wish to report the findings of researchers who have conducted important studies on the question of how preemies develop into childhood. First, however, it might be useful to have a general overview of the respects in which low-birth-weight infants have traditionally lagged behind their full-term brethren.

❧

Science is still attempting to come to grips with the extent to which prematurity influences the development of a child's health, intellectual capacity, and behavior. However, before we get into what may seem to be grim details, it is important to note that the vast majority of premature infants have normal outcomes. A major study of 878 low-birth-weight, premature infants sponsored by the Robert Wood Johnson Foundation showed that by the thirty-sixth

Famous Preemies through History

Winston Churchill

Samuel Clemens (Mark Twain)

Albert Einstein

Isaac Newton

Charles Darwin

Napoleon Bonaparte

Auguste Renoir

Anna Pavlova

Sidney Poitier

Richard Simmons

Stevie Wonder

month of life, 87 percent of premature infants have a normal neurological outcome. So when we generalize about the problems that premature infants are at risk for, by no means are we saying that your baby will necessarily have those problems.

Of course, outcomes are not always good. Long-term studies of children born in the 1960s confirmed the occasional detrimental effects of prematurity, which are sometimes measurable into adolescence. As a group, premature infants have a higher incidence than full-term infants of subnormal physical growth, illness, and neurological developmental problems. The frequency and severity of problems (if any) has been generally correlated to the infant's birth weight and gestational age. The lower the birth weight and gestational age, the more likely developmental problems are and the more severe they tend to be.

And science has not always helped matters, either. Sometimes the use of new high-tech therapies for premature infants has brought unintended negative consequences. In the 1940s and 1950s several new treatments had detrimental effects on the children's development. The withholding of feeding in the first weeks of life sometimes led to dehydration and hypoglycemia. The aggressive use of oxygen is thought to have caused retinopathy of prematurity and even blindness. Heavy doses of antibiotics sometimes led to deafness. Brain damage due to severe jaundice (called *kernicterus*) was linked to the use of sulfa drugs.

Today, of course, the side effects of neonatal care are being managed more effectively. Many very-low-birth-weight children are surviving today where they once would not have. But as we review the statistics on the later-life development of premature infants, please keep in mind that your baby's fate does not lie in the statistics—or biology. Even where evidence of abnormality exists, you have the capacity to influence your child's development. It has been determined over and over again that socioeconomic and environmental factors appear to have at least as great an effect on a child's long-term cognitive development as do biological factors. This may be heartening news, for it suggests that involved, loving parents who understand their premature infant's medical status and make sure she receives regular medical care throughout infancy and childhood can stack the deck in their child's favor.

To accurately track the incidence of major neurological problems, children need to be followed closely until they are at least eighteen to twenty-four months old. The detection of subtler abnormalities in learning ability, social competence, or fine motor skills requires close follow-up into early school age.

Health

The most common health problems experienced by premature infants in later life include asthma, upper and lower respiratory infections (including bronchiolitis and pneumonia), and

AGES AT WHICH DEVELOPMENTAL PROBLEMS BECOME EVIDENT IN VERY-LOW-BIRTH-WEIGHT INFANTS	
Age	*Developmental Disorder*
6 months	Attachment, eye-hand coordination, language problems
6–12 months	Retinopathy of prematurity, cerebral palsy, mental retardation
12 months	Minor neurological dysfunction
18 months	Slight cerebral dysfunction, attention deficit disorders, language problems
3 years	Mild mental retardation, behavioral problems
3–6 years	Learning difficulties
6–9 years	Developmental lags diminish

Source: Levene & Tudehope, *Essentials of Neonatal Medicine,* 381.

ear infections. While respiratory problems tend to decrease after twenty-four months, health difficulties can persist for many children, leading to restricted physical activity, school absences, and subpar academic performance. These problems have been shown to be more severe for children who come from disadvantaged socioeconomic backgrounds. Children who have residual respiratory complications as a result of prematurity may eventually be able to participate in the usual activities of an active childhood. Such problems can sometimes persist into a child's teenage years.

Respiratory difficulties are a common cause of rehospitalization for low-birth-weight infants. Very-low-birth-weight babies have been shown to average from one to three readmissions before they finally stabilize. Preemies also face a higher incidence of rehospitalization for problems with the eyes (such as strabismus), ears (recurring infection, which may necessitate ear tubes), nose (infected or overgrown adenoids), and throat (infected tonsils, tracheal complications). Most of these problems (strabismus, ear tubes, airway problems) are not common in the preterm infant except for those who may have had numerous or prolonged intervention. For example, the preterm infant with severe ROP is at highest risk for strabismus (lazy eye, cross-eye) compared to those with the milder stages of ROP. Treatment is usually patching of one eye, but early intervention is crucial. Follow-up with the ophthalmologist is so important. Problems with recurrent ear infections or hoarseness may be related to prolonged need for an endotrachael tube. Both problems are usually amenable to surgery, but early identification of these problems by you

and the pediatrician is important. Children who suffer from cerebral palsy may have to be hospitalized for orthopedic surgery or other therapy.

The smaller and more immature the preemie is at birth, the more severe the potential health consequences in later childhood. Environmental factors can exacerbate health problems a preemie might have, particularly household exposure to irritants such as cigarette smoke or to the increased risk of infection found in public settings such as day care centers.

Growth

Intrauterine growth retardation (IUGR) and complications of prematurity such as respiratory distress syndrome (RDS) can inhibit the growth of the premature infant initially. But current research suggests no long-term or permanent detriment arising from that fact. The genetic potential of the child, which is set before birth, is the ultimate determinant of a child's size. The latest studies support the encouraging finding that premature infants eventually realize their full potential for growth. The duration and severity of the initial growth failure influences the length of time for the catch-up growth to take place.

Neurological Disorders

Abnormalities in neurological health include hydrocephalus, mental retardation, microcephaly, blindness, deafness, seizures, and cerebral palsy. Of these, cerebral palsy is by far the most frequent neurological abnormality seen in premature, low-birth-weight children. As many as 85 percent of the abnormal neurological diagnoses made in premature infants are for cerebral palsy. The frequency of disorders increases as birth weight decreases. The following table shows the percentages of school-age children born prematurely who were found to have a neurological disorder by birth weight.

Birth Weight	Rate of Neurological Disorder
less than 1,000 grams (2 lbs. 3 oz.)	approx. 20%
1,000–1,500 grams (2 lbs. 3 oz. to 3 lbs. 5 oz.)	14–17%
1,501–2,499 grams (3 lbs. 5 oz. to 5 lbs. 8 oz.)	6–8%

The percentage of neurological disorders in full-term, normal-birth-weight children is reported to be 5 percent.

Blindness occurs in 5 to 6 percent of children born below 1,000 grams (2 pounds 3 ounces). Deafness occurs in 2 to 3 percent of low-birthweight babies and does not seem to disproportionately affect the most premature babies.

A major randomized clinical trial was sponsored by the Robert Wood Johnson Foundation and administered by Stanford University and the University of North Carolina at Chapel Hill. Published in 1997, the results showed that a child's neuromotor ability at thirty-six months of age was strongly correlated to birth weight. The study graded 878 thirty-six-month-olds on seven scales: motor strength and tone; posture and spontaneous motor activity; reflexes; gross motor development; gait; cerebellar function; and cranial nerves. The children were graded on

each of these seven scales as either normal (no concerns about neuromotor ability), suspicious (no diagnosis made, but evidence of developmental difficulty), or abnormal (a specific diagnosis of neurological deficit is made). The results of the study clearly showed the developmental benefits three years later of higher birth weights:

Overall Population	Normal	Suspicious	Abnormal
	87%	8%	5%
By birth weight:			
Less than 1,500 grams	78	14	8
1,501–2,000 grams	88	9	3
2,001–2,501 grams	92	6	1

A similar correlation was found between birth weight and the incidence of respiratory distress syndrome (RDS), as shown in the following chart:

Birth Weight	% Developing RDS in the First 36 Months
Less than 1,500 grams	74
1,501–2,000 grams	37
2,001–2,501 grams	19

Cognitive and Psychological Development

If cerebral palsy, seizures, and blindness are at one end of the neurological spectrum, then less severe deficits such as subnormal IQ, language disability, attention deficit, difficulty with balance and coordination, and reduced memory are at the other. Children who were born as premature, low-birth-weight infants are at higher risk of these lesser forms of neuromotor dysfunction than are children who were born at

Cerebral Palsy

Cerebral palsy (CP) is a rare disorder that involves the permanent impairment of motor function arising from injury to the brain during pregnancy or delivery. The exact cause is usually unknown. Affecting between 5 and 15 percent of premature infants weighing less than 1,500 grams at birth, the disorder is nonprogressive, meaning that it does not get worse over time. But because it involves neurological damage it is incurable, though the symptoms can be managed. It varies in degree from barely discernible muscular weakness to severe impairment that makes movement impossible.

SYMPTOMS: Given CP's wide range of possible severity, the symptoms are diverse. They can range from a poor attention span, hyperactivity, and learning disabilities to seizures and spastic movements of the extremities.

TREATMENT: Because CP is caused by permanent neurological damage, treatment efforts are aimed at improving motor function rather than curing the disability. Physical and occupational therapy are the primary components in such treatment. Physical therapy targets the large muscle groups such as the legs and arms. Occupational therapy involves treatment of the fine motor skills, focusing on the hands, which enable activities such as eating, dressing, and hygiene. It may also be necessary to employ a speech or language pathologist. But again, the variability of symptoms may mean that a child with CP will have no speech impairment.

PROGNOSIS: The goal is to help the child gain as much motor control and personal autonomy as possible. A child with CP might walk with a splint, or he might be confined to a wheelchair. CP more commonly affects lower rather than upper extremities and may or may not affect intelligence.

---

normal birth weight. The risk has been found to be especially great in children born below 1,000 grams.

Low-birth-weight infants who have had extended stays in the NICU due to complications tend to have more serious developmental problems. Complications that can have a significant effect on a premature infant's development include intrauterine growth retardation (IUGR), intrauterine or intrapartum infection, severe asphyxia, neonatal meningitis/encephalitis, intracranial hemorrhage, seizures, or severe bronchopulmonary dysplasia, which requires the infant to receive prolonged mechanical ventilation. However, the extent of developmental problems is always difficult to predict accurately. Infants with similar neonatal histories can have very different outcomes.

Cognitive differences among premature newborns can be noticeable in an infant's first years of life. Generally visual recognition and information processing are significantly slower in premature infants with developmental difficulties than they are in full-term normal-birth-weight newborns. Research has shown that high-risk premature infants tended to manipulate objects less frequently or less vigorously—that is, without the looking, active handling, banging, mouthing, turning, or transferring from hand to hand that is typically found in infants during their first year. The researchers established a link between the ability of a nine-month-old and his later cognitive ability at twenty-four months. Similarly, the play behaviors a baby exhibits at twenty-two months have been shown to correlate with that baby's cognitive proficiency at five years.

A 1989 study compared two groups of 65 nine-year-olds. One group consisted of children who had been born at very low birth weights but were free of neurological impairment. The children in the second group were born at normal birth weight and were matched to the first group's age, gender, ethnicity and social class, intelligence quotient (IQ), visual-motor and fine motor abilities, and academic achievement. This study found that very-low birth-weight infants scored lower on general intelligence, even though both groups' mean intelligence was in the average range. It also showed a pattern of lower academic achievement among the children who were born prematurely at low birth weight. Their deficit tended to be especially pronounced in mathematics and in visual or spatial skills.

In a series of neuropsychological tests performed on school-age children who had been born across the range of prematurity, a group of researchers found that infants with birth weights below 750 grams performed significantly more poorly than children who were born prematurely at birth weights between 750 and 1,499 grams. The difference between these two groups of premature infants on some criteria was found to be twice the one that existed between the 750- to 1,499-gram group and full-term infants. IQ can also be affected by extreme prematurity, insofar as extremely premature infants have a higher incidence of medical complication. In the study just mentioned, 20 percent of the children born at birth weights below 750 grams were found to have subnormal IQs (between 70 and 84). By comparison, just 8 to 13 percent of children who were born weighing less than 1,000 grams had subnormal IQs. Even very-low-birth-weight infants of average general intelligence tended to have selective difficulties with mental arithmetic, visual-motor and fine motor skills, spatial ability, language, and memory.

Behavior and Social Competence

Prematurity brings with it an increased risk for behavioral problems, particularly among boys. These problems can include hyperactivity, acting out, and attention deficit hyperactivity disorder (ADHD). A study of five-year-olds published in 1990 showed that 16 percent of children with birth weights below 1,000 grams had ADHD, compared with just 6.9 percent in a normal-birth-weight control group. Since the two groups of children had roughly equivalent incidences of other types of behavioral problems, the researchers concluded that the children born prematurely had biological causes for their attentional disorders. Another study involving five-year-olds who had been born prematurely, published in 1988, linked prematurity with shyness, passivity, withdrawn emotional states, and subnormal social competence.

The incidence of social and behavioral problems tends to be greater the lower the birth weight of the child in question. Very-low-birth-weight infants who have undergone complicated treatments have exhibited higher rates of gaze aversion, tended to interact less with others, and have shown less enthusiasm for playing or vocalizing. Children with behavioral problems have also tended to have other cognitive or neurological abnormalities.

Behavioral disturbances have tended to hold through the first year of life, thereby sometimes influencing the parents' way of interacting with their child. The high degree of frustration parents can feel in attempting to connect with their behaviorally limited premature baby can reinforce those problems. So it is important to surround your child with an atmosphere of love and acceptance, even when she doesn't appear to be reciprocating.

Behavioral problems tend to be significantly greater among boys who were born at very low birth weight. A study of nine-year-old boys who had been born at very low birth weights revealed a more pronounced tendency toward both "internalizing" behaviors such as depression and anxiety and "externalizing" behaviors, which include hyperactivity and aggressiveness. These results were not a function of intelligence or social class, the researchers found. Girls did not demonstrate a significant behavioral disturbance by birth weight.

School Performance

A range of research studies from the 1980s onward have found a higher incidence of learning problems among low-birth-weight children compared with full-term, normal-birth-weight children. As with other developmental problems, their frequency has tended to increase with lower birth weights. Levels of achievement in reading, spelling, and math have been shown to be lower in very-low-birth-weight children than for full-term children. A study of eight-year-olds published in 1991 in the *Journal of Pediatrics* did not find explicit learning disabilities in children born at very low birth weight. However, the study did find that children with birth weights of less than 1,000 grams were more likely than their normal-birth-weight counterparts to be getting special help with their studies. Very-low-birth-weight children of normal intelligence and without neurological abnormality also tended to score lower on achievement tests, with problems being particularly acute in math, studies have shown.

A 1990 study found that 34 percent of very-low-birth-weight children were having difficulty in school, as manifested by their being kept back a grade or by placement in special education programs. Just 14 percent of the normal-birth-weight control group had similar problems—a difference the researcher determined was not attributable to socioeconomic factors. Other researchers have placed the special education rate for preemies far higher than 34 percent, and their findings have revealed an increased incidence of special education placement as the children progress from one grade to the next.

A Caveat for the Concerned Parent

But one can take statistics only so far. You may find that trying to make sense of the data and percentages presented in this chapter is a bit like looking at a battlefield from thirty thousand feet in the air. Though you can get a sense of the big picture, the fortunes of individuals remain as hard to predict as fortune itself. In the face of all of these potentially frightening numbers, it is important to reiterate that more than four out of five premature babies have none of the developmental problems described in this chapter. They grow into childhood like any other infant. A year or two from now, you may be hard-pressed to notice any difference between your baby and his full-term, normal-birth-weight peers. In the end, statistics are just numbers, and it turns out that parents may not be so powerless after all.

What a Parent Can Do

There is additional encouraging news, even for parents of preemies who do have some developmental disturbance: The power of social and environmental factors is strong enough on infant development to suggest that parents *can* sometimes improve the developmental prognosis for their low-birth-weight, premature infants in some respects.

Social disadvantages such as low levels of parental education and low socioeconomic class have been shown to exacerbate the detrimental effects of prematurity on newborns. The reason appears to be that parental education level is often a proxy for a number of other factors important to infant development: these factors include income, the frequency and quality of medical care, and the quality of attention and variety of stimulation provided by the parents to their infants. In fact, for most low-birth-weight children, social and environmental factors seem to have a greater long-term effect than do biological risk factors. It also appears that cognitive problems associated with environmental or social factors become more pronounced over the long term.

Conversely, those factors can be turned to your child's advantage if they are positive. The quality of the home environment can play a significant role in improving your premature infant's behavioral development. Environmental factors that are within the control of a parent include the following:

• Sensitive child rearing that recognizes what may be the limitations of your premature infant's behavioral development. A warm, loving, accepting home atmosphere is a step in the right direction here.

• Active participation in your child's learning activities. This encompasses a variety of interactive learning experiences that parents can participate in with their infants, including reading, singing, and talking.

• Providing your baby with a variety of experiences every day. Just breaking up the boredom by taking your baby outside stimulates her senses and thus her developmental growth in ways that are significant. Music is an excellent stimulant for your baby, possibly promoting neurological development. Selecting a variety of toys for your baby can be a simple way to enable her to practice the motor skills that can improve her physical development.

- Protecting your baby from detrimental environments, such as smoke-filled rooms and public spaces known to have a higher incidence of infection.

The message we would like to close with is simple and straightforward: Parents need not be passive in the face of biology or statistics. The minority of premature, low-birth-weight children who do have some developmental disturbance can be greatly assisted by the loving, attentive care of a committed parent. The following story from AnnMarie from Massachusetts, the mother of twins who survived twin-to-twin transfusion syndrome and were born at twenty-seven weeks, amply illustrates how the loving care of a concerned parent can alleviate even the most serious of developmental problems.

❦

"Miracles happen every day. You just have to believe. I believe that all children are miracles. I know this and I believe this with all of my heart," AnnMarie wrote. After confronting problems with infertility, AnnMarie and her husband became the parents of a full-term daughter, Sarah. Two years later AnnMarie found that she was pregnant again—with triplets. This pregnancy would test her in ways she could never anticipate.

"[W]ithin two weeks, I was certain something was very wrong. . . . I asked the doctor if he would see me. He agreed. I asked him to please check the babies right away. He did, and that is when we discovered that one of the triplets had died in utero. I was told that day I would have to carry the baby, knowing he had already died, until the other two were delivered.

"I was angry, hurt, and above all disappointed in myself for not having been persistent enough to stand up two weeks prior and ask the doctor to see us. At times I wonder if I had been more diligent, perhaps my little one would have survived. My faith tells me that these things happen and they are God's will. And I know that is how I am supposed to accept it.

"At week twenty of the pregnancy, our twins were diagnosed with twin-to-twin transfusion syndrome [TTTS; see chapter 1 for further details]. . . . The death rate for twins who develop TTTS at midterm of their pregnancy is 80 to 100 percent. Babies may die in utero, at birth, or years later from the effects of TTTS. Those who do survive often suffer from an array of serious challenges, including cerebral palsy, developmental delays, cardiac and pulmonary difficulties. Some challenges are transient, some are long-term. . . .

"When we received this diagnosis, I began to research everything I possibly could on the syndrome. There was not very much information available, and I began to see just how resourceful I had to be. I asked a friend who was working for the University of Massachusetts Medical Center to help me search data. Together we researched Medline and many other Internet medical information services. I found myself getting very aggressive and more determined with each piece of information I came across. When I would get to a dead end in the way of pertinent information, I would start getting very creative in my strategies. I amazed even myself with the avenues I found accessible.

"At twenty-two weeks we discovered that our daughters were monochorionic [they shared the outer sac], monozygotic [one egg that has divided into two exact living beings], monoamnionic [one amniotic sac was shared also], identical with a TTTS going on in utero. This represented many other serious concerns. One of the main causes of death from being monoamnionic was entanglement. I was starting to feel incredibly vulnerable. I thought, What else could go wrong? I should have never asked that question! I was frightened and felt as though I needed more information. I needed a real miracle. I followed my doctor's orders to the letter. We were having ultrasounds weekly to keep a close eye on the syndrome's progression. The syndrome had stopped and started a few times during the pregnancy. I felt like this was the first ride of the perpetual emotional roller coaster.

"I have always been a woman of strong faith, but this was more than even my faith could handle. I began to ask my family and friends to pray for the children. My mother-in-law had asked the children from the Catholic school that she taught at to also pray for them. Surely God would listen to the children! I felt so hurt and so angry that this was happening to us. This was such an injustice in my eyes. Still, I would not give up on them. After all, if their mother gives up on them, then whom can they count on? I guess this may be hard for some to understand, but the love a mother feels for her child (unborn or born) is one of the strongest forms of love possible. I loved them, wholeheartedly and completely.

"I continued to talk to them and sing and read to them while they were in utero. I would listen to peaceful music when I felt that their movements were strong and active, and fast-tempo music if they seemed to be slower in their daily movements. I spent time stroking my tummy and just loving each moment of my pregnancy, fully understanding that this might be the only time I would share with them. I wanted them to know that they were loved and wanted, hoping that they might feel it and hold on to their lives. Perhaps sharing with them my strength and faith. I know that may sound crazy, but it is what I felt. I believe that when there is real love, honest love, that it can be felt even by an unborn child. I believe my love was so strong that they could feel it. So because of that deep feeling, I just kept on talking and singing and praying out loud, knowing that as long as there was life, there was surely hope.

"Well, the weeks dragged on and on. The Thanksgiving holiday had passed, and I was holding on to the hope that they would make it to Christmas. It was like a mental milestone for me. This was a very important time, one of the holiest days of my faith. My thought was, If they die at this time, it will be a glorious time to enter heaven. If they survive, what a blessing at this time of year to be forever reminded of. You see, I am Catholic and have always had a special devotion to the Blessed Mother Mary. Many times I had prayed for her intercession in this craziness. I felt, Who would better understand the fear of losing her child? So as we approached Christmas week (the twenty-seventh week in the pregnancy) I felt perhaps we would make it to a 'safe' time of delivery.

"With twenty-five weeks being the time of real viability, I thought that we were on our way to a real possibility of at least being able to see them alive. And maybe if I prayed harder, more would be possible.

"On Christmas morning 1991, at twenty-seven weeks' gestation, our identical twin girls were born. Christina Victoria was born weighing 2 pounds 9 ounces, measuring 15 inches long. Mary-Katherine Yolanda was born weighing 1 pound 12 ounces, 13 inches long. They had many complications during their very long neonatal intensive care unit stay.

"They came home with many medical and developmental issues. Mary-Katherine was born profoundly hearing impaired. She also has cerebral palsy, broncopulmonary dysplasia, restrictive airway disease, some growth and nutritional problems, and immunological and developmental problems. Christina was born with serious lung problems. She also had some neurological problems that impact her tactile sensory integration. Simply, her sense of touch and sound were so oversensitive that she was unable to cope, and this affected her on many physical and emotional areas of her life. Some of these difficulties for both have resolved with the help of early intervention, occupational therapy, physical therapy, speech therapy, and surgeries. I believe that much of their progress can be attributed to the efforts of the unity of our family. We have all worked endlessly and diligently to assist the twins to overcome things that were possible. The road ahead is going to be long, with many unexpected turns, I am sure. I was grateful that they were alive and that a road ahead actually existed.

"I love being 'Mommy.' It is a very natural role for me to have. Mothers love and protect their children. This I know from experience in my life. I thank my mother, grandmother, aunts, uncles, and brother because they taught me so much about a loving family. I learned how to love by being loved. I was able to accept others by loving the good I saw in them. I learned many lessons with love as my foundation. They had always

told me that there wasn't anything that I could not do, as long as I put my mind to it. I believed what they told me, because I trusted them. It just took a major life trauma for me to see it in myself. I'd heard these words of confidence and encouragement throughout all of my growing years. Those, along with many of the typical proverbs and clichés, that Mom and Nonie [grandmother] were well-known for. These were such words of wisdom. Life's lessons, if you will. They built a foundation of incredible strength inside of me of self-confidence, one that I hope to pass on to my children as their legacy. I have learned in life that we should strive for excellence . . . not perfection.

"Having to become an advocate for my children allowed me to grow in many ways. It was far more important to be certain about what I needed to do than it was to give a hoot about what other people thought of me and my choices. I am stronger, happier, and a lot more self-confident now than I have ever been. I had to look inside of myself, and when I did, I found out that I really like me. I learned a lot about myself and a lot about the people around me. I had people who loved me. I was going to have to know that the love I had learned was what I was using in return. I have learned to trust in myself and in my choices. I am sure I will make my mistakes along the way. But they will be just that: my mistakes. I can accept that, because I am careful about my choices. Everyone makes good and bad choices. I am no different. Sometimes we cannot see or understand why bad things happen. No one wants these types of things to happen in their lives. I do think that all things, both bad and good, affect us.

"My favorite quote is, 'The longer I live, the more I realize the impact of attitude on life. Attitude, to me, is more important than facts. It is more important than the past, than education, than money, than circumstance, than failures, than successes, than what other people think or say or do. It is more important than appearance, giftedness, or skill. It will make or break a company, a church, a home, a person. The remarkable thing is we have a choice every day regarding the attitude we will embrace for that day. We cannot change our past . . . we cannot change the fact that people will act in a certain way. We cannot change the inevitable. The only thing we can do is play on the one thing we have, and that is our attitude. I am convinced that life is 10 percent what happens to me and 90 percent how I react to it. And so it is with you. We are in charge of our attitudes.' That was written by Charles Swindoll.

"Never has a more truthful statement ever been made. I will continue to work hard with and for all of my children. This is my choice. I believe that they will be positive and productive and happy children because we teach them with God's love and his blessings. We teach them about family and about love.

"Now almost seven years have passed. Christina and Mary-Katherine have made such tremendous progress. Christina's tactile sensory issues have for the most part been completely resolved. Developmentally she is age appropriate. Though she will always have restrictive airway disease and some tactile defensiveness, she lives a very healthy, normal life. She is very bright and loves life. She is a sensitive, loving, and ambitious little girl.

"Mary-Katherine now hears within normal ranges. Her growth and development are progressing at an incredible pace. Her immune system is beginning to get stronger. Mary-Katherine is an energetic, inquisitive, intelligent, and happy little girl. Both girls will be attending Catholic school in the fall with their sister Sarah. The school they will attend is the one where the children prayed for them when they were first born. . . . They have come full circle. They will now pray with the children at St. Mary's for other people who will need prayer. We believed in miracles, and now our little miracles will help others to believe in them, too."

12

PREMATURITY AND THE SPECIAL NEEDS CHILD

WHAT YOU'LL FIND IN THIS CHAPTER

- "Will my child be able to live a full life?"
- Another baby?
- Parenting the special needs child

As any parent of a child with special needs will tell you, life is what you make of it. There is victory to be won out of seeming disaster, joy to be found in disappointment, and celebration to be found in the midst of despair. It's all a matter of time, perspective, and attitude. This comes home to us anytime we encounter a brave parent whose baby faces a physical or mental disability as a result of complications of pregnancy.

Cathy is the mother of Alex, a spirited seven-year-old boy who was born with cerebral palsy. He is able to walk on his own using braces and crutches and custom-made shoe inserts known as *ankle-foot orthotics,* or *AFOs*. Alex has learned well the value of perspective and attitude.

On the first day of school one year, one of his classmates walked up to him and asked (in the straight-on way that schoolmates seem naturally given to), "So, what's wrong with your legs?"

Alex didn't skip a beat. He answered, "It's just an old war wound."

"What war?" the classmate countered.

"Oh, you know, the big one," he said.

"Oh," the classmate said, and the conversation ended as crisply as it had begun, with all parties holding on to their pride.

The buoyant, good-humored outlook of children such as Alex has much to teach their parents. The overriding sense of spirit and joy exhibited by a child who from a distance might appear to be a tragic figure is a testament to the irrepressibility of the human spirit. It persists in

A Struggle with Anger

"After the birth of my twin boys and the discovery of some of their physical disabilities and limitations, I really began doubting my religion. I didn't understand how this could happen to me. I wanted to ask God, 'What have we done to deserve this? What have our boys done to deserve this?' I am working through this, but some days are more difficult than others. . . . Today my boys are older and I still struggle with my religious convictions. I want to teach them to believe, but it's difficult when I am still unresolved about my own feelings and my own faith has been so badly shaken."

the face of the most daunting obstacles. Where children have known nothing else, they have not had the opportunity to acquire the talent for self-pity that would be more likely to beset an adult in that same situation.

Of course, this may sound much easier to say than to do. The fact is that most parents of a special needs child face many of the same reactions that parents of stillborn children do. When the news first comes that something is wrong with the pregnancy, there is denial, followed by anger, bargaining, and finally acceptance. The delivery of a child with a significant physical or mental disability can entail feelings similar to those that perinatal loss involves. Parents of special needs children may feel that not only has their dream of having a healthy, normal child been shattered, but an additional burden has been placed on their shoulders as well.

As we pointed out earlier in the book, there is an unfortunate irony to the great progress obstetrical and neonatal medicine has made in the past twenty years: While today babies born as young as twenty-four weeks' gestation are surviving, thereby reducing mortality rates, the overall rate of disability has increased slightly as a result of their survival. The tiny babies who once would have died are living today. But their extreme prematurity is not always free of permanent consequence. As a result, more parents today than in previous generations are faced with the challenge of coping with a disabled child. The earlier the gestation, the higher the risk of such occurrences.

"Will My Child Be Able to Live a Full Life?"

Just because a child is born with special needs does not mean he can't live a happy and fulfilled life. Parents and children of today have a great advantage over those of a generation ago in terms of the resources available to them. Today there are more programs available for the child with special needs, and children with special needs, be they emotional or physical, are being given a head start in school. They are being mainstreamed into classrooms of their peers, with the ultimate goal to integrate them into the real world. At the same time, normal kids are being taught about dealing with others who have a disability. They are learning that a physical disability doesn't necessarily mean a mental handicap. And mental disabilities don't necessarily mean a person can't learn or is unteachable.

Just a few generations ago parents were told to institutionalize disabled children because they were considered a burden on family life and society. In the 1990s each and every child has a place and a right to live in our society.

AnnMarie delivered her twins at twenty-seven weeks, and they survived a dangerous condition called twin-to-twin transfusion syndrome (read her story in chapter 11). Mary-Katherine was born profoundly hearing impaired and has cerebral palsy, bronchopulmonary dysplasia, restrictive airway disease, growth and nutritional problems, and immunological and developmental problems. Christina was born with serious lung problems. She also had some neurological problems that cause her senses of touch and sound to be so oversensitive that she was unable to cope, and this affected many physical and emotional areas of her life. Some of these difficulties have resolved with the help of early intervention, occupational therapy, physical therapy, speech therapy, and surgeries. But the problems persist, as do the labels.

"I get upset, infuriated, with the label 'handicapped,'" AnnMarie said. "I guess my problem with it is that I don't believe you should ever say 'I can't.' I remember one day my girlfriend came over to the house and told me that I was horrible mother because I made that 'poor handicapped child' do chores around the house.

"I said to her, 'The only handicap that this child has is the one that you just placed on her. There isn't anything she can't do. She has legs, so she can walk. She has hands, so she can carry dishes to the sink.' I set her straight, and we're still friends today.

"Having that attitude has been my daughters' saving grace. Once they asked me, 'Why are we seven years old and still in kinder-

---

A Few Things to Remember If Your Child Has Special Needs

- Having a special needs child is not a failure.

- While it is disappointing and hard to deal with initially, ultimately it is an opportunity to become a deeper, more empathetic person and parent.

- Everything happens for a reason, but reasons are not always plain to see.

- Out of adversity can come great strength. Franklin Roosevelt and Helen Keller are just two examples, but there are thousands of unsung heroes for every one you have heard of. You and your child could be among them.

- Even the most seriously handicapped children can find triumph in the small activities of everyday life. They can be sources of inspiration to their loved ones. Love knows no bounds.

---

garten?' I responded, 'I don't know, but aren't you lucky? You're the tallest girls in the class. I'll bet you get the best grades, too.' And you know what? They do."

Getting to this kind of comfortable, confident place is not an overnight process. It takes time. And during that time you will probably experience some very raw, painful emotions as part of your own journey of acceptance and healing. As the Chinese proverb goes, the longest march begins with a single step. One mother said, "After discovering that one of my twin daughters had Down's syndrome, I was numb, in total shock. I asked my husband what we were going to do. He simply said, We're going to take her home and love her. What else is there to do? That is what we did, and though there have been trials and tribulations over the years, we took her home and loved her and she loved us back, one day at a time. Can parents really ask for more than that?"

Another Baby?

Having a special needs baby means accepting a loss—the loss of the perfect child of your dreams. Many parents have an overwhelming desire to have another baby after such a loss. But this is something that you should think about carefully. Give yourself time to grieve for your loss; you can't replace this child by having another so quickly. Pain and grieving over what you've lost is never easy, but it is necessary in order to come to terms and acceptance and eventually move forward.

Once you have found some form of acceptance, you will be much more able to move toward having your next child. The new child will bring his own identity into your family. As parents, we are aware of how special each child is and just how miraculous it is that life can still be created and grow and thrive, especially after such difficulty. Hopefully, in time we will come to realize that all things happen for a reason; we are just here to be the best parents that we can to the children that we are lucky enough to be blessed with.

As one mother of a special needs child put it, "It's like planning nine months for an exciting winter vacation on the slopes of Aspen, but instead you arrive on a tropical island. The journey is the same, but you end up in a foreign and unexpected place. This may be confusing, shocking, and frightening at first, the journey that you had dreamed about and anticipated for so long would not be realized, but then you realize that your journey with a special needs or disabled child is still a wonderful place to be. And you come to realize it's not the journey or unexpected destination that you are left to enjoy and appreciate over the years, but the special gift that you have been entrusted with."

Parenting the Special Needs Child

Most of us feel that we can handle whatever life throws at us. But not everyone has it within themselves to care for a child with a disability or handicap. Some people simply don't have the emotional or psychological resources to raise a child with a mental or physical disability. However, many parents who discover they are having a child with special needs feel so strongly about the calling to provide a loving home for a handicapped child that they go out and adopt another child with special needs. Many who open up their own hearts and homes to children with special needs feel they are pursuing a calling, doing what they are meant to do. But the reality is they have chosen their path. They have analyzed and carefully chosen their path and are where they want to be.

We are not being judgmental in stating this, only pointing out that knowledge is power. Discuss your feelings openly with your spouse or other family members. Everyone has a different tolerance for misfortune and the unexpected.

Being prepared and knowing how each other feels about these and other parental issues will serve you and your family well.

Through this whole process you will gain knowledge about your family, strengthen your relationship with your spouse, and find clarity on what really matters—and the level of obligation and hardship that you can ultimately live with. There will always be surprises in life, but this will limit a few. Our children are the biggest emotional investment we as parents make in our lives. Better understanding of our family history, the odds that we face, and the statistics will helps us better prepare for any curveballs that life might throw us.

Cathy turned her experience with Alex into a resource for her community. She founded Texas Advocates Supporting Kids with Disabil-ities, Inc., a group for parents with children with disability. "It's a common bond we share," she said. "We started because insurance was giving us trouble and we wanted to pool our resources and our know-how. But it has evolved into a wonderful resource for all of us. Those of us with a common need have such strength in numbers. We have lobbied for our children's rights at the Texas capital. We put out a quarterly newsletter, called *TASK Force,* with up-to-date information on legislative issues and so forth. There is no better cause than to fight for those who have so much potential but who can't fight for themselves. As a parent I have found this a very healing experience. I am very proud of this project and very happy that we were able to build our experiences into such a project that has helped so many."

13

WHEN THINGS GO WRONG

WHAT YOU'LL FIND IN THIS CHAPTER

- What you should expect from your hospital
- The stages of grieving
- Common emotions felt by bereaved parents
- Accepting and integrating your loss
- Bereavement and your relationships with friends, neighbors, and co-workers
- The grieving child

There is probably no subject more difficult to think, read, or write about than the death of a child. There is certainly no tragedy that strikes more deeply into the heart of our hopes, fears, and expectations than such an unexpected outcome. So although our overall aim in this book is to provide information on high-risk pregnancy and prematurity in a way that reflects the encouraging progress medicine has made in preventing and treating high-risk pregnancies, we would ultimately be performing a disservice to our readers if we did not acknowledge and discuss the sadder side of the issue. As painful a topic as it is, it is important not to pretend it does not exist.

Hundreds of thousands of women get preg-

nant every year. Some seem to do so without even trying. Others succeed only after years of anguish, infertility treatment, frustration, and large medical bills. The frequency of problem pregnancies varies with age, race, socioeconomic status, and overall health. But one thing is clear: A pregnancy that involves serious maternal complications or fetal disabilities leading to death can happen to anyone. Although advances in prenatal care over the past few decades have saved innumerable women's and infants' lives, sometimes things just go wrong. As often as not, the cause is never known.

Perinatal death is defined as any loss that occurs from the twentieth week of gestation to the twenty-eighth day after birth. Sometimes

> "I hated my body because it had failed me. I hated my breasts for producing milk when there was no baby to feed. I hated the doctor who had failed to revive my baby after she was born. I hated all those women who had live, healthy babies to feed and care for. I hated the sad faces of people who came to see me. Most of all, I hated God for letting this awful, unimaginable thing happen."
>
> —a parent quoted in *When a Baby Dies,*
> by Nancy Kohner and Alix Henley (1997)

miscarriages are included in this definition as well. But since this is the most painful experience a parent can ever face, it is not an issue of definitions. It is an issue of dashed hopes and unexpected sadness, of dreams that will be delayed or perhaps even put out of reach. As such, it does not matter to most parents whether their pregnancy terminates by miscarriage in the tenth week or via stillbirth at term. The impact is significant regardless of the stage of pregnancy at which it occurs.

Sometimes it happens without warning. Other times it is the end point of a long and agonized period of waiting. A critically ill infant may fight for survival in a special care nursery for a few days or several months. Some parents will face the sudden shock of an unexpected loss, whereas others may have to endure a burden of uncertainty that lasts for an extended period of time. Either before or after an infant's death, parents have time to reflect on their every move during pregnancy and question whether they are to blame. Second-guessing

oneself becomes so easy and natural that a bereaved parent will normally find any number of reasons to blame him- or herself.

When an infant dies, a life is lost that was no less valuable than any other life. Although the baby did not have a chance to grow and find her place in the world, and although her parents may not have developed all of the parental bonds with the baby that they would have developed over time, the baby already had a distinct identity. Parents may have posted sonogram images of the baby on their refrigerator. They may have bought baby name books and spent many evenings trying different combinations of names. Friends and relatives may have already given baby showers for the couple. Given all of this acknowledgment of the baby that may have already taken place, it is essential—and healthy—to recognize the extent of the loss that has taken place. It is a loss no less significant, no less heartrending, than any other.

In certain respects, it is an even greater loss. It is a loss of a future that will never become. For parents, the death of an infant represents the loss of part of themselves. We naturally invest our children with our own hopes and aspirations. If the baby was a first child, parents return to being a "mere" couple. The loss of parenthood itself is a significant secondary loss. If the couple is in their thirties or older, they may be feeling time pressure to have a family. The looming sense of disappointment can root itself deep in the psyche and color all aspects of the parents' lives.

No words that a friend or relative can say will relieve the pain. In fact, sometimes parents who have lost a child prefer that nothing be said at all. Perhaps the best starting point, then, is to recognize the value of what has been lost. Out of this grief will come, in time, healing.

Spenser's Story

"People tend to hear stories," said Liz, "about how there was this baby who was born so small—and now he's a rocket scientist. They don't hear about what can go wrong." The Maryland clinical laboratory researcher and her husband, Greg, lost their thirty-week son, Spenser, two months after he was born. He developed hydrocephaly following a bout with full-blown spinal meningitis. For all the pain their story entails, it also shows how hope can spring out of the darkest of times.

Liz was thirty-eight years old when she became pregnant with Spenser. Given her age, she saw a perinatologist at fifteen weeks for an amniocentesis. The perinatologist found a partially separated placenta and a subchorionic bleed. Something was said about bed rest, but the perinatologist seemed to defer to the obstetrician, Liz said, who didn't take the lead in putting her on bed rest. "I continued to bleed. It was pretty heavy," she said. "It would come and go. At one point I remember calling about the bleeding. They thought I was miscarrying, and since I wasn't experiencing any pain, they told me to come in Monday for a D&C [dilation and curettage—see glossary]. I came in, and he was alive and kicking."

Liz was a competitive swimmer who swam six days a week, 2½ miles a day, until the complications began. When the bleeding persisted into her twelfth week, the doctor advised her to stop swimming, concerned about the impact of such rigorous exercise on her pregnancy. Liz second-guesses the decision not to take her off work, but since her clinical job did not entail a great deal of physical strain, it seemed advisable at the time. When the bleeding stopped at around twenty-four weeks, she was allowed to resume swimming. "Everything was okay," she said.

With her doctor's permission, she made plans in the twenty-ninth week of her pregnancy to fly to the Northeast to see her mother. By this time she was having panic attacks. "I would get in my car to go to work and I would just start to panic. I didn't want the window up, because I was claustrophobic. But I couldn't put it down, either, because I couldn't stand the feeling of the air on me. . . . There were so many frightening things about my pregnancy, and nothing was ever really addressed. All the books recommend that pregnancies like mine be handled as high-risk—very close management, testing, and all that. I just kind of slipped between the cracks. That's why I started having these panic attacks. Even now I get really stressed whenever I think about it.

"I ended up getting on this plane. Physically I thought everything was fine; but emotionally I was getting all worked up. The plane was sitting there on the runway at nine-thirty P.M. and I felt this gush. I ran to the lavatory just scared to death. I was wearing white pants, and I was bleeding all over the place. I went to the stewardess and they took me off the plane and called the paramedics." It was three A.M. before her husband, who had returned home from the airport, and her mother, who was waiting for her in Boston, discovered that Liz had been taken to the hospital. She was released the next day to her parents-in-law's home and promptly started bleeding heavily again. When she was readmitted to the hospital, a transvaginal ultrasound showed that her membranes had ruptured. She went into labor shortly thereafter and delivered her son at thirty weeks, at 2 pounds 11 ounces, via a cesarean delivery.

When Spenser was just three weeks old, he developed full-blown spinal meningitis from an *E. coli* infection. "From that point on, he just went downhill," Liz said. Magnetic resonance imaging (MRI) and computerized tomography (CAT) scans showed massive neurological damage. The doctors said he would never survive infancy. Liz was told Spenser would be "technologically dependent" for the short remainder of his life. A do not resuscitate (DNR) order was placed in effect. Spenser was baptized right there in the NICU. The neonatologist extubated him. And still Spenser clung to life.

"He would take a bottle," Liz said. "He would open his eyes. They said that was just a reflex, because he was still on a feeding tube. They transferred him to a pediatric hospital and told us to rescind the DNR. We were able to bring him home.

"This was my first child, so I really didn't know what behavior to expect," Liz said. "He fussed, he took his bottle, he didn't like having his diapers changed or taking a bath—we thought maybe things would be okay. We knew he would be developmentally disabled, but we thought he might survive."

By the middle of October 1996 Spenser lost the ability to regulate his temperature. When it dropped to 92 degrees Fahrenheit, his head showed its first sign of swelling. Another MRI revealed that Spenser had advanced hydrocephalus and that very little brain tissue was left. Spenser was transferred to a hospice. A DNR order was put into effect again as his temperature fluctuated between 90 and 107 degrees.

"He could lie on his stomach and was still taking his bottle. But we knew he was not going to be with us much longer. One weekend he just started to crash. His lungs filled with fluid. The hospice team came out. He spent his last days at home with us. They didn't think it was going to be as quick as it was. The nurse and the social worker came out and spent a whole day with us. He died on Monday afternoon, Veterans Day.

"He was with us when he died. That was important. If somebody told me this had happened to them—that their baby died in their house—I would have thought it would have been the worst thing in the world. But I was glad he was with us and that we were able to keep him with us for the three or four hours until he was taken to a funeral home. It was actually very peaceful. If I hadn't been through it myself, I wouldn't have felt that way. I would've thought that I never could have gotten through it. But we did. The hospice was very good; they were part of our family. They were all crying, too. They and three of the NICU nurses came to the funeral. It meant a lot."

It meant so much to Liz and Greg that they decided to create a legacy in Spenser's memory. Vowing that women with high-risk pregnancies should have access to better information than they had, they followed up on the head neonatologist's suggestion and created a parents' resource room on the NICU floor of their hospital. "We probably have sixty or seventy books there now," Liz said. "There are some wonderful resources out there. We have videos on everything from acquainting parents with the NICU to multiples, single mothering, infant massage, and taking care of your preemie. It's very important for me to do this. It's a big part of my life."

Other aspects of Liz's life have been deeply affected by the experience. "I feel like I can't do anything right," she said. "I haven't been able to swim the way I could before." But she remains undaunted and has turned her pain into passion for activism in her community. She is trying to start a local support system for women who are having complicated pregnancies. It will have resource guides giving high-risk, expecting mothers information about and access to grocery stores that deliver, Meals on Wheels programs, transportation services so they can make doctors' appointments, and home health care aides to help out with other kids.

Talking about Spenser, and the activism his short life inspired, is something Liz has come to enjoy doing. "It keeps him very much alive in my memory," she said. "Even though he's no longer with us, I love to show people pictures. I know that all parents want their kids to shine. I feel like this library is Spenser's way of shining."

Liz's stepdaughter, Jessica, who was seven when Spenser died, has weathered this trial surprisingly well. "This turned her whole life upside down. But she came through well. She wrote a story about Spenser for school. When she got a puppy, she took it out to see Spenser's grave. She blames him for her messy room, saying that he's her guardian angel and he just comes down and messes it up. If anything unexpected happens to her, she says, 'Spenser did it. I'd be blaming things on him if he was alive, so I might as well do it now, too.' "

What You Should Expect from Your Hospital

Kimberly recalled the final hours in the life of her infant daughter, one of twins. Though the pain had softened by the time we spoke to her, the vividness of her memory spoke to the poignancy of her little girl's first and final days.

"We called our family so that they could see her one last time. It was midnight before a lot of them got there. They came in one or two at a time and saw her for a few minutes. Afterward we went home and got a good night's sleep so we could be sure we were doing the right thing. The next morning her meds were lowered. She passed away that morning, still on the vent.

"We went into the office of one of the neonatologists and we held her as she died. My husband took the tubes off her. We stayed there for a couple of hours. You have a lot of doubts in a situation like that. You know she felt pain. You know she did. You wonder if you have the right to keep her alive for those eight days. You wonder if it's for our sake rather than hers. My husband and I are both religious. This wasn't a spur-of-the-moment decision."

The difficulty of making life-and-death decisions, which often involve hard ethical considerations (discussed in chapter 14), is only heightened by the need to make them amid the bustle of a hospital. The NICU is not a hospice. It is a busy, high-tech environment where major life events such as birth and death are business as usual. Hospitals—and NICUs in particular—are generally sensitive to the needs of parents facing the death of a baby.

Following is what you should expect from your hospital when the worst happens and you are facing the loss of a child.

INFORMATION

A common tendency of health care personnel, whether your baby is near death or otherwise, is to shield you from the pain of having too much information. They are concerned that detailed information can frighten or confuse you, exacerbating an already stressful situation. The fact of the matter, however, is that during a time of crisis you need information to help orient you and help you make decisions. This might include the following:

- the cause of the baby's death or an explanation of why there isn't one.
- where the baby will be kept.
- when you will be able to be with your baby and take a photograph, if you so desire.
- if, when, and by whom an autopsy will be performed.

- whether a religious ceremony can be performed in the hospital.
- how a funeral and burial or cremation arrangements are to be handled.
- what kinds of support and follow-up care are available.
- what this means for your chances for a future pregnancy.

TIME

The grief and shock of losing a baby will never go away, but it can be ameliorated by the opportunity to spend time with and hold your baby and to take away a photograph as a memento of the short time you had together. The feeling of closeness that comes from being with your baby after death can ease the pain of saying good-bye. Hospitals are such loud public spaces that private time alone with your spouse and baby is essential for you to give voice to your grief. This can be a hard balance to strike. You don't want to feel alone or abandoned by the hospital professionals. Yet you need to have someone at the ready to answer the questions that will come up. Making good decisions requires perspective, and gaining perspective is a matter of time. Many hospitals have special rooms situated away from the rooms where new parents stay, designated for use by bereaved parents. Ask the hospital staff—a nurse, social worker, or doctor—about the availability of private space, so that you can begin to work through your grief alone with your baby, spouse, and family.

FOLLOW-UP

To ensure that you have the opportunity to ask questions that will invariably arise as time passes, it is important to arrange a follow-up appointment with your physician. These are usually scheduled for four to six weeks after your baby's death. At this appointment, the results of the autopsy (postmortem) will be available to you, and if an explanation of the cause of your baby's death wasn't possible initially, there may be one now. Waiting several weeks to get this information may be difficult for you. But the wait affords you time to reflect on the experience and to compose a list of questions that you'll want to ask your doctor or social worker.

The Stages of Grieving

A traditional way of understanding grief has been to view it as progressing in stages. Elisabeth Kübler-Ross, in her famous work *On Death and Dying,* counted five: denial and isolation, anger, bargaining, depression, and acceptance. She described how a bereaved (or dying) person moves from one to the next, each of which has definable phases and characteristics. Today other psychologists have slightly different views that probably correspond more faithfully to your experience, if you have faced significant bereavement. Mara Tesler Stein, Ph.D., a Chicago-based psychologist who is the co-author of a forthcoming book on the emotional dimensions of high-risk pregnancy and mother to thirty-week preemie twins, told us, "Many people think grieving is a linear process. But it's really more like a spiral. Imagine a spiral standing upright. Moving in a circle around that spiral are different issues: denial, grief, anger, frustration, confusion, a whole array of emotions that flood people who are bereaved. You move through one emotion, then overlap, and

go through another phase, then backtrack and do it all over again. At any point you might say to yourself, I thought I was over this. You might be shocked that you're reexperiencing feelings you thought were behind you.

"But grieving is not a process of 'getting over' something. It's a process of *integrating.* You knit the painful experience into the fabric of who you are, and you're never the same again. You look in a mirror and you don't recognize yourself. How could you possibly? Why should you? I think people, in time, come to value the change."

Common Emotions Felt by Bereaved Parents

SHOCK, DENIAL, AND ISOLATION: "THIS CANNOT BE HAPPENING TO ME"

The mind has a way of protecting us from pain, so in the early stages of grieving it is likely that you will experience a feeling of detachment, as if the loss happened to someone else. One mother put it, "I had no idea how to react. I felt so detached from it all. I sometimes felt as if I were watching someone else play a role in a very sad movie." Faced with the unexpected reversal of your hopes and dreams, you may go into a virtual state of shock when the anticipation of birth is unexpectedly transformed into the reality of death. The reality of the death may not hit you for days or weeks after its occurrence. Another defense your mind may put up is denial of the reality of the situation. If you have been told you have miscarried, you may find yourself insisting upon a second medical opinion in the hope that there has been some kind of misdiagnosis. You may find yourself harboring irrational beliefs about cause and effect. You may root their denial in either science ("This is impossible—there is no history of birth defects in my family") or faith ("This is impossible—God would not do this to me").

ANGER: "WHAT DID I DO TO DESERVE THIS?"

Anger has been said to be a by-product of guilt, the entirely natural response to the deep sadness of losing the one person a mother most urgently needs. Unlike the death of an elderly person, which can be an occasion to reflect on and appreciate a well-lived life full of accomplishment and meaning, the death of a child is valid reason to express rage and anger born of plans that will go unfulfilled and dreams that will go unrealized. Disruptive and painful though it is, angry feelings often mark the end of denial and another step toward integrating the death into your life. In this stage you may find yourself asking, "Why me?" You may feel resentment toward parents of healthy children—they possess the thing you want most— or toward your doctor, who you may feel should have been able to save your baby—and you—from this fate.

"When my baby died, my first reaction was anger," one parent said. "I was angry with my OB/GYN for taking me so far in the pregnancy without warning me that this could happen. I was angry with the doctor who broke the news to me. Why couldn't he have done more? I thought. What was that fancy medical diploma on his wall for if he couldn't bring back my baby?" At the same time you may face an all-encompassing sense of inadequacy.

As Elisabeth Kübler-Ross has observed, the feeling of rage can be difficult to cope with because it is often directed "in all directions and projected onto the environment at times almost at random." It is a very natural reaction to loss. Friends and families, even if they are targets of the anger, need to understand its source. Kübler-Ross wrote: "Maybe we too would be angry if all our life activities were interrupted so prematurely; if all the buildings we started were to go unfinished. . . . What else would we do with our anger, but let it out on the people who are most likely to . . . rush busily around only to remind us that we cannot even stand on our two feet anymore. People who order unpleasant tests and prolonged hospitalization with all its limitations, restrictions and costs, while at the end of the day they can go home and enjoy life."

SENSE OF LOSS AND DEPRESSION

It is natural for a deep sense of loss to set in once some time has gone by and the reality of the bereavement takes root. At a certain point you can no longer plausibly deny the loss or comfortably forestall sorrow with anger directed at other people or the world in general. The plain reality of the death of a child stands there, finally, for contemplation. This realization can lead to depression, during which bouts of anger can resurface. If you are suffering from depression, you need to allow yourself to express your grief and mourning. Hard though it may be, you should try not to lock others out, be it your spouse, a friend, or a counselor. At the end of the day, there is no easy shortcut. You are not likely to want to hear the sunny reassurances from people who are not close enough to you to truly empathize. You have been through denial already and don't need any more of it.

On the Loss of a Twin in Utero

Mary's bout with twin-to-twin transfusion syndrome led to the death of one of her twin boys. It taught her about the importance of medical professionals acknowledging the loss of a twin at the same time that they celebrate the birth of a new life. She told us:

"Steven always made himself known in the middle of the night. On this night, he gave me the most profound kick. I knew that he wasn't saying good-bye, only 'I love you, Mommy.' Two months later I delivered both of my twins. It has been ten years ago this week since my little Steven passed away.

"One Thursday morning, two days after Steven's kick, we were at our appointment with the perinatologist. He said he heard the heartbeats at the same rate. He wanted an ultrasound done. That afternoon, with the same high-risk doctor peering intensely at the screen, I heard the words 'I'm sorry, honey, his heart isn't beating anymore.' They had to hold me down, I was crying and screaming so hard. All I could think of was Jesus' resurrection, and I said, 'Maybe it will beat again.' And he said, 'No, honey. I am so sorry.'

"Two days later I went into preterm labor, which was stopped with an intense dose of IV ritodrine. This happened three more times, with the fourth delivering by C-section. Each time I came back from the hospital, every day seemed like a year. I had no one to talk to. I lay in bed and watched the sun go up and the sun go down. I isolated myself from everyone in my life, including my doctor. I felt that I needed to concentrate solely on Matthew's movements. I would not eat the same food I ate when Steven was alive, because I thought that it would kill Matthew, too. I was deeply depressed and suffering from obsessive-compulsive disorder. Instead of getting help, we were told by one doctor that we had to stop thinking about death or we would end up in a psychiatrist's office. He had seen it before, he said.

"That one statement did the most damage. The delivery could have been planned for. It could have been a compassionate delivery, performed with the appreciation that we are still the parents of twins and always would be. He might have said, 'It is okay to cry. Let me find someone for you to talk to.' But we were treated as though that status had been taken away from us, as though there really weren't two babies anymore. But the reality of both of their lives came home to me every time Matthew would move. Whenever he moved, I would feel Steven move, too. It felt like Steven was in a car that was underwater, like he was pounding on the window, crying for Mommy to save him. I was running toward Steven, running and running and reaching my arms out to him, never able to get close enough, though I had to watch. I have never been quite able to put my experience into words, but that is what it felt like and always will.

"After six and one-half months on bed rest, more than twenty ultrasounds and twenty nonstress tests, over a month in the hospital, four episodes of preterm labor, three amniocenteses, and ten weeks after my son Steven passed away, I delivered my twins on December 7, 1989. Matthew Steven was born to a room filled with laughter and cheers. Steven James was born five minutes later to a room filled with piercing silence. I cried for him. But the medical staff barely talked about my loss. In the couple of months leading up to it, a time when everyone knew it would be bittersweet, not one word was said, not one plan was made. This was so very wrong.

"On the day that they were born, I made a promise to Matthew and Steven: that they would be known and remembered and that I would find the answers. This promise has become my life's conviction. Twin-to-twin transfusion syndrome is a terrible, evil disease. But it is not stronger than a mother's love."

Mary Slaman-Forsythe has made good on her promise. She is the founder and president of the Twin-to-Twin Transfusion Syndrome Foundation, an international nonprofit organization dedicated to providing educational, emotional, and financial support to families, medical professionals, and other caregivers before, during, and after a pregnancy diagnosed with twin-to-twin transfusion syndrome.

DISORGANIZATION, APATHY, AND VULNERABILITY

Having lost a child, you may find yourself unable to cope with the demands of your busy life. You might have trouble concentrating on routine tasks, forget important details, or just stop caring about life the way you once did. Apathy, pessimism, powerlessness, and vulnerability may overcome you.

If you are in this phase of grief, it is important to open up to someone you trust—be it a friend or a professional counselor—so that you can acknowledge your emotions.

PHYSICAL SYMPTOMS OF GRIEF

An emotional trauma this strong often has a physical dimension as well. Physical symptoms of grief can include the following:

- illness, including fatigue, allergies, muscle or joint pain, or recurring infections.
- anxiety, including rapid heartbeat, nausea, rapid breathing, perspiration, headaches, insomnia, or irritability.
- compulsive/addictive behavior, including drug use, excessive television viewing, gambling, spending, sleeping, or sexual activity.
- depression, including boredom, lack of concentration, crying, indecisiveness, or guilt.

Accepting and Integrating Your Loss

Every person in the bereaved family needs to be allowed to grieve in his or her own way and at his or her own pace. Some will progress quickly through these stages; others will need more time to complete this emotional journey. Most likely, each member of the family will find a different way to deal with the loss. This may have to do with individual differences in how loss or bereavement was handled in their own families while they were growing up. Men and women also tend to have different ways of handling the grief of loss. Each situation is unique because of the complex combinations of personalities involved.

Some people may choose to seek professional counsel in dealing with their loss. In other cases, informal support groups consisting of other bereaved parents may be more helpful. Well-meaning family and friends can be comforting, but sometimes it is difficult to discuss painful issues with people who haven't "been there" themselves. Parents typically benefit most from the companionship of a friend or relative who has a quietly reassuring manner, someone who will neither dwell on the negative nor offer unrealistic, Pollyanna-ish encouragements.

If you have had enough time and help in adjusting to the loss of a baby, you may reach a stage where you feel neither depressed nor angry. Granted, you are not joyfully happy. But the struggle is over, and you are ready to accept the reality of the death or disability of your child. The loss of your child has become integrated into the fabric of your life. It has changed the core of your being, made you a different person. You see the world differently. You react to situations, handle people, differently. Sadness and grief can become transformed into deep aspects of your character and personality.

In her excellent book about infant loss, *Empty Cradle, Broken Heart* (1996), developmental psychologist Deborah L. Davis describes several ways to help yourself work

It's Normal

It is easier to cope with grief once you realize that the wide range of reactions and feelings of loss that you may be experiencing are *normal.*

- Grief takes time to work through.
- Everyone responds to grief differently.
- Give yourself the time and, more important, the permission to grieve.

through the grieving process (the bulleted items that follow are abridged from what appears in her book):

- Do not let others decide how you should feel. Don't measure your grief against anyone else's. You need to find your own path and do what is best for you.

- Give yourself permission to experience all your emotions and thoughts. . . . By burying or avoiding them, you only give them more power to compromise your life and your happiness. By expressing them constructively, you empower yourself to get through grief and eventually make life meaningful again.

- Label your emotions specifically—anger, guilt, anxiety, despair. Once you do this, you can start finding relief from them.

- Dwell on your memories and your hopes and dreams of what might have been. By reviewing your experiences and your fantasies, you can identify what you have lost and then gradually let go of your emotional investment.

- Identify the things you regret not doing with your baby and find appropriate ways to have closure. . . . You may want to talk about how you feel with supportive friends or other bereaved parents, write a letter to your baby, or go to the grave or the place where you scattered or keep the ashes and talk to your baby.

- Give yourself opportunities to be alone and cry. . . . For at least the first year, try to avoid making significant changes in your life. Major changes may only increase your stress and multiply the adjustments you must make.

- Let others help and nurture you. . . . Find people who can listen and accept your feelings and thoughts.

- Have realistic ideas about what resolution means. Remember that you aren't giving up or forgetting your baby. . . . Continued suffering and misery are not proof of your devotion to your baby. Healthy grief and resolution mean adjusting to a new future while remembering and finding appropriate ways to feel connected to your baby.

The bereavement that goes with the loss of an infant is hard enough to deal with all by itself. The difficulty of dealing with other people can magnify the pain. Friends, family, and co-workers may want to help. But often their inability to relate to the experience of infant loss limits their helpfulness.

Bereavement and Your Relationships with Friends, Neighbors, and Co-Workers

The emotional pain of loss can change the dynamics of bereaved parents' relationships with friends and neighbors or anyone else who might find it suddenly awkward to interact with someone who has suffered a tragic loss. Greg, the father of Spenser (see box, page 293), recalled how his neighborhood was full of pregnant mothers when he and Liz were pregnant with Spenser. After Spenser died, their relationships with their neighbors changed. "Only one or two couples have spoken to us since [Spenser died]," Greg said. "I want to tell them, 'This isn't a disease!' But they don't seem to know how to relate to us now. They have healthy families. Some of them have a child who would have been Spenser's age. They don't seem to know how to talk to you. They alienate themselves to comfort themselves."

At work, Greg found that a similar awkwardness pervaded his interactions with colleagues. "I was constantly asked, 'How's Liz? How's the baby?' Apparently I wasn't supposed to feel anything. Well, I suffered a loss, too. They weren't treating us like a pair. Just some acknowledgment, just being included, just some recognition that I was part of the grieving process—that would have helped."

The Grieving Child

If you have lost a baby and have other children at home who are old enough to comprehend what has happened, you face the additional trauma of having to shepherd your other child or children through the very same trauma you are still struggling with yourself. Elizabeth's story, which follows, is extraordinarily sad and moving, but not without a ray of light at the end.

Elizabeth was the mother of children ages three, four, and five when she became pregnant for the fourth time in six years back in the early 1970s. She thought it would be educational and fun to involve her oldest child, Michael, in the pregnancy. "I had whizzed through my previous pregnancies and never stopped to see how wonderful they really were," she said. "I didn't want to wait ten years to explain all of this to him, by which time he would know everything anyway."

It was a sensible enough idea. Michael seemed fascinated by her swelling belly and all the talk of another sibling on the way. When Elizabeth gave him a little blue book all about pregnancy, he pored over it every day, memorizing diagrams and doing somersaults across the floor to demonstrate his understanding of the baby's position within the womb. He showed it to neighborhood children—which promptly brought phone calls from parents who weren't so eager for their young ones to share his advanced knowledge of human reproduction. "We had to keep the book in the house after that," Elizabeth told us.

As time went by, Michael showed his helpful side, looking for places to put the baby in the house, rearranging beds, getting involved, asking a lot of questions. He was curious about what his sister would be like: "Will the baby eat mucky oatmeal? Will she dig worms in the garden?" Elizabeth said, "I told him that she would be a part of all of us. He wanted her to be good at pluses—at addition—because that's what he was good at. He had talked about her counting

the stars with him." Because the baby was due right before Christmas, he wanted to hang a fourth stocking on the fireplace. He asked Santa to bring extra toys.

New Year's Day came and still there was no baby. "I had to explain to him that she would make up her own mind when she was coming," Elizabeth said. On January 11, when Elizabeth began to feel some cramping, which she thought might be contractions, she went to the hospital in Baltimore. The doctor who examined her wasn't sure she was in labor. (This was before the advent of the sonogram.) But they kept her anyway because she was more than a month late.

"I began to have continuous pain," Elizabeth said, "but it wasn't like a contraction. The nurse said it was nothing. But I finally convinced her several hours later to get a doctor, and a resident came over. He discovered that I was bleeding and rushed out of the room to get assistance. They had a hard time detecting a heartbeat. They asked me how I felt, and when

I had last felt the baby move. I said that I was sure I had felt movement, though there were no big kicks or anything. I thought I would have noticed an absence of that."

The delivery room was subdued as the implications of these symptoms sank in. The baby hadn't survived. It turned out that the umbilical cord had become wrapped around the baby's neck and had tightened as she descended. "The room was very quiet. I was pretending at that point that they were talking about someone else. I imagined myself eavesdropping on another person. They told me I had a girl, and I was overjoyed, as if I had actually had a girl. Then reality set in that she was gone. But I didn't ask to see her. I was pretending that they were talking about someone else. I really regret that.

"Her life was snuffed out by the cord that gave her life. The cord from page five of Michael's little blue book. He didn't understand my pain. He only understood his own. He withdrew. I wanted to hold him and hug him, but he kept pushing me away. I quickly realized that I'd set him up for this loss, and I felt guilty about that. If I hadn't gotten him that little blue book, he wouldn't have been in such pain."

At school Michael stopped talking about how his mommy had gone to the hospital to have a baby. When the teacher asked whether he had his new sister yet, he shook his head and didn't say anything. "He didn't go to recess, he didn't play, and I began to worry about him."

Children have their own ways of dealing with loss, and in time a transition took place in Michael. Eight weeks later, on back-to-school day, looking for a way to help Michael, the teacher had decided to have a class during which the children would talk about their families. Michael loved school still, and she encouraged him to participate. Michael described his family as consisting of three boys and an angel. "She's good at pluses," he said. "And she counts the stars in the sky."

Though involving her son in her pregnancy caused her a great deal of pain at the time, Elizabeth said that Michael, age thirty-four today, has grown to be a very sensitive person who has a particularly strong bond with his mother. "Maybe involving him in my pregnancy wasn't such a wonderful idea," she said. "But in life you have to do what seems right at the moment and hope for the best. This was one of life's lessons that we shared."

14

HARD QUESTIONS, TOUGH DECISIONS—RESOLVING ETHICAL ISSUES IN NEONATAL CARE

WHAT YOU'LL FIND IN THIS CHAPTER

- A historical perspective
- Good information: the foundation of ethical decision making
- When your doctor must say "no"
- Mediating your dilemma: the hospital biomedical ethics committee
- Common ethical issues in the neonatal ICU

Kimberly and her husband faced the toughest choice parents can confront. At twenty weeks they found out that their twins had twin-to-twin transfusion syndrome, a grave condition that, untreated, has a mortality rate for the infants of 80 to 100 percent. She began seeing a perinatologist, but complications along the way, including a bladder infection and preterm labor, led to the cesarean delivery, at twenty-four weeks, of twin girls, one weighing 1 pound 8 ounces and the other just 11 ounces, and 8½ inches in length.

The smaller baby, McKenzie, was simply too small to survive. It was later found that her umbilical cord was not attached very well. "She did well the first day or two, but then they started having to increase her dosage on all of the medications she was taking. We felt like they were experimenting on her. They said that they didn't really know what they were doing. They kept saying, 'Ten years ago, this is how we kept 500-gram babies alive.' This wasn't acceptable to us. We told them, 'You're not coming home with us and you're not going to be with us ten years down the road, living in our shoes living with this [likely handicapped] child." McKenzie's agonized parents searched their hearts, talked to their doctor, and decided to place a DNR (do not resuscitate) order. Her meds were reduced to normal levels, and she died within two hours, eight days after she was born.

"I'm confident that we made the right move,"

Kimberly said. "Just because medical science *could* keep her alive didn't mean we wanted them to. We felt she should be allowed to die without suffering. We met with the neonatologist several times. The weekend before she died, he was very understanding. I told him, 'We can keep her alive, but if she's going to spend her life in the hospital, or spend her life in a vegetative state, we don't want to be a part of that.' This was a parental choice. He agreed. We had reached the limit."

Some of the hardest ethical questions a parent can face involve issues that arise in the course of a preemie's neonatal care. Many thick books have been written on the topic of medical ethics, including several that treat the specific ethical dilemmas that we will touch on in this chapter. Controversies over medical ethics tend to get extensive coverage in the media as well. Because we have limited space in a comprehensive book such as this to deal with such a broad and often profound topic, we will attempt to present the most frequently confronted neonatal ethical issues along with a commonsense approach for dealing with them. We won't try to provide you with answers to particular questions. Answers to individual ethical situations are highly situation-specific, so the "right" decision in any given situation will depend upon a unique combination of factual and moral (and sometimes legal) circumstances. Rather, we will give you a sense of what to expect from your doctor and the hospital when an ethical issue arises and give you some guidelines for approaching these issues in a constructive way. We hope that understanding the institutional processes that most hospitals have established for resolving difficult ethical issues will empower you to make use of them if the worst happens and you find yourself faced with a difficult choice to make.

A Historical Perspective

The relatively new subspecialties of neonatology and perinatology have seen tremendous growth in their knowledge bases over the last three decades. This increase in understanding has brought about wonderful new treatments for mothers and newborn infants. When they first developed, something as simple as sterile technique during delivery and using incubators to keep premature infants warm were viewed as radical. More recently, breakthroughs such as the development of artificial surfactant to treat lung immaturity have produced a tremendous improvement in newborn survival, especially in the very small premature infant. However, with every advance, small or large, there have been questions raised as to the benefits and costs to the patients receiving the treatment. And by "costs" we do not refer only to the fiscal considerations.

Insightful neonatologists and perinatologists have welcomed open discussion of the ethical considerations generated by newer therapies such as in utero surgery or the use of antenatal steroid administration. Medical ethicists and parents and legalists have also contributed to the continuing dialogue about therapies and their implications. The issues are never the same owing to the uniqueness of each mother, father, infant, family, illness, or treatment. Although seasoned physicians may have encountered similar ethical and clinical scenarios in the course of their careers, no two situations are the same.

The answers, of course, won't and shouldn't be the same. The questions that get asked, however, are another story. The resolution of ethical issues requires consistently asking the same questions. Asking the same questions forces any variety of circumstances into a consistent analysis. Such an approach ensures that nothing is left out, assumed away, or ignored out of bias.

Good Information: The Foundation of Ethical Decision Making

To arrive at a reasonable and ethical approach—to be able to answer meaningfully the same questions in each situation—depends upon both parent's and doctor's obtaining and understanding all of the medical facts particular to the situation. This means that 1) the information about the medical condition of the patient and the possible treatments is reliable and presented to you in a nonbiased fashion; 2) the medical and ethical issues are fairly represented; and 3) all considerations, both pro and con, have been addressed.

The physician's willingness to communicate with you has a great impact on whether the information you need is available to you as you wrestle with whatever ethical question is facing you. We believe that a physician has both a professional and ethical obligation to give you medical facts to an extent that enables you to participate fully in making important decisions about your or your preemie's care. The physician's presentation of that information should be truthful and balanced. She should outline all of the possible alternatives. Of course, since the

JOE GARCIA-PRATS: "When I was a young intern, in the early stages of my career, a very small and critically ill premature infant was admitted to the neonatal intensive care unit. The mother was fifteen years old and one of eight children from a very poor family. Though my supervisory resident and I worked diligently to stabilize this infant, he did not respond to the treatments. We worked hard to save him for most of the night and into the next morning. At one point during that long night, I commented to my supervisory resident that maybe it would be best if the infant didn't survive, since the future did not look very bright for him. I reasoned that the baby's mother was so young, and his family was so poor, that bringing another mouth to feed into the mix would only produce greater stress for the family and leave fewer resources for the other members of the family. My supervisory resident replied, 'You've been taking care of sick infants in this unit all month long. Since when has a family's ability to care for a child been used as a criterion to select how much effort we make to save a baby's life?'

"I matured a lot that evening because I realized the importance of carefully reasoning through the issues used to make decisions. I also realized the importance of always addressing the same issues in each case. Always asking the same questions insures that a consistent approach is used when addressing each situation. I recognized, however, that the answers to these questions change with each situation."

JOE GARCIA-PRATS: "Though I agree that generally a physician should be as unbiased as possible, I do believe it is a doctor's duty to make recommendations to the family and not just dump tough decisions on them to confront alone. It's not enough for a doctor to say, 'Here are your choices. What would you like me to do?' The good judgment of your baby's physician is one of the most important sources of support you have at your disposal. Of course, it is also important to seek support from other family members, your religious resources, social workers, friends, and so forth. Good and loving advice can come from many sources. The better the support, the better the parents' ultimate decision. The physician is an important part of that equation."

doctor is an expert, she will have her own well-informed opinions, too. Indeed, spelling out all of the options can be difficult for a physician who has already formed a strong opinion about the best course of treatment. However, as long as the alternatives have been presented, with pros and cons for each scenario, we feel that the physician should be free to give you an honest opinion. Additionally, your physician should offer you the option of seeking a second opinion when appropriate.

In most medical contexts, after you have been presented with all of the information relevant to your or your baby's medical condition, the wishes of the patient will be considered. Of course, since a newborn's wishes cannot be known, another question arises: Who makes the determination about what a baby would want? In most cases it is the parents who decide for their infant. Since making a decision for another can be extremely difficult, with factors other than the other's well-being playing a role, your physician will listen closely to your thoughts and try to determine whether factors aside from the actual well-being of the infant are at work. If your baby's physician articulates such questions, try not to take them personally. Remember the importance of the same questions being asked in every situation. In the spirit of that consistency, these are questions physicians will ask in *all cases.* The fact that they ask them does not imply any type of judgment about you or your infant. The physician's mental checklist may include questions such as the following:

- Is the parents' decision in the best interest of the infant?
- Who is looking out for the rights and best interests of the infant, the parent or the physician or both?
- What pressures (religious, financial, and so on) are the parents facing at the time they are called upon to make a tough decision regarding their infant?
- If the parents choose to continue a treatment that may yield little benefit to their infant, how significant are the implications—to society, to the availability of scarce resources, and to the neonatal team that is forced to continue the therapy?

Likewise, in evaluating the way a physician is approaching an ethical dilemma, you should bear in mind the following, similarly nonjudgmental questions about the doctor's approach to the situation:

- Is the physician being motivated by the potential for financial gain or the pursuit of research interests?
- Have all of the realistic (or merely possible) alternatives for treatment been put on the table?
- Are treatments available at other institutions not being offered because these other institutions are my hospital's competitors?
- Will my insurance carrier be willing to pay for the therapy my doctor is recommending?

When Your Doctor Must Say "No"

Parents should understand that there are times when their physician simply cannot honor their wishes. In certain situations a requested medical procedure simply may not be medically or physically possible. For example, asking for a lung transplant is not a realistic option for a preemie. Other situations are governed by federal law. If a family requests that medical support of their infant be withdrawn solely because the baby would be handicapped if she survived, "Baby Doe" regulations passed by Congress in 1984 would block the request. This federal statute states that withholding or withdrawing care from children with handicaps constitutes discrimination against the disabled and is thus illegal. This federal regulation arose in the early 1980s when two sets of parents decided to refuse treatment for what they considered handicapping conditions that their infants were born with. One infant had Down's syndrome, and one infant was born with spina bifida. Both infants were not treated, and both died. In the ensuing furor, Congress received significant lobbying pressure from advocates for the handicapped. Subsequently Congress passed protective regulations establishing three classes of patient for whom withholding treatment would be permissible:

1. the infant whose condition was hopeless and for whom life support only prolonged the inevitable demise;

2. the infant who would remain in a permanently vegetative state;

3. the infant whose proposed therapy would be excessively painful and not reasonable in light of the infant's condition.

At the time, many observers thought that these regulations would have a tremendous effect on how neonatologists practiced their profession. Most neonatologists, however, don't feel that it changed how they practice. Many, however, do grant that the new law made them more sensitive to the ethical issues in decision making for critically ill infants.

As we have mentioned earlier, doctors aren't the only parties concerned with medical ethics. When difficult issues like these arise, there are numerous resources that can be tapped to assist in these difficult times. You should consider asking your rabbi, priest, or minister to help in counseling. Many hospitals also have medical social workers who may point a family toward other resources as well as assist in the family's process of coming to a decision. Your obstetrician or pediatrician may also be of assistance. Another resource is the hospital's biomedical ethics committee.

Mediating Your Dilemma: The Hospital Biomedical Ethics Committee

More often than not, physicians and parents agree about the approach to take when a difficult question arises. However, when a resolution can't be found, one alternative is to seek the input of the hospital ethics committee. In this section we will give you some background on when and how it is supposed to function. We hope that you will take advantage of this important ethical resource whenever a tough issue arises that does not get answered through discussions with your baby's physician.

The Joint Commission on the Accreditation of Healthcare Organizations (JCAHO), a federal accrediting agency for hospitals, has required that a structured ethics process be in place for all accredited hospitals. Administration of this process usually takes the form of a biomedical ethics committee at each hospital. The role of the committee requires attention to patients' rights as well as the ethics of the institution. It is important to note that *the committee's goal is to make recommendations, not binding mandates.*

Examples of conflicts that could arise include differences about what treatments to pursue or disagreements about when to limit or withdraw care. When parents and their physician find a major area of conflict regarding the level or type of treatment, the biomedical ethics committee can be called upon to review the circumstances of the case. Often these types of disagreements are simply the result of miscommunications between the parties. In such cases the committee can perform the valuable service

of objectively explaining one party's position to the other. In other cases communication is clear, but there is an impasse over an ethical issue. In this latter scenario the committee's role is to review the case and make a recommendation that either doctor, parent, or patient has the discretion to follow or disregard.

Most biomedical ethics committees operate according to certain general guidelines: 1) the presumption of goodwill by all members of the committee; 2) strict confidentiality in all situations; 3) a patient-centered decision-making process; and 4) an equal voice for each member of the committee. One of the committee's ongoing tasks is the education of the hospital's medical, nursing, and administrative staffs about its own existence. In order for it to be effective, hospital personnel must know that it exists. And to ensure diversity and a broad base of perspectives, it is usually recommended that the makeup of the committee reflect the entire hospital community. Thus physicians, nurses, social workers, chaplains, housekeepers, patient advocates, attorneys, and members of the business community will be asked to sit on the committee. In most instances the composition of the committee is set by the hospital or medical staff policy.

Anyone involved in the care of a patient or the patient's family may bring an issue before the ethics committee. However, each committee handles a request for consultation differently, and not every request will result in a full committee review. Often a request for consultation can be handled by a subset of the committee's members. Such is the case especially when the conflict that arises is due to the unfamiliarity of physician or patient/parent with hospital policy. Many times the resolution of a straightforward communication problem can be brought about by the committee members initially assigned to look into the case.

When a case is brought to the committee by a nurse, physician, or parent, the process may involve several steps: 1) identification of the person bringing the request for a consultation; 2) clarification or restatement of the ethical problem; 3) gathering of information regarding the clinical situation; 4) listing of each option and its pros and cons; 5) identification of any legal issues; and 6) recording and communication of the options. It is usually the goal of the committee to address the issues promptly, within twenty-four hours of the request, although in certain instances delays may be necessary in order to allow for family members to participate in the committee's review of the situation.

Once this formal consultation has been accomplished, one or more recommendations are written down, reviewed by all members of the committee, and forwarded verbally to the parties involved—for example, the patient's family and physician. The written copy of the recommendations is kept in a confidential file for review. *While implementation of the recommendations is not mandatory for either party,* appropriate use of the committee usually provides helpful direction for everyone involved.

Common Ethical Issues in the Neonatal ICU

Many volumes have been written on medical ethical issues. We will attempt here to give you a general sense of three of the most common ethical considerations that arise in the course of

JOE GARCIA-PRATS: "In my experience, it is usually medical personnel who request the involvement of the biomedical ethics committee. Perhaps this is because families are less aware of the ethics committee's existence than medical personnel. Parents should be aware of this resource and not hesitate to make use of it when an ethical issue arises. While ethics committees have no formal authority to force either side to accept their recommendations, the recommendation carries authority and credibility and can therefore have a powerful impact on a disagreement between a physician and parents."

neonatal care: 1) the limits of viability; 2) quality of life considerations; and 3) withdrawal of support.

LIMITS OF VIABILITY

Even in the early 1900s physicians who cared for premature infants were criticized for trying to change outcomes that some felt should be left to nature to decide. In that early era of neonatal care, the standard practice was to leave the newly born infant alone. If he were sufficiently mature, he would survive. Otherwise he would not.

As neonatology developed as a subspecialty, critics of neonatal care, who often believe that neonatologists are meddling in situations better left to nature, have continued to protest research into newborn physiology and disease processes and to the use of newly discovered medical interventions to improve the overall survival for preemies. Indeed, there has been a price to pay for this improvement: an increase in the proportion of survivors who have been left with disabilities. Over the past three decades this criticism of neonatology has persisted from certain quarters.

In the beginning of the "modern" era of neonatal care, during the 1970s, controversy surrounded the question of what the appropriate threshold gestational age or birth weight was where a physician should begin considering to intervene with neonatal care. Thirty years ago the patients who were the object of this discussion were premature infants who weighed 3 to 4 pounds at birth. By today's standards they were relative giants. With all of the recent advances in neonatal and perinatal medicine, however, today these same discussions and arguments now apply to the 1.5- to 2-pound "micropreemies" who are born as early as twenty-two to twenty-four weeks. Compelling questions arise: When should nature be permitted to take its course? When are physicians overreaching, "playing God in the nursery"? As long as there are decisions of care to be made by parents and physicians, these issues in neonatology are both appropriate and essential to address. We must not forget, however, that although most of these decisions will be made by parents and physicians, they must be made within state and federal law.

In most neonatal ICUs in the United States, a gestational age of twenty-four weeks is the threshold level of maturity where most neonatologists would consider offering the full range of neonatal treatments and support. Prior to this gestational age opinions vary widely, since the mortality of the twenty-three-week or less gestational age infant may be greater than 60 to 70 percent. Dr. Julian De Lia, an obstetrician and surgeon who has gained renown as the first physician to perform successful in utero laser surgery on twins who had an often fatal condition known as twin-to-twin transfusion syndrome (TTTS—see chapter 1), is frustrated that many physicians and parents prefer the certainty of death to the possibility of life with (or without) a handicap. Since most of the one-hundred-plus procedures Dr. De Lia has performed since 1988 have been on infants who had not yet reached viability, he has sometimes conflicted with doctors and parents who would prefer to leave high-risk multiple pregnancies to nature and to fate.

Styles of neonatal care vary from place to place and doctor to doctor. Like most critical care subspecialists, however, neonatologists tend to prefer an aggressive approach. One medical ethicist has called this aggressive style of treating the very premature infant the "wait until certain" approach. Under it, every infant who is thought to have any chance of survival receives continuing treatment until it is *certain* that survival is not possible. Until it is certain that the infant's lungs are not mature enough to sustain life, or that the heart is not mature enough to provide sufficient blood pressure, or that the kidneys are not mature enough to function, the baby gets full support and treatment. This approach errs on the side of supporting life even when survival carries with it a fairly high probability that the survivor will have a handicap or eventually die. This approach is concordant with a society in which individualism is a strong value. In addition, we must acknowledge that the United States is a very litigious society. In view of these considerations, such an approach in neonatal care is understandable.

At the other end of the ethical spectrum are those whose approach to treatment aims to maximize the probability of a good outcome based strictly upon the reported survival statistics broken out by birth weight or gestational age. By reviewing the survival statistics, a decision is made about who should be resuscitated and who should receive only "comfort care"— that is, warmth and touch but no ventilator or other intensive care treatments. This "statistical approach" has a goal of avoiding severe handicaps, even at the cost of the deaths of some potentially normal infants.

The third approach to the immature infant is known as the "individualized strategy." Under this approach intensive care is begun for any infant who appears to have a chance of survival. With this approach it is urgent to determine as quickly as possible whether pursuing such care would be in the best interests of the child, even before all of the medical information is available. This differs from the "wait until certain" approach by attempting to make determinations as to viability by using less "certain" criteria. These criteria may be the physician's clinical assessment of the infant at delivery or the quality of the infant's response to treatment or resuscitation. Such an approach does raise some concerns. How certain must an outcome be before treatment is withdrawn? Would the variability between one physician's assessment and another's, or one neonatal unit's and another's, be within an ethically acceptable range?

As you might expect, these discussions about what style of care is appropriate in a given circumstance are difficult and heartwrenching for both the parents and physician.

Whenever possible, discussions about the treatment approach taken by the hospital should take place *before* having to confront this situation in an emergency situation. More often than not, when such a decision has to be made in an emergency situation, most neonatologists will support the baby until good information can be ascertained about the baby's viability.

We cannot emphasize enough that although there may be decisions that the physician and parents feel are correct and ethical, state and federal law may not see them as such. For example, the state of Texas requires that all live births (defined as a newborn infant born with a heart rate) receive appropriate support. Such a mandate cannot be ignored since the legal repercussions to physicians and parents are significant.

The Decision Maker's Burden

What would the patient want? Legally children are patients with their own rights, not merely the property of their parents. In the case of the newborn infant, however, it is impossible to know the patient's preferences for medical treatment. The standard guide for medical decision makers is the question "What is in the 'best interests' of the infant?" This boils down to "What steps best protect the infant's welfare?" The ethical question here is "Who is best suited to deciding what is in the infant's best interests?"

Parents don't have a blank check. While parents are always the primary decision makers for their children, they do not have the sole right to refuse treatment for their infant where the doctor believes there is hope. In a situation where a critically ill infant was in need of a lifesaving surgical procedure and the parents refused, a physician would be acting unethically

> JOE GARCIA-PRATS: "Several decades of practice have convinced me that parents almost always genuinely want what is best for their baby. In most cases where a disagreement arises with the treating physician, once all parties can sit down and explain their reasons for their decisions, a plan of action is almost always arrived at that considers the best interests of the infant and satisfies the concerns of parents and doctor alike."

if he or she did not try to convince the parents of the importance of the procedure and, if this did not change their mind, take steps to obtain temporary legal custody in order to provide the procedure for the infant. In this set of circumstances the parents would probably be seen as not seeking the best for their infant.

QUALITY OF LIFE CONSIDERATIONS

As we stated earlier in this chapter, one of the cornerstones of good ethical decision making is the importance of always asking the same questions in difficult situations. One of these questions is "Will treatment insure a high quality of life for the patient?" This question, while essential, is problematic because the definition of "quality of life" varies widely from person to person. For some, to live life visually or hearing impaired, or walking with a limp, would not be an acceptable quality of life. For others with a different point of view, it would be perfectly acceptable. "Quality of life" is not a bio-logical or medical phenomenon; it is a subjective condition. Quality of life considerations are further complicated with respect to newborns because infants are not able to express their view of what they consider an acceptable quality of life.

Because of these difficulties, we don't believe that "quality of life" considerations alone should be the decisive factor in a life-or-death decision. Every such case should be reviewed with great care and consideration. Also bear in mind, as we mentioned earlier, that quality of life justifications for the withdrawal of support may be outside the criteria established by federal and state legislation applicable to such situations.

WITHDRAWAL OF SUPPORT

One of the most difficult situations that parents and physicians can be forced to deal with involves withdrawing support from an infant. In most instances this issue is initiated by the medical team. In a minority of situations the parents put the issue on the table. Before a DNR order can be placed, the baby must meet the criteria defined in the "Baby Doe" regulations:

1. continued care will be medically futile; that is, it will only delay the patient's death;

2. the patient is in a persistent vegetative state; that is, the patient's vital functions are stable but there is no cognitive function detectable and the patient's condition will not change from this state;

3. the therapy that is offered to the patient will cause excessive pain and discomfort.

JOE GARCIA-PRATS: "I remember quite vividly a discussion I had on rounds in our newborn intensive care unit about the level of medical support that an infant with numerous malformations (none life-threatening) should receive. One of our young pediatric residents strongly believed that support should be limited, since the malformations, in his view, would reduce the infant's quality of life. Our postdoctoral fellow in neonatology turned to the resident and asked quietly, 'Who has a better quality of life? This infant with a loving family and many physical malformations, or the healthy infant in that crib over there whose father is a dope dealer and whose mother is a prostitute and who both have AIDS and who both are abusive to their children? If we're considering quality of life in making medical care decisions, then the presence of malformations should not be our only focus.' I agree. When withdrawal of therapy is at issue, I think that quality of life considerations deserve to be only very small modifiers in the decision-making process."

In most instances the physician will usually use the first two criteria as the basis for a DNR recommendation. Both criteria lend themselves to verification with objective medical information. They offer clear guidelines to a physician who is morally and legally compelled to oppose a family that asks for withdrawal of support when none of the three criteria are met, even if the parents believe that their baby is undergoing procedures without benefit or that their child will survive but not be "normal" in some respect. When these criteria are met, physician and family alike must realize the legal and ethical issues involved. As in any case where medical authority opposes their wishes, the family may want a second medical opinion or perhaps a transfer of the baby to another institution or to the care of another physician who is more in line with the family's wishes. Review by the hospital biomedical ethics committee may help bring clarity and conviction, if not ease and certainty, to such a decision. As with all bioethical issues, the answers will vary from case to case. Just remember to always ask the same questions.

Glossary

ABO incompatibility—A blood incompatibility that may occur when the mother's blood type is O and the baby's blood type is either A or B.

AGA (appropriate for gestational age)—Label given to a baby who weighs between the 90th and 100th percentile by weight for his gestational age.

Alpha Feto Protein (AFP)—A protein normally produced by a fetus, which can be measured prenatally to identify possible birth defects.

alveoli—Tiny sacs in the lungs where the exchange of oxygen and carbon dioxide take place.

amniocentesis—A procedure for removing a sample of amniotic fluid from the uterus by way of a needle inserted through the mother's abdominal wall in order to obtain information about the fetus.

amniotic fluid—The fluid surrounding the fetus in utero, which serves to protect the fetus during pregnancy.

anemia—An abnormally low number of red blood cells, which carry oxygen to the tissues.

anomaly—A malformation of a part of the body.

anoxia—Absence of adequate levels of oxygen.

antepartum—Before birth.

antibodies—Proteins produced by the body that fight infections caused by bacteria and viruses that have entered the body. Many helpful antibodies are found in a mother's breast milk, and can be passed onto a baby through nursing. Premature babies have very low antibody levels in their blood since the protective antibodies from mother are usually passed on to the baby in the last trimester of pregnancy.

Apgar score—A score first introduced by Dr. Virginia Apgar to assess the newborn's need for resuscitation. Apgar scores range from 0 to 10, evaluating newborn's heart rate, breathing effort, muscle tone, reflexes, and color.

apnea—Absence of breathing for longer than fifteen to twenty seconds that may be accompanied by a low heart rate and turning blue.

arterial blood gases (ABG)—A sample of blood obtained from an artery in order to analyze its oxygen, carbon dioxide, and acid content.

asphyxia—The interruption of blood gas exchange, causing low oxygen and high carbon dioxide and acidosis to accumulate in the body.

aspiration—Breathing a foreign substance such as meconium or formula into the lungs.

audiologist—A trained professional who tests for hearing loss, assists in determining the cause of such hearing loss, and plans a program to address hearing impairment in infants.

betamethasone—A steroid medication given to mothers when a premature delivery is anticipated. Helps mature the baby's lungs and reduce the incidence of numerous problematic conditions in the preterm infant.

bili-lights—Special lights used to treat neonatal jaundice.

bilirubin—A substance produced when red blood cells break down. When excessive amounts are present in the bloodstream, jaundice, a yellowing of the skin and whites of the eyes, can occur. When very high levels are present, brain damage can result. (See **kernicterus**.)

bonding—The process of attachment between infants and parents.

BPD—See **bronchopulmonary dysplasia.**

bradycardia—A slower than normal heart rate.

breech delivery—When a baby is born buttocks or feet first.

Brethine—See **terbutaline.**

bronchial tubes—The tubes that lead from the trachea (windpipe) to the lungs.

bronchioles—Small tubes that branch off from the bronchial tubes.

bronchiolitis—An inflammation or infection of the bronchioles.

bronchitis—An inflammation of the bronchial tubes.

bronchopulmonary dysplasia (**BPD**)—Damage to the lungs (airways, blood vessels) thought to be caused by severe immaturity and possibly by prolonged use of a respirator.

cardiopulmonary resuscitation (**CPR**)—A method of reviving a person whose heartbeat and breathing have stopped.

CBC—See **complete blood count.**

central line—An intravenous line that is threaded through the vein until it reaches a position close to the heart. Central lines are used to administer 1) solutions containing high concentrations of sugar or protein or 2) medications that must be given for a prolonged period.

cerebral palsy (**CP**)—Brain damage that can result in difficulty with coordinated movements. Intelligence may be normal in those with CP.

cerebrospinal fluid (**CSF**)—Fluid produced in the ventricles of the brain that circulates around the brain and spinal column.

cervix—The lower section of the uterus, which dilates (opens) and effaces (shortens) during labor and delivery to allow for the passage of the infant.

chest tube—A tube surgically inserted through the chest wall and into the chest cavity to remove air or fluid that has caused a lung to collapse and allows the lung to reexpand.

colostrum—Breast milk produced in late pregnancy or in the early days after delivery. This milk is usually yellowish in color and is especially rich in nutrients and antibodies.

complete blood count (**CBC**)—A blood test to determine the number and types of cells found in blood. This test checks for cells that may be associated with infection as well as determining the percent of red blood cells when considering anemia as well as other important diagnostic laboratory values.

conductive hearing loss—A temporary or permanent type of hearing loss caused by middle ear problems.

congestive heart failure (CHF)—Failure of the heart to perform efficiently because of a circulatory imbalance. This condition can occur in patent ductus arteriosus (PDA).

continuous positive airway pressure (CPAP)—Pressurized air, sometimes with additional oxygen, that is delivered to the baby's lungs to keep them from collapsing as the baby inhales and exhales.

corrected age—The age of a premature baby determined by adding his postnatal days to his gestational age at birth. A baby who is fourteen days old and was born at twenty-six weeks would have a corrected age of twenty-eight weeks.

CP—See **cerebral palsy.**

CPAP—See **continuous positive airway pressure.**

CPR—See **cardiopulmonary resuscitation.**

CSF—See **cerebrospinal fluid.**

cyanosis—A dusky blue discoloration of the skin caused by lack of oxygen.

cytomegalovirus (CMV)—A type of virus transmitted from the mother to the child in utero that may infect an unborn baby. In some cases CMV causes severe illness and birth defects.

DES—See **diethylstilbestrol.**

dexamethasone—A steroid medication that may be used to reduce swelling in the brain following a brain injury or may be given to a baby who has BPD to enable the physicians to wean the respirator.

dextrostix—A screening blood test used to measure levels of sugar in the bloodstream.

DIC—See **disseminated intravascular coagulation.**

diethylstilbestrol (DES)—A synthetic estrogen drug prescribed for pregnant women from the 1930s to the early 1970s to prevent miscarriage and premature labor. The drug was found to cause physical abnormalities in the genitalia of the daughters of women who took it. So-called DES daughters are also at increased risk of infertility, ectopic pregnancy, miscarriage, and preterm labor.

disseminated intravascular coagulation (DIC)—A problem in the ability of the blood to clot that may be caused by severe infection or prolonged low blood pressure.

diuretic—A medication that increases the excretion of body water through the urine.

Down's syndrome—A chromosomal abnormality, characterized by the presence of an extra chromosome 21, that can include certain physical manifestations as well as varying degrees of mental retardation.

DTaP—See **diphtheria, tetanus, pertussis.**

dyspnea—Shortness of breath.

electrocardiogram (EKG)—A tracing of the electrical pattern of the heart that may show problems of the size of the pumping chamber or receiving chambers of the heart, as well as any problems with the electrical conduction of the rate of the heart.

embryo—The term used to describe the early stages of fetal growth, approximately the fourth to ninth week of pregnancy.

endotracheal tube—A tube inserted into the trachea to allow the delivery of oxygen into the lungs.

fetus—The developing baby from approximately the ninth week of pregnancy until birth.

fraternal twins—Twins formed when two eggs are simultaneously released and fertilized.

full-term (FT)—An infant born between the thirty-eighth and forty-second weeks of gestation.

GA—See **gestational age.**

gavage feeding—Feedings given through a tube passed through the nose or mouth and into the stomach.

genetic abnormality—A disorder arising from an anomaly in the chromosomal structure that may or may not be hereditary.

genetic counseling—Advice and information provided by trained professional counselors on the detection and risk of occurrence of genetic disorders.

gestational age (GA)—The baby's age in weeks from the first day of the mother's last menstrual period before conception until the baby's birth.

hernia—A weakness in the abdominal wall that causes a portion of the intestines to protrude into the umbilical or inguinal area. This may also occur with a problem of the diaphragm that causes the bowel to enter the chest cavity, resulting in underdevelopment of the lung.

HMD—See **hyaline membrane disease.**

hyaline membrane disease (HMD)—Also known as respiratory distress syndrome (RDS), respiratory distress that affects premature babies. It is caused by a lack of surfactant, the substance that keeps the lung alveoli from collapsing.

hydrocephalus—An abnormal accumulation of cerebrospinal fluid in the ventricles of the brain.

hyperalimentation—See **total parenteral nutrition.**

hyperbilirubinemia—Excess bilirubin in the blood.

hypertension—Elevated blood pressure.

hypotension—Abnormally low blood pressure.

hypothermia—Abnormally low body temperature, a frequent problem with low-birth-weight premature babies.

indomethacin—A medication sometimes used in the treatment of patent ductus arteriosus.

intracranial hemorrhage (ICH)—Bleeding in or around the brain.

intrauterine growth retardation (IUGR)—Refers to a baby who is smaller by weight than normal for her gestational age at birth. This can be caused by various fetal or maternal complications.

intraventricular hemorrhage (IVH)—Bleeding within the ventricles of the brain.

intubation—The placement of a tube into the trachea to allow air to reach the lungs to assist with breathing.

in utero—Within the womb.

isolette—A type of incubator, an enclosed, heated bed.

IUGR—See **intrauterine growth retardation.**

jaundice—The yellowing of the skin and whites of the eyes caused by elevated bilirubin blood levels.

kernicterus—A rare condition caused by prolonged elevated levels of bilirubin in the blood of certain high-risk babies. Can lead to mental retardation, seizures.

lactation—Milk production by the breast.

lanugo—The fine downy hair that covers the body of a fetus.

lumbar puncture (LP)—The procedure of withdrawing a sample of cerebrospinal fluid (CSF) between the vertebrae of the lower back. The sample will be sent to the laboratory for analysis.

meningitis—Inflammation or infection of the meninges, the membranes surrounding the brain and spinal cord.

naso-gastric tube (NG tube)—A small plastic tube inserted through the nose or mouth and into the stomach. This tube is used for gavage feedings when an infant is unable to bottle- or direct breast-feed.

necrotizing enterocolitis (NEC)—A condition that can involve the intestinal tract of premature infants, where the bowel becomes inflamed and possibly necrotic. The cause of this condition is unknown.

neonate—A baby during the first month of life.

neonatologist—A pediatrician who specializes in the care of neonates.

neurologist—A physician who specializes in the conditions of the brain and nervous systems.

oligohydramnois—A condition of too little amniotic fluid.

ophthalmologist—A physician specializing in diseases of the eye.

orthopedist—A physician specializing in diseases of the bone.

otolaryngologist—A physician specializing in diseases of the ears, nose, and throat.

patent ductus arteriosus (PDA)—A blood vessel present in the fetus that allows blood coming from the placenta that is rich in oxy-gen to bypass the left side of the heart and lungs and flow through this blood vessel to the rest of the body. It usually closes in the first two weeks of life in term infants but may remain open in the preterm infant, requiring treatment to close it.

perinatal—The period from the twentieth week of gestation through the first twenty-eight days after delivery.

perinatologist—A physician who has completed training in obstetrics and takes further training in the care of high-risk pregnancies.

periodic breathing—A cyclic pattern of reduced frequency of breathing followed by a pause in the respiratory rate that can be followed by a normal to fast rate. This pattern is then repeated. This is a normal finding in a preterm infant but may lead to apnea.

periventricular leukomalacia—Small cysts found in the brain that, if they persist, may result in cerebral palsy. The cause is not known, but may be associated with maternal infection or periods of low blood flow to the brain.

petechiae—Small pencil-lead-size red dots noted on the infant's skin that are usually associated with trauma at delivery but may also indicate a bleeding problem.

phototherapy—Special green or blue lights that convert bilirubin into a water-soluble form that can be eliminated in the kidneys.

placenta abruption—A separation of the placenta from the wall of the uterus, causing pain and bleeding in the mother. If the separation is large, and the bleeding large, this may be life-threatening to the mother and infant.

placenta previa—Painless vaginal bleeding

caused by the location of the placenta over the os or opening of the uterus. If delivery of the infant occurs through the placenta, there may be significant bleeding to mother and baby. This may be life-threatening to mother and baby.

pneumonia—An infection of the baby's lungs.

polyhydramnios—An excessive amount of amniotic fluid, usually over 2.5 liters of fluid. May be associated with problems of the fetus swallowing the amniotic fluid.

positive end expiratory pressure (PEEP)—Usually administered through an endotracheal tube and connected to a respirator to provide the infant pressure to keep his airways open.

postpartum—After delivery.

preeclampsia—A medical term to define the maternal condition of elevated blood pressure, edema of the hands and feets, and the presence of protein in the urine during a woman's pregnancy. Also known as toxemia or pregnancy-induced hypertension.

pregnancy-induced hypertension (PIH)—See **preeclampsia.**

premature infant—An infant who is less than thirty-seven completed weeks' gestational age at birth.

pulse oximeter—A monitoring device used as a general indicator of a baby's oxygenation. This noninvasive device is taped to the skin, usually a finger or foot, for oxygen level readings.

radiant warmer—An open-air bed with a heat source above it. This type of bed is used in the NICU immediately after delivery to allow easy access to the baby and also to help maintain a baby's body temperature.

red blood cells (RBC)—RBCs are a part of the body's blood that contains hemoglobin and carries oxygen to all the cells and tissues of the body.

respirator—See **ventilation.**

respiratory distress syndrome (RDS)—A condition that affects the lungs of preterm infants. This is caused by lack of surfactant. Also referred to as hyaline membrane disease.

retinopathy of prematurity (ROP)—A disease affecting the retina of a preterm baby's eye. ROP can lead to serious eye complications and even blindness.

sepsis—An infection in the blood.

small for gestational age (SGA)—A term used for a baby born below the tenth percentile for height and weight per standard gestational age guidelines.

special care nursery—See **step-down unit.**

spinal tap—See **lumbar puncture.**

step-down unit—A nursery for babies that provides less intensive care than that given in an NICU; may also be called an intermediate care nursery, a level II unit, or a special care nursery unit.

surfactant—A substance produced by the lung that serves as a coating in the air sacs and keeps the tiny air sacs open between breaths. Surfactant is often lacking in preterm babies, and this can lead to respiratory distress syndrome or lung immaturity in the premature baby. Today there are man-made surfactants on the market that can dramatically improve a preemie's respiratory status.

terbutaline (Brethine)—A tocolytic medication used to stop preterm labor.

term infant—An infant born between approximately thirty-eight and forty-two weeks of gestation.

tocolytic drugs—Medications that are given to suppress labor, indicated for use when a woman is in preterm labor.

TORCH—A group of maternal infections that can cause serious effects on the fetus: toxoplasmosis, other viruses, rubella, cytomegalovirus, and herpes simplex virus.

total parenteral nutrition (TPN; hyperalimentation)—A type of nutrition that is administered through intravenous infusion. TPN provides all of the essential nutrients needed.

tube feeding—See **gavage feeding.**

twin-to-twin transfusion syndrome (TTTS)—A condition of the placenta that can occur in identical twin pregnancies. TTTS results in blood passing disproportionately from one twin baby to the other through connecting blood vessels within the shared placenta.

ultrasound (sonogram)—A diagnostic imaging technique where high-frequency sound waves are used to evaluate fetal well-being.

umbilical cord—The connection between the baby and the placenta.

ventilation—Mechanical breathing assistance.

very low birth weight (VLBW)—An infant, of any gestational age, who weighs less than 1,500 grams at birth.

vital signs—Term that refers to temperature, pulse, respiration, and blood pressure.

warmer—See **radiant warmer.**

wean—To slowly decrease and then stop an intervention. This could be used when stopping a medication or when removing certain technological support such as a ventilator.

white blood cells (WBCs)—WBCs are a part of the body's blood responsible for fighting against infection.

X-ray—A diagnostic technique where an electromagnetic wave produces an image of internal body parts.

APPENDIX A

Developmental Milestones

If you're a parent of a preemie, you may feel like a world record holder who has an asterisk next to her name in the record books. Whenever you proudly watch your child reach an age milestone—six months, a year, or what have you—you will have to remind yourself to subtract the length of his prematurity from his age in order to determine his "real," or gestational, age. A simple question from an admiring stranger at the grocery store can thus become an occasion for more conversation than you may be in the mood for:

Stranger: "Oh, what a cute little boy. How old is he?"

You: "Well, he's six months old, but actually he was two months premature, so his real age is four months, I guess. . . ."

It's a pleasant enough exchange. But after going through it a few dozen times, you may find yourself, for simplicity's sake, automatically adjusting your baby's age for his prematurity—and disappointing yourself that you're not giving his "real" age.

When your baby visits the pediatrician and has his height and weight pegged on the percentile charts, you may have similar feelings. The growth charts published by the American Academy of Pediatrics are geared to full-term infants. Therefore your child will in all likelihood significantly lag behind the mean, or average, for his age range. Since charts calibrated to a baby's prematurity are not generally available, you may find yourself unsure of how your baby's growth is tracking with that of his peers—at least for the first year or two, before he finishes playing the game of catch-up.

"It helped us greatly when we adjusted our point of view with respect to the percentile charts," said a mother of an eight-week-premature baby boy. "When the pediatrician told us that he was at the thirtieth percentile for height, we focused on the positive, not the negative. Instead of worrying that he was smaller than 70 percent of all babies his age, we turned the equation the other way around: we focused on the fact that *he* was bigger than three in ten babies his age, even though they were born at *full term.* When you look at your baby's growth that way, it puts you in a much better frame of mind."

In using the chart below, which was developed for full-term infants, be sure to make the adjustment for your baby's prematurity. For example, if you have a thirty-two-week preemie (two months premature) who is six months old, you would use the chart for four-month-old babies.

Full-Term Infant Growth and Development Chart

2 Months

Nutrition

Formula or breast milk is still all your infant needs.

Feeding intervals vary from 3 to 4 hours during day and, hopefully, longer at night.

Try to resist adding solid foods until approximately 4 months of age.

Sleep

Some infants will sleep through the night, but most will awaken every 3–4 hours.

Limit daytime sleeping periods to less than 3–4 hours.

Bowel Habits

Usually becomes less frequent, 1–2 times a day or sometimes once every 3 days. Grunting and groaning are normal.

Development (High Variable)

Usually can hold head upright, but still unsteady.

May grasp rattle placed in hand and may hold briefly.

Begins to respond to human face, especially parents. Social smiles.

Coos and squeals.

Startles to loud noises.

Increasing drooling.

Stimulation/Parenting

Hold, cuddle, rock, sing to the infant.

Play copycat with infant by repeating infant's sounds and actions.

Offer different objects for infant to touch and hold.

Go for walks or just sit outside.

Social

Both parents should spend time with infant and together without infant.

Share responsibilities at home. Bath time can be fun.

Spend time playing with, or reading to, other children in the family.

Begin to find baby-sitters you can be comfortable with.

Immunizations

Arrange for DTaP (diphtheria, tetanus, pertussis), HIB, and oral polio, hepatitis B vaccines. (These immunization schedules change as new information and new vaccines are developed. Check with your pediatrician for updated information.)

For fever and fussiness, use Tylenol every 4–6 hours for 3 doses as necessary.

4 Months

Nutrition

Breast or bottle feedings average every 4–5 hours during day and about 32 ounces per day.

May start solid foods. Use spoon and cup. Avoid putting solids in bottles.

Try not to use the bottle as a pacifier, and do not prop bottle in bed.

Sleep

Most infants can sleep through the night now.

Put infant to bed while awake so he can learn to fall asleep by himself instead of having to be rocked to sleep each night.

May discontinue nighttime feedings.

Allow infant to fuss for widening intervals

(5, 10, 15 minutes) as necessary to allow him to fall back asleep.

Development (Highly Variable)

May hold head high and raise body on hands while on belly.

Fairly good head control.

May roll from front to back.

May smile, coo, laugh, squeal.

Follows fairly well with eyes and orients to sounds.

Begins thumb sucking.

Stimulation/Parenting

Allow and encourage infant to play alone in playpen.

Talk to infant and respond to crying.

Begin reciting nursery rhymes and playing peek-a-boo and other games.

Allow infant to handle and play with objects.

Allow infant to bear some weight and push off.

Show pictures and place infant in front of mirror.

Immunizations

DTaP, HIB, oral polio, hepatitis B (The immunization schedules change as new information and new vaccines are developed. Check with your pediatrician for updated information.)

For fever and fussiness, use Tylenol; 2–3 doses and then as necessary for 1–2 days.

6 Months

Nutrition

Continue breast or bottle feeds, but no more than approximately 1 quart per day.

Avoid use of milk or juice as a pacifier, and avoid putting bottle in bed with infant.

Begin serving water, juice, or milk from a cup.

May start eating finger foods.

Sleep

Use favorite toy, blanket, or dolls when infant resists sleep.

Expect some nighttime awakenings. Reassure infant, but try to keep her in crib. Avoid restarting nighttime feedings.

Development (Highly Variable)

Rolls over.

Improving head control.

Bears some weight.

Reaches for and grabs objects.

May begin stranger anxiety.

Responds to sounds and follows with eyes.

Begins to laugh and squeal.

Unhappy when toys are lost.

Stimulation/Parenting

Allow to finger-feed and to manipulate objects.

Play pat-a-cake and imitative games.

Allow to play with measuring cups, pans, lids, toys.

Explain to infant what you are doing while eating, working, and so on.

Make up games, make facial expressions at infant.

Immunizations

DTaP, HIB, oral polio, hepatitis B (The immunization schedules change as new information and new vaccines are developed. Check with your pediatrician for updated information.)

For fever and fussiness, use Tylenol; 2–3 doses and then as necessary.

Nutrition

Begin soft table foods at the dinner table.

Allow self-feeding, drinking from cup.

Begin to wean from bottle if infant wants to.

May begin to show some drop in appetite.

Feedings average 4 times per day.

Sleep

Set a bedtime routine.

Try to take nighttime awakenings in stride. Use favorite toy or possessions to reassure infant. Allow some fussing before responding.

Development (Highly Variable)

Sits without help.

Crawls, creeps, hitches—or may begin to walk.

Finger-feeds partially.

Imitates vocalizations.

Understands a few words.

Plays social games.

May show stranger anxiety.

Separation anxiety is common; play "leaving and coming back" games to reassure.

Stimulation/Parenting

Encourage vocalization and communication.

Initiate sounds and actions.

Allow some exploration and independence.

Begin to set some limits; say "no" and distract by removing infant from the situation.

Use discipline as a rule teacher and for limit setting rather than as punishment.

Play hide-and-seek, sing to your infant; ignore messes, pay attention to good behavior.

Nutrition

Increase use of table foods.

Whole or 2 percent milk is fine.

Continue to wean from the bottle.

May begin to get picky with meals; decreasing appetite.

Avoid snack foods and desserts.

Development (Highly Variable)

Pulls to a stand. May walk without support.

Begins good pincer grasp.

Points. May place objects inside each other.

May say a few specific words.

Plays games.

Knows to look for hidden or dropped objects.

Stimulation/Parenting

Encourage speech development by naming objects, body parts. Talk while feeding or bathing your infant.

Use picture books with 1 picture/1 word per page.

Encourage self-stimulation and playing alone as well as playing with others.

Dance and laugh with your infant.

Stay calm and unattentive when infant has a tantrum, and pay attention to good behaviors.

Make a house or car out of an old box.

Set some limits on undesired behavior.

Immunizations

Tuberculin skin test. (The immunization schedules change as new information and new vaccines are developed. Check with your pediatrician for updated information.)

15 Months

Nutrition
Phase out use of the bottle.

Make mealtime a family time.

Allow children to feed themselves with a spoon or fingers. Don't worry about tidiness or manners.

Give 3 meals a day and nutritious snacks (vegetables and fruit instead of chips and candy).

Avoid juice or sugary substances in bottles, and do not use bottles in bed.

Picky eating habits are common at this age.

Sleep
Adopt a bedtime routine.

Naps usually once or twice a day.

Development (Highly Variable)
Walks alone, stoops, explores.

Self-feeds, drinks from a cup.

Three- to 6-word vocabulary, lots of babbling and scribbling.

Understands simple commands, points to a few body parts.

Will listen to part of a story being read.

Begins to communicate his desires in various ways.

Hugs and smiles.

Pacifier and finger sucking are normal activities.

Stimulation/Parenting
Use toys for stimulation: stuffed animals, books, cars, blocks, balls, household items such as pots and pans, cups and spoons, empty boxes.

Encourage activities that infant can imitate such as cleaning house, chasing each other, making facial expressions, playing ball, and so on.

Use favorite objects (blanket or toys) as transitional objects for sleeping or when frightened.

Stimulate speech by reading to, naming common objects and explaining what you are doing throughout the day.

Limit TV time.

Discipline
Pay attention to and praise good behavior and ignore acting-out behavior.

Remove from temptation.

Allow some autonomy and self-exploration.

Discipline means teaching. Begin to set limits.

Be consistent.

Immunizations
MMR (measles, mumps, rubella) and HIB (may develop a fine rash and fever 7–10 days after the vaccine). (The immunization schedules change as new information and new vaccines are developed. Check with your pediatrician for updated information.)

Use Tylenol for discomfort or fever.

18 Months

Nutrition
Use mealtime as family time.

Eating habits may be variable and inconsistent. Avoid battles.

Avoid frequent snacks in place of meals.

Wean from bottle if this isn't already accomplished.

Sleep
Use bedtime ritual.

Fear of the dark is common. Use transitional objects, reassurance, and night-lights.

Try not to regress to nighttime feedings or

parental bed sleeping for middle of the
night awakenings.

Development (Highly Variable)

Walks, runs, climbs stairs with one hand held,
sits in chair.

Stacks 3–4 cubes.

Kicks and throws ball.

Vocabulary of 4–10 words; may begin to use 2-
word phrases.

Feeds self; holds and uses cup.

Imitates crayon strokes.

Kisses parents.

Stimulation/Parenting

Read simple stories.

Do not expect toy sharing yet.

Encourage play with building blocks.

Begin to use "pretend play," and encourage
both quiet and active play.

Begin to suggest "picking up" and "orderly" activities.

Praise good behaviors.

Discipline

Allow some independence and decision making.

Consistency among caregivers.

Set limits and use removal to different loca-
tions, or short "time-out" intervals, for mis-
behavior.

Praise good behaviors.

Self-Comforting Behaviors

Thumb sucking, feeling different parts of the
body, and favorite toys are all normal development activities at this stage.

Toilet Training

May begin to show signs of readiness.

Encourage, but do not force.

Average age of readiness is about 2½ years.

Immunizations

DTaP vaccine. (The immunization schedules
change as new information and new vaccines are developed. Check with your pediatrician for updated information.)

24 Months

Nutrition

Make mealtimes happy times.

Avoid struggles and mealtime battles; save leftovers for later without making a big issue
out of it.

Use few, nutritious snacks. Use small quantities for meals if child is a picky eater.

Sleep

Variable naps (0–2 per day). Encourage staying
in room for nap time to allow some time for
parents to finish chores and stimulate self-
play.

May want to move to regular bed, especially if
infant is able to get out of the crib.

Use bedtime routine.

Development (Highly Variable)

May climb and go down steps alone.

Uses spoon/cup; kicks and throws overhead;
may open doors.

Stacks 5 or 6 cubes and aligns objects.

Vocabulary of about 20 words, although may
be quite variable. May use 2-word phrases.

Responds to commands; imitates actions and
speech.

May use a toy appropriately.

May have mild stuttering or mispronuncia-
tions.

Interest in self-dressing.

Body curiosity is common.

Temper tantrums are very common.

Stimulation/Parenting

Use assembly toys and musical toys.

Read together as much as possible.

Encourage talking.

Encourage play with other children of same age; do not expect true sharing yet.

Recite nursery rhymes and leave key words for child to say.

Watch children's shows together, but avoid too much TV.

Begin to encourage helping with household chores.

Begin to brush teeth with small dab of toothpaste.

Praise good behaviors and minimize attention to bad.

Toilet Training

Look for signs of readiness.

Praise and reward accomplishment and minimize attention to mishaps.

APPENDIX B

Conversion Charts

CONVERSION OF POUNDS AND OUNCES TO GRAMS

Pounds \ Ounces	0	1	2	3	4	5	6	7	8	9	10	11	12	13	14	15
0	—	28	57	85	113	142	170	198	227	255	283	312	340	369	397	425
1	454	482	510	539	567	595	624	652	680	709	737	765	794	822	850	879
2	907	936	964	992	1,021	1,049	1,077	1,106	1,134	1,162	1,191	1,219	1,247	1,276	1,304	1,332
3	1,361	1,389	1,417	1,446	1,474	1,502	1,531	1,559	1,588	1,616	1,644	1,673	1,701	1,729	1,758	1,786
4	1,814	1,843	1,871	1,899	1,928	1,956	1,984	2,013	2,041	2,070	2,098	2,126	2,155	2,183	2,211	2,240
5	2,268	2,296	2,325	2,353	2,381	2,410	2,438	2,466	2,495	2,523	2,551	2,580	2,608	2,637	2,665	2,693
6	2,722	2,750	2,778	2,807	2,835	2,863	2,892	2,920	2,948	2,977	3,005	3,033	3,062	3,090	3,118	3,147
7	3,175	3,203	3,232	3,260	3,289	3,317	3,345	3,374	3,402	3,430	3,459	3,487	3,515	3,544	3,572	3,600
8	3,629	3,657	3,685	3,714	3,742	3,770	3,799	3,827	3,856	3,884	3,912	3,941	3,969	3,997	4,026	4,054
9	4,082	4,111	4,139	4,167	4,196	4,224	4,252	4,281	4,309	4,337	4,366	4,394	4,423	4,451	4,479	4,508
10	4,536	4,564	4,593	4,621	4,649	4,678	4,706	4,734	4,763	4,791	4,819	4,848	4,876	4,904	4,933	4,961
11	4,990	5,018	5,046	5,075	5,103	5,131	5,160	5,188	5,216	5,245	5,273	5,301	5,330	5,358	5,386	5,415
12	5,443	5,471	5,500	5,528	5,557	5,585	5,613	5,642	5,670	5,698	5,727	5,755	5,783	5,812	5,840	5,868

To Convert Pounds and Ounces to Grams:
Find the baby's weight in pounds down the left side of the table. Find the ounces across the top of the table. The intersection of the two measurements equals the equivalent weight in grams. For example, 3 pounds, 8 ounces equals 1,588 grams.

To Convert Grams to Pounds and Ounces:
Find the number that's closest to your baby's weight in grams on the chart. Look to the far left line for the pound measurement and to the top of the gram column for the ounces.

Conversion of Centimeters to Inches

Centimeters	Inches	Centimeters	Inches
25.4	10	52.1	20½
26.7	10½	53.3	21
27.9	11	54.6	21½
29.2	11½	55.9	22
30.5	12	57.2	22½
31.8	12½	58.4	23
33.0	13	59.7	23½
34.3	13½	61.0	24
35.6	14	62.2	24½
36.8	14½	63.5	25
38.1	15	64.8	25½
39.4	15½	66.1	26
40.6	16	67.4	26½
41.9	16½	68.7	27
43.2	17	69.9	27½
44.4	17½	71.2	28
45.7	18	72.5	28½
47.0	18½	73.8	29
48.3	19	75.1	29½
49.5	19½	76.4	30
50.8	20	77.6	30½

Conversion of Temperature (Fahrenheit and Centigrade)

To convert degrees Fahrenheit to degrees centigrade, subtract 32, multiply by 5, and divide by 9. To convert degrees centigrade to degrees Fahrenheit, multiply by 9, divide by 5, and add 32.

Fahrenheit	Centigrade
96.1	35.6
96.4	35.8
96.8	36.0
97.7	36.5
98.6	37.0
99.5	37.5
100.4	38.0
101.3	38.5
102.2	39.0
103.1	39.5
104.0	40.0
104.9	40.5
105.8	41.0
106.7	41.5
107.6	42.0

APPENDIX C

Helpful Resources on Prematurity and High-Risk Pregnancy

It is staggering how much information is available today on pregnancy in general and prematurity and high-risk pregnancy in particular. Surfing the Internet for just a few minutes is proof enough of that. The Internet puts a world of information at your fingertips, from the official Web site of the American Academy of Pediatrics to the personal Web pages of mothers who have been through what you're experiencing—and have the digitized photos to prove it. A question that once may have required several trips to the library to answer can now be answered with a few well-chosen clicks of a mouse button from the comfort of your own home (or hospital bed, if you have a laptop). If you are interested in doing further research on your pregnancy but aren't yet a driver on the information superhighway, we encourage you to become one as soon as possible. If you don't have Internet access, most public libraries offer computers which can be used to access the Internet.

The caveat, of course, is that on the vast Internet there is a high degree of variance in quality of information. Some Web sites are maintained by professional associations or government agencies. These are generally reliable, authoritative, and often peer-reviewed. Other sites offer information that is anecdotal, personal, experimental, or just flat wrong. On the Internet, the operative phrase is, let the buyer beware.

Here we give you some starting points for further investigation of prematurity and high-risk pregnancy in general, and your condition in particular. Most of the resources below are available on-line. Since new pages are always being added and removed from the Internet, it is hard to keep all of this information up-to-date. Invariably, one or more of these Internet addresses will have moved or changed or ceased to be by the time this book reaches you. Of course, your Internet searching will likely take on a life of its own, and so you will find useful resources that aren't listed here. (If you find helpful resources that aren't mentioned here, we would be grateful if you would write to us, care of Crown Books, 299 Park Ave., New York, NY 10171, so that we can consider adding your suggestion to future editions of this book.)

U.S. GOVERNMENT RESOURCES

Centers for Disease Control and Prevention
The CDC maintains a valuable on-line resource called the National Clearinghouse for Health Statistics, which warehouses all types of data on health issues and concerns.

600 Clifton Rd.
Atlanta, GA 30333
(800) 311-3435, (404) 639-3534
www.cdc.gov/nchs

National Institutes of Health

The NIH's Health Information page is an on-line gateway to a wide range of authoritative medical information. The site provides an index to information on diseases currently under investigation by NIH, major NIH research areas, and other important health-related topics.

National Institutes of Health
Bethesda, MD 20892
www.nih.gov/health

National Library of Medicine

The NLM operates a medical search service called PubMed, a search service that provides access to over 10 million citations in MEDLINE, PreMEDLINE, and other related databases, with links to participating online journals.

www.ncbi.nlm.nih.gov/PubMed

ASSOCIATIONS AND ORGANIZATIONS

American Academy of Pediatrics

From the AAP's Web site, you can search back issues of the academy's excellent journal, *Pediatrics* (dating back to 1948), for information on a wide variety of pediatrics- and childbirth-related topics. The current electronic edition of the journal is free to access. The full print version is also available electronically, but requires either a subscription payment, or a per-article payment.

www.pediatrics.org
www.aap.org

American College of Obstetricians and Gynecologists

A valuable resource for pregnancy information, news releases, legislative bulletins, and physician referrals.

409 12th Street SW, Washington, D.C. 20006,
(202) 863-2518
www.acog.org

March of Dimes National Resource Center

From the March of Dimes home page, you can access their Resource Center, which maintains a staff of trained professionals who can provide prompt personal responses to questions about pregnancy and infant health problems and other relevant subjects.

1275 Mamaroneck Ave.
White Plains, NY 01605
(888) 663-4637, (914) 482-7100
www.modimes.org
e-mail: resourcecenter@modimes.org

OTHER INTERNET RESOURCES

WebMD

An on-line medical news organization that features health news, medical reference databases, "ask the experts" features, message boards, chat rooms, and information sorted by medical topic, including pregnancy. The impressive content here is prepared by WebMD's full-time staff, or culled from AP and Reuters.

www.webmd.com

Medscape

Designed for doctors but useful for the layperson as well, this is one of the Web's largest collections of free, full-text clinical medicine articles enhanced with keyword searches, graphics, and annotated links to Internet resources. Medscape's searchable databases include MEDLINE, Medscape's full-text articles, news sorted by medical specialty, patient information, medical images, and more.

www.medscape.com

Childbirth.org

A collection of links to a variety of pregnancy-related articles written by nurses, doulas, childbirth educators, and others who advocate natural childbirth methods. Motto: "Birth is a natural process, not a medical procedure."

www.childbirth.org

Pregnancy Today

Information about pregnancy, parenting, babies, and more, including a bed rest bulletin board.

www.pregnancytoday.com

ParentsPlace.com

Information and support for pregnant women and parents. E-mail and other interactive services provided, including a pregnancy bed rest support group.

www.parentsplace.com

Baby.com

Links to many other interesting sites about babies, including baby names, reviews of baby books, and e-mail service.

www.baby.com

PREEMIE-SPECIFIC SITES

Preemie-L Mailing List and Homepage

Preemie-L is a listserv, an automated mailing list that delivers to you daily discussion on all types of prematurity-related topics. It is a well-established community on the Internet, and should be of interest to anyone with a premature infant or high-risk condition of pregnancy. The Preemie-L Web site provides:

- Archives of past listserv messages
- A discussion forum
- A monthly electronic newsletter called *Early Edition,* and
- Links to other preemie resources and Web pages.

www.preemie-l.org
The *Early Edition* newsletter
www.vicnet.net.au/~earlyed/welcome.htm

University of Wisconsin's "For Parents of Preemies" Website

This very useful preemie site is maintained by the University of Wisconsin's Meriter Hospital.

www.medsch.wisc.edu/childrenshosp/
parents_of_preemies/index.html

It is even available in Spanish:

www.medsch.wisc.edu/childrenshosp/
Preemie_Parent_Sp/spindex.html

ComeUnity's Premature Baby Site

An excellent compendium of information on preemies, with links to other helpful sites for parents of preemies.

www.comeunity.com/premature/index.html
www.comeunity.com/premature/preemie-child/index.html

American Association of Premature Infants

A.A.P.I. is a nonprofit advocacy organization dedicated to improving the quality of health, developmental, and educational services for premature infants, children, and their families.

P.O. Box 6920
Cincinnati, OH 45206
(513) 956-4331
www.aapi-online.org

BREAST-FEEDING

La Leche League International

An international, nonprofit, nonsectarian organization dedicated to providing education, information, support, and encouragement to women who want to breast-feed.

(847) 519-7730
www.lalecheleague.org

Bed Rest Support Groups, Pregnancy Chat Rooms, and Other Direct Support

Sidelines National Support Network

A national volunteer network for women on bed rest and with high-risk pregnancies. The organization provides support via telephone and e-mail. The Sidelines Web site contains news reports on prematurity and high-risk pregnancy, chat rooms, and useful information on other resources for mothers with high-risk pregnancies.

www.sidelines.com

Schedule of weekly chat sessions on high-risk pregnancy:

www.sidelines.org/chat3.htm

National Office:
P.O. Box 1808
Laguna Beach, CA 92652
(949) 497-2265

ParentsPlace

A general pregnancy and parenting Web site that also includes a bulletin board for women on bed rest.

www.parentsplace.com

BabyCenter

This site offers guidance for new and expectant parents, and also maintains a bulletin board for women on bed rest.

www.babycenter.com

Go directly to the bed rest bulletin board at

www.babycenter.com/bbs/3369/

ParentSoup

This highly interactive general pregnancy site offers information and support to parents at every stage of parenthood. Dozens of bulletin boards (including a great one exclusively for bed rest), games, ask the experts, and more.

www.parentsoup.com

Go directly to the bed rest bulletin board:
http://boards.parentsoup.com/messages/get/psbedrest17.html

Twins/Multiples Resources

Mothers of Supertwins

A nonprofit organization devoted to education, information and resources for families expecting triplets or more. Free quarterly magazine, parent pack, networking resources.

P.O. Box 951
Brentwood, NY 11717
(631) 859-1110
E-mail: maureen@mostonline.org
www.mostonline.org

Twins Magazine

A bimonthly publication for families of multiples. Features, reference information, and resources. You can subscribe on-line, or call.

(800) 328-3211
www.twinsmagazine.com

Triplet Connection

A nonprofit, tax-exempt organization that provides information, encouragement, and resources to families who are expecting triplets, quadruplets, quintuplets, or more. The Triplet Connection offers an expectant parent's packet containing information on preterm birth prevention and multiple-birth pregnancy and a quarterly newsletter where the organization's 9,000-plus members and health professionals share the joys and challenges of having and raising multiples.

P.O. Box 99571
Stockton, CA 95209

e-mail: tc@tripletconnection.org
(209) 474-0885
Fax: (209) 474-2233
www.tripletconnection.org

Twin-to-Twin Transfusion Syndrome Foundation

An international nonprofit organization dedicated to providing educational, emotional, and financial support to families, medical professionals, and other caregivers before, during, and after a pregnancy diagnosed with twin-to-twin transfusion syndrome.

www.tttsfoundation.org
(440) 899-TTTS (899-8887)

Grief and Loss Support

Pen Parents, Inc.

An international referral and support network for grieving parents.

P.O. Box 8738
Reno, NV 89507-8738
(702) 826-7332
www.penparents.org
e-mail: penparents@penparents.org

Share

An organization providing support, information, and resources for parents experiencing pregnancy and infant loss.

National SHARE Office
St. Joseph Health Center
300 First Capitol Drive
St. Charles, MO 63301-2893
(800) 821-6819, (636) 947-6164
www.nationalshareoffice.com
e-mail: share@nationalshareoffice.com

A Place to Remember

"Uplifting support materials and resources for those who have been touched by a crisis in pregnancy or the death of a baby."

1885 University Avenue, Suite 110
St. Paul, MN 55104
(800) 631-0973, (612) 645-7045
www.aplacetoremember.com

Other Sources for Help

American Diabetes Association

A nonprofit health organization founded in 1940 to prevent and cure diabetes, and to improve the lives of all people affected by diabetes. Funds research, publishes scientific findings, and provides information and other services to people with diabetes, their families, health care professionals, and the public.

1701 North Beauregard Street
Alexandria, VA 22311
(800) DIABETES (342-2383)
www.diabetes.org

DES Action

A national nonprofit consumer organization dedicated to informing the public about DES (diethylstilbestrol) and helping DES-exposed individuals. The organization produces a quarterly newsletter, *The DES Action Voice,* and other information on DES exposure. The organization also maintains a national physician referral list, which is available free of charge.

615 Broadway, Suite 510
Oakland, CA 94612
(800) DES-9288 (337-9288), (510) 465-4011
e-mail: desact@well.com
www.desaction.org

Group B Strep Association

Information, resources, and support for parents of children with GBS infection. Advocates prevention of neonatal GBS through routine prenatal screening.

P.O. Box 16515
Chapel Hill, NC 27516
(919) 932-5344
www.groupbstrep.org

PREGNANCY-RELATED SHOPPING WEB SITES

The Preemie Store and More

Mail order catalog with an assortment of preemie clothing for hospital or home, as well as birth announcements, pacifiers, diaries, and preemie books.

(800) O-SO-TINY (676-8469)
www.preemie.com

Maternity Mall

Online shopping for maternity and nursing wear, baby clothes, baby toys, and more.

www.maternitymall.com

Baby Gap

Baby clothes and gifts for your baby.

www.babygap.com

Motherwear

"The complete catalog for the nursing mother."

www.motherwear.com
(800) 633-0303 for a free catalog.

Tiny Bundles

Handmade preemie clothing, diapers, and specifically designed pacifiers for the premature or low-birth-weight baby. Free brochure.

11468 Ballybunion Square
San Diego, CA 92128
(619) 451-9907
www.tinybundles.com

OTHER BOOKS ON HIGH-RISK PREGNANCY AND PREMATURITY

Chism, Denise M. *The High-Risk Pregnancy Source Book*. Lowell House, 1997.

Davis, Deborah L. *Empty Cradle, Broken Heart*. Fulcrum, 1996.

Gilbert, Elizabeth Stepp, and Judith Smith Harmon. *Manual of High-Risk Pregnancy and Delivery*. 2nd ed. Mosby, 1998.

Hales, Dianne, and Timothy Johnson. *Intensive Caring: New Hope for High-Risk Pregnancy*. Crown, 1990.

Kohner, Nancy, and Alix Henley. *When a Baby Dies*. Thorsons, 1997.

Ludington-Hoe, Susan, and Susan K. Golant. *Kangaroo Care: The Best You Can Do to Help Your Preterm Infant*. Bantam, 1993.

MacArthur, Barton, and Anne Dezoete. *Early Beginnings: Development in Children Born Preterm*. Oxford, 1992.

Manginello, Frank P., and Theresa Foy DiGeronimo. *Your Premature Baby*. Wiley, 1991.

Merenstein, Gerald B. *Handbook of Neonatal Intensive Care*. Mosby, 1993.

Novotny, Pamela Patrick. *The Joy of Twins and Other Multiple Births*. Crown, 1994.

Rich, Laurie E. *When Pregnancy Isn't Perfect*. Larata Press, 1996.

Van der Meet, Jason, Janine and Antonia. *Parenting Your Premature Baby*. Henry Holt, 1989.

Zaichkin, Jeanette. *Newborn Intensive Care: What Every Parent Needs to Know*. NICU Ink, 1996.

Index

NICUs and, 175, 196, 178, 215–16, 219, 222

pregnancy-induced conditions and, 24, 32–33, 36

tips on management of, 18

tocolytics and, 72

ultrasounds and, 61–62, 178

heart monitors, 132–33, 141, 179, 238, 240

heart rates:

anesthesia and, 113

and bringing preemies home, 243

in determining EDC, 61

discharge and, 231

and first twenty-four hours after delivery, 117–20, 133–34

gestational age and, 157–58, 162, 164, 167, 169

high-risk pregnancies and, 56, 95

intermediate care nurseries and, 234

monitoring of, 66–68, 70, 110–11

NICUs and, 186, 196, 212, 216–17, 219, 222

pregnancy-induced conditions and, 44

self-care and, 262

tocolytics and, 72–73

HELLP syndrome, 27, 89, 105, 142

hemoglobin levels, 222–23

hemolyic anemia, 27, 142

Henley, Alix, 292

heparin, heparin locks, 20, 132, 135, 141

herbs, herbal drinks, 49, 264

herpes, 6, 53–54

high blood pressure (hypertension), 69, 83, 199, 224

definition of, 11

and first twenty-four hours after delivery, 140–43, 147

high-risk pregnancies and, 5–7, 10–16, 48, 94, 97

kidney problems and, 12–13, 17–18

and listening to your body, 15–16

medical attention for, 12–16

pregnancy-induced, *see* pregnancy-induced hypertension

rest and relaxation for, 12–14

self-care and, 262

tips for management of, 13–16

tocolytics and, 72

treatment of, 12–15, 81

and when to go to hospital, 104

high-risk pregnancies, 3–100

accidents and, 49–50

autoimmune disorders and, 19–24

bed rest and, 56, 59, 77–96

causes of, 3–56

choosing medical facilities for, 98–100

confronting and coping with shock of, 3–10

and determining length of pregnancies, 60–63

diabetes and, 16–17, 48, 55, 59

fact vs. fiction on, 11

guilt and, 5, 7–10, 14

HELLP syndrome and, 27

high blood pressure and, 5–7, 10–16, 48, 94, 97

at home, 77–78

infections and, 50–55, 59, 94

management of, 57–100

as numbers game, 59–60

planning and, 102–3

preexisting conditions leading to, 10–18

pregnancy-induced conditions leading to, 5–6, 9, 11–13, 15–16, 23–47, 58–59, 97–98

premature labor and, 6, 8–9, 49–50, 55, 57, 67–79, 81, 83, 89–90, 94–95, 97

prenatal care and, 3–6, 48–49, 56, 95

resources on, 335–40

special procedures in, 93–97

TORCH diseases and, 53–54

holding, 190

home, 77–78

breast-feeding vs. bottle-feeding at, 249–53

bringing preemies, 241–58

discharge and, 229–30

dressing at, 256–57

environment of, 243–49, 280–81

preemie support groups and, 257–58

home apnea monitors, 231–32

home uterine activity monitoring (HUAM), 83, 95

and labor and delivery areas, 110–11
NICUs and, 178–79, 186, 190–92, 212, 216–17, 224, 226–28
pregnancy-induced conditions and, 24, 26, 28–29, 31–32, 35, 40–41, 43–45
premature labor and, 66, 70–72, 74, 76–77
self-care and, 259, 263, 268
types of, 66–68
and when to go to hospital, 104–5
see also specific tests and monitors
morning sickness, 46–47
multiples, multiple pregnancies, xviii, 295
bed rest and, 79, 81, 85
breast-feeding and, 254
and bringing them home, 244, 248, 253–55
C-sections and, 107–8
ethical decision making and, 305, 312
and first twenty-four hours after delivery, 124–26, 147
as high-risk, 3, 29–38, 40, 45, 60, 93–94, 98
later-life development of, 281–84
NICUs and, 184, 193
perinatal death of, 299–300
PIH and, 24
premature labor and, 68
resources on, 338–39
special needs children and, 286–88
tips for parents of, 254
treatment of, 32–33
see also quadruplets, quadruplet pregnancies; triplets, triplet pregnancies; twins, twin pregnancies
muscles, muscle tone, 22, 159, 251, 277, 300
discharge and, 230, 238
and first twenty-four hours after delivery, 118–19, 140
gestational age and, 155–57, 161–62, 166
NICUs and, 175, 179–80, 190–92, 215
self-care and, 261–62
tocolytics and, 74
Musco-Garcia-Prats, Catherine, xx, 267
myasthenia gravis, 19, 22

myometrium, 43–44
myopia, 220

narcotics, 49
nasal continuous positive airway pressure (NCPAP), 137, 179, 217
nasal prongs, 137
naso-gastric (NG) tubes:
gestational age and, 157–58, 164, 168
NICUs and, 177–78, 217–18
National Center for Health Statistics, xix
National Institute of Child Health and Human Development, 97, 213
nausea, *see* vomiting and nausea
necrotizing enterocolitis (NEC), 112, 196, 250
and bringing preemies home, 246
causes of, 217
gestational age and, 131
intermediate care nurseries and, 234
NICUs and, 206–7, 217–18
treatment of, 217–18
neonatal care:
ethical decision making in, 305–16
historical perspective on, 306–7
Neonatal Health Index, 272
neonatal intensive care units (NICUs), ix–x, xvii–xviii, xx, 115–16, 171–230
apnea and, 179–80, 206–7, 209–10, 216–17, 222, 224, 230
babies' charts in, 192
and bringing preemies home, 241–43, 246–47, 249, 252–57
childbirth classes and, 104
common medical procedures in, 174–80
C-sections and, 108, 188
discharge and, 237, 239–40
doctors vs. nurses of, 189
emotions and, 127–30, 171–74, 181–84, 196, 199–200
equipment of, 132–37
ethical decision making and, 307, 311–15
and first twenty-four hours after delivery, 118, 120–30, 132–42

pregnancy-induced conditions and, 45–46
premature labor and, 63, 66, 68, 70
vasodilan (Isoxsuprine), 69, 71, 73
vegetables and fruits, 266
venereal disease research laboratory (VDRL) tests, 52
ventilators (mechanical respirators), 136
ventriculo-peritoneal (VP) shunts, 215
viability, limits of, 311–14
viral meningitis, 211–12
vision, vision problems, 6
  examination of, 175–76, 237–38, 240
  and first twenty-four hours after delivery, 139, 141
  gestational age and, 160, 162, 165, 168–69
  high blood pressure and, 13, 16
  infections and, 52
  and later-life development of preemies, 274–76, 278
  NICUs and, 175–76, 206–8, 220–22
  pregnancy-induced conditions and, 24–26
  as side effect of tocolytics, 74
  see also retinopathy of prematurity
visitors:
  accommodation of, 146–47
  and bringing preemies home, 243–46, 249
  self-care and, 260–61
vitamins, 64, 242
volunteers, NICU, 138–39
vomiting and nausea, 83
  and bed rest, 81, 90
  and gestational age, 164
  and GER, 231
  and high-risk pregnancies, 96
  and infections, 51
  and intermediate care nurseries, 234
  and NICUs, 210, 214, 217

and planning, 102
and pregnancy-induced conditions, 46–47
and tocolytics, 72–75
vulnerability, 300

"wait until certain" approach to treatment, 313
WebMD.com, 203, 258, 336
weeks of gestation, 60
weights, xvii–xx
  autoimmune disorders and, 21, 23
  bed rest and, 82, 85–86
  at birth, see birth weights
  and bringing preemies home, 255
  diabetes and, 16
  discharge and, 229–30, 232–33
  high blood pressure and, 13, 16
  high-risk pregnancies and, 3, 6, 9, 13, 49
  infections and, 51
  intermediate care nurseries and, 234
  and later-life development of preemies, 272
  pregnancy-induced conditions and, 24–25, 28–30, 36–38, 45–47
  self-care and, 261, 263–65
When a Baby Dies (Kohner and Henley), 292
Wisconsin, University of, 203, 337
withdrawal of support, 311, 314–15
Women, Infants and Children (WIC) programs, 146

X-rays, 180, 212, 216, 218–19

yeast infections, 53
Yutopar (ritodrine), 69, 71–73, 299

Zantac, 244
Zestril, 141